2019

To Linda,

Enjoy the journey &

Love, Kay

Perfect Hor-Mo-Nē

A Woman's Gift: Hormone Harmony

Cover design & interior illustrations © 2018 Bernadette Lund

Printed in the United States of America

First Printing, 2018
ISBN: 978-1-79017-595-6

Kay Smith, P.A.C.
15721 Pomerado Rd.
Poway, CA 92064-2021

perfecthormone.com

Perfect Hor-Mo-Nē

A Woman's Gift: Hormone Harmony

Kay Smith, P.A.C.

Dedicated

To

My patient husband, Guy

To

Our precious daughter, Ashlee Mary

To

My two supportive sisters, Maureen and Janet

To

My Great-Grandmother Molly for her love of medicine

To

My beloved mother Mary, for inspiring & teaching me values

To

My beloved father Richard who believed I had a gift for medicine

To

My loyal patients, colleagues & friends who gave me encouragement

To

All women who read this book
as they journey through midlife & beyond

Thank You!

Acknowledgements

A special thank you to the following colleagues who volunteered their time to review this material:

Andrew M. Blumenfeld, MD., Diplomate American Board of Psychiatry and Neurology. Certified in Headache Medicine and Director of the Headache Center of Southern California. San Diego, California.

Janice Baker, Registered Dietician. Certified Diabetes Educator and Nutrition Support Clinician. Board Certified in Advanced Diabetes Management. Poway, California.

Thomas Dayspring, MD., FACP, FNLA, NCMP, Cardiologist. Director of the Cardiovascular Education for Health Improvement and Technology. Fellow of both the American College of Physicians and the National Lipid Association. Certified in Lipidology and as a Menopause Practitioner by the North American Menopause Society. Richmond, Virginia.

Daniel Einhorn, MD., FACP, FACE. Endocrinologist and Diabetologist. Medical Director of the Scripps Whittier Diabetes Institute and a Clinical Professor of Medicine at the University of California San Diego. Poway, California.

Dr. Christopher M. Herman, D.D.S., Cosmetic and Family Dentistry. Oceanside, California.

S. Douglas Klein, M.D., Diplomate, American Board of Internal Medicine, Diplomate, American Board of Addiction Medicine. Poway, California.

Michael A. Kosmo, M.D., Hematologist and Oncologist. San Diego, California.

Dr. Tracey L. Lysander, DDS, Dentist. Rancho Bernardo, California.

Dr. Bonnie Marblestone, RN, FNP, PH.D. Internal and Family Medicine at Scripps Clinic in San Diego, California

Timothy Maresh, MD., Obstetrics and Gynecology, Retired. Poway, California.

John J. Martin, MD., Urologist, Retired. San Diego, California

Maureen Fleming-Mullins, PA-C, Primary Care Physician Assistant. San Diego, California

Smitha C. Reddy, MD., Board Certified in Rheumatology and Internal Medicine. Founding Physician of Arthritis Care and Research Center in San Diego. Poway, California.

Ronna Semonian, P.T., Physical Therapist, Performance F.A.S.T.—Functional Advanced Sports Training—"Physical And Mental Literacy Faster." San Diego, California.

William Shapiro, MD., Board Certified in Emergency Medicine and Internal Medicine. Kaiser Permanente in Maui, Hawaii.

Richard J. Snyder, MD., Diplomate American Board of Gastroenterology. San Diego Digestive Disease Consultants Medical Group. Gastroenterology and Liver Diseases. San Diego, California.

Dr. Shelby J. Thorpe, Ph.D., Psychologist, Retired. Oregon.

Neil W. Treister, MD., MBA, FACC. Board Certified in Internal Medicine and Cardiology. Founder of the Salus Heart and Wellness Center at Sharp Memorial Hospital in San Diego.

Elizabeth E. Vierra, MD., Board Certified Dermatologist. Poway, California.

David W. Westinghouse, MD., Board Certified in Internal Medicine and Cardiology. Retired, Escondido, California.

INTRODUCTION

This purpose of this book is to help women gain a better understanding of how hormones influence the various stages of their lives.

We begin the roller coaster ride with puberty, when our hormones take center stage and follow them through to the grand finale of menopause, when they take their final bow.

Hormones can impact our health in many ways. I will explain the midlife challenges we may encounter and the effects different hormones can have on each system of our body.

The goal is to achieve "BALANCE" in order to maintain a healthy body and restore perfect harmony ("PERFECT HOR-MO-NE")!

Many women find themselves arriving at their menopausal years not certain about the changes occurring within their mind and bodies, which can create fear and frustration. I believe the more knowledge one gains, the better understanding one will have of the journey that lies ahead. Knowledge can help alleviate the stress and fear associated with menopause. Having less fear enables you to maintain control and restore balance in your life.

This book was written not only to help educate, but to empower women so they can make informed decisions regarding their health.

The K-I-S-S format "keep it simple sweetheart" is for those of us whose memory and patience are challenged these days.

This light, detailed, but easy to read format using bullets with larger print should help in case you don't have your reading glasses handy.

I hope you will find the information helpful in understanding the changes we encounter on our journey through midlife and beyond.

I encourage all women who read this book to embrace and enjoy every day of your life. Life is the most precious gift of all and passes much too quickly. Cherish it!

FOREWORD

BY STUART DOUGLAS KLEIN, M.D.

PERFECT HOR-MO-NE IS THE ESSENTIAL GUIDE FOR ALL WOM-EN TO LEARN HOW TO MAINTAIN THEIR HEALTH DURING MID-LIFE AND BEYOND. This book educates women about the female anatomy and how hormones influence your health from adolescence through to menopause and beyond.

Kay provides valuable information about the many changes that can occur in your body early in midlife when hormone levels begin to decline. She outlines common medical conditions associated with these changing levels of female hormones that can occur during perimenopause, menopause and postmenopause in an easy to understand format. She emphasizes how beneficial proper nutrition and exercise can be in helping women take care of themselves from the inside out, especially during this time of transition.

She discusses in great detail the associated health risks and what you can do to prevent and treat these conditions before they progress. Kay shares my philosophy that patient education and prevention go hand in hand. I am a strong believer in lifestyle modification in preventing diseases such as diabetes, heart disease and cancer. You will find information on prevention, lifestyle modifications and treatment measures you can implement early on to help prevent diseases and progression of many diseases throughout the different stages of life.

Kay has spent several years studying natural alternatives for treating conditions associated with the hormonal changes that occur with menopause. She will guide you through hormone replacement options, explore alternative therapies and provide insight to help you identify and understand the many midlife changes. She is a very caring clinician with added humor which is reflected in this book. This is truly a fun read while covering serious topics to help you gain a better understanding of "women's midlife challenges." Kay has consulted with many medical experts and colleagues to help provide you with up-to-date medical facts in this cutting edge book.

Kay Smith, P.A.C., obtained her Physician Assistant degree from the University of Southern California, School of Medicine in 1982. She is board-certified in Primary Care Medicine and has her own private practice in Poway, California and practices with her sister Maureen Mullins, PA-C. Kay enjoys teaching and has served as a student preceptor for the Physician Assistant and Nurse Practitioner programs at George Washington and Stanford Universities. I am honored to be serving as her supervising physician.

TABLE OF CONTENTS

Hormones & How They Affect The Female Body

Chapter 1

BEGINNING WITH THE BASICS

The Anatomy of the Female Genitalia

In order to understand how hormones influence the various stages of our lives, it is important to be familiar with the female anatomy. After thirty plus years of practicing medicine, I have come to realize that many women have a limited understanding of the female genitalia and the associated internal organs.

My mother always told me, "A picture is worth a thousand words," so let's dive right in and review the female anatomy as a prelude to understanding how our female hormones work. Let's begin with *Figure 1.1* on the following page.

The *vulva* consists of folds of delicate sensitive tissues, which form the *labia* or "lips" at the opening of the vagina. There are two sets of labia:

- The outermost folds are called the *labia majora* and are covered with pubic hair.

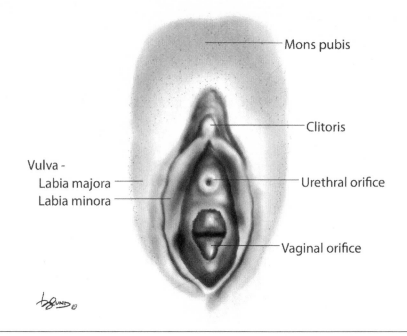

Figure 1.1

- The inner folds are called the ***labia minora*** and some women have very little expression of them. We refer to this at the office as "the two door opposed to the four door model vulva."

The ***mons pubis*** or ***mons veneris*** (mound of Venus) is the fleshy area covering the pubic bone.

The ***clitoris*** is a very sensitive small round organ about the size of a pea.

The mouth or opening of the vagina is called the ***introitus*** or ***vaginal orifice.***

The opening where urine passes through to exit the body is called the ***urethral orifice.***

The ***vaginal orifice*** is the entrance to the vaginal canal which measures about six inches in length and provides a passage way from the outside of the body to the uterus (womb). It is also called the birth canal during childbirth. This canal receives the penis during intercourse and provides an exit for the uterine lining to shed during menstruation, commonly known as your period.

The ***uterus,*** or womb *(Figure 1.2)*, is a hollow pear-shaped organ with thick muscular walls. It typically measures around 3 inches in length, 2 inches in width and one inch in thickness, prior to childbirth.

The lining of the uterus is called the ***endometrium*** and this tissue builds up monthly with the influence of your female hormones. If an egg does not become fertilized, the lining will shed and menstruation will begin.

The ***myometrium*** is the middle layer of the uterine wall, consisting mainly of uterine smooth muscle cells. The main function of the myometrium is to induce uterine contractions.

The ***cervix*** is the lower part of the uterus, which opens into the vaginal canal.

The ***ovaries*** are almond-shaped and usually measure one and one-half inches by three quarters of an inch.

The ***fallopian tubes*** transport the egg from the ovary to the uterus. Fallopian tubes are lined with small hair-like projections called cilia, which help move the egg through the tube into the uterus. Typically once a month, one of the fallopian tubes will transport an egg from the ovary to the uterus.

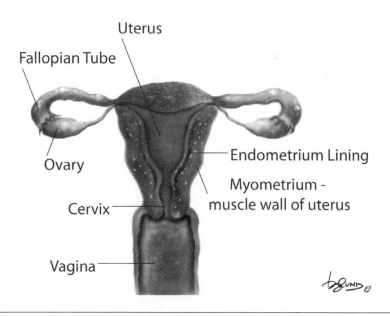

Figure 1.2

Conditions and Infections of the Vagina

It is important to take proper care of your vagina and vulva. Be sure to avoid irritants that can cause swelling, redness and pain. Be aware of any changes in sensation, pain, odor and discharge.

Your vagina is self-cleaning in the form of normal vaginal discharge. Throughout the month, the discharge will change in character and amount. During mid-cycle the discharge becomes clear and stretchy, resembling an egg white, allowing sperm to travel easily into your cervix and uterus where it may become fertilized.

There are various conditions and infections which can affect the vagina. Symptoms such as redness, odor, swelling, discharge or a rash can appear which require different forms of treatment. Be sure to consult your clinician if you develop any of these symptoms.

Vulvovaginitis

This is the name used to describe "inflammation" of the vulva (vulvitis) and the vagina (vaginitis). These two areas of the genitalia are in close proximity and therefore inflammation of one structure can precipitate inflammation of the other.

Vulvovaginitis may occur at any age and will affect most females at some time in their life. It is important to identify the cause so treatment can be recommended.

Vaginitis

A healthy vagina contains "good" bacteria called *lactobacillus* along with other bacteria and fungi. Vaginitis is the term used when an infection or inflammation of the vagina is present.

Causes

A vaginal infection occurs when the bacterial organisms or fungi grow out of control or when new ones are introduced into the vagina through unsafe sex or poor hygiene.

Viral infections are a common cause of vaginitis and can be introduced through sexual intercourse.

Vaginitis occurs more often in females who take the birth control pill. Birth control pills prevent the normal hormone-generated mucous from being produced. This mucous is protective.

Symptoms

Typical symptoms to look for would be redness, swelling, itching, rash and a foul smelling discharge. Be aware that some home remedies can be harmful and even make an infection worse.

NOTE: Do not douche before seeing your clinician, because you will wash away the evidence of any infection and create a diagnosis dilemma.

Allergic Vaginitis

The vulva can be especially sensitive to perfumed soaps, detergents and fabric softeners.

Causes

Allergic Vaginitis can occur after exposure to:

- Hygiene sprays and toilet paper
- Douches and detergents from clothing
- Chemical irritants from spermicidal products
- Lubricants which are used in the vaginal area
- A retained foreign body such as a tampon or diaphragm can also cause irritation and a possible infection.

Symptoms

These products can cause burning, itching and a vaginal discharge.

Treatment

The symptoms usually resolve once the offending agent is stopped. Cool *Aloe vera* gel (stored in the refrigerator) can be applied topically to sooth the discomfort.

Atrophic Vaginitis

Atrophic vaginitis can occur after menopause due to vaginal dryness and decreased mucus production. As we age, our estrogen diminishes and vaginal discharge can decrease becoming almost non-existent. The vagina becomes very dry and this is called atrophic vaginitis. Estrogen keeps the vagina moist and elastic.

Vaginal Changes Associated with Decreased Estrogen:

- The vagina now becomes less acidic and more bacteria friendly due to less mucus production. The normal pH of the vagina is less than 4.5.

- Your vagina becomes more susceptible to tears due to thinning of the lining.
- Sexually transmitted diseases can invade your body more easily through open tears. *Think protection!*
- Loss of estrogen can cause the vagina to become drier, thinner and actually shrink in size.

Symptoms
Vaginal irritation and dryness

Vaginal soreness and pain with intercourse

Treatment
Practicing regular sexual activity will help stimulate blood flow and lubrication.

Vaginal lubricants like Replens, Astroglide and KY Jelly can help relieve vaginal dryness and discomfort with intercourse.

(See Chapter 3 for more detail on vaginal lubricants)

Try using a vitamin E capsule as a lubricant. Break or cut open the capsule so the gel can flow easily and insert into the vaginal canal and let it dissolve.

Topical vaginal estrogen creams seem to be more effective than oral hormonal treatments for relieving vaginal dryness, pain and irritation. Hormone vaginal treatments can be prescribed in lower doses than oral forms and there is less systemic absorption, which may lower the risk for developing endometrial and/or breast cancer. Ask your clinician if this treatment would be right for you.

Natural estrogen cream called *"Estriol",* or prescription estradiol cream, can provide relief by restoring hormonal balance thus keeping the vagina more acidic. These estrogen creams can also help restore the friendly acidic bacteria called Lactobacilli, while decreasing the risk for developing infection.

Natural progesterone may be an option for individuals who are unable to take estrogen.

(In Chapter 3, "Championing the Change," hormonal therapy is discussed in greater detail.)

Drinking more water helps keep your entire body hydrated. Try drinking half your body weight in ounces per day. If you weigh 140 pounds, you would need to drink about 70 ounces throughout the day. This may sound like a lot, but remember your body is comprised of 70% water.

Bacterial Infections

Bacterial Vaginosis

Bacterial vaginosis (BV) is the most common vaginal infection among women of child bearing age and may also affect women after menopause.

Causes

Bacterial vaginosis is caused by a bacterial overgrowth when the vaginal *ph* is not in balance and becomes less acidic. The microorganisms involved include Gardnerella vaginalis, Mobiluncus bacteroides and mycoplasma. BV can be associated with intercourse although there is no clear evidence of sexual transmission and sexually inactive individuals can also become infected. Sexual intercourse creates a more basic (alkaline) environment that promotes bacterial and fungal overgrowth.

Symptoms

• A copious watery, milky or grayish frothy discharge which can have a "fishy" odor, most commonly noticed after intercourse. We refer to this as the "positive whiff test!"

• Vaginal swelling, itching, soreness and at times can cause burning with urination (dysuria) due to increased irritation of the vaginal tissues.

Treatment

This infection responds well to oral and vaginal cream antibiotics. Consult with your clinician if you have any of the above mentioned symptoms.

Chlamydia

Chlamydia is the most commonly reported bacterial sexually transmitted disease in both women and men in the U.S. Chlamydia vaginitis is the most common cause of cervicitis (inflammation of the cervix).

Causes

Chlamydia trachomatis is a bacterial infection which, when introduced through the vagina can infect the urethra, cervix and upper reproductive organs in women. Chlamydia can also infect the rectum and eyelids (conjunctiva).

Chlamydia commonly occurs in females between the ages of 18 and 35 who have multiple partners.

Screening Recommendations

You should be screened for chlamydia annually if you are sexually active and are:

• 25 years of age or younger

• 25 years of age or older and at increased risk with a new partner or multiple partners.

Symptoms

Women commonly DO NOT experience symptoms with this infection, so you must be screened for this if you are sexually active, especially if you have multiple partners!

Some women may experience a mucopurulent vaginal discharge and/or increased pain and frequency in urination. In some women, the only symptom could be bleeding with intercourse.

Pregnant women may pass this infection to their newborns during delivery!

Treatment

Once you have been diagnosed with chlamydia, you and your partner, or partners, need to be treated at the same time.

A single dose antibiotic may be taken by mouth for treatment of chlamydia or a seven day course of antibiotics may be given. You should abstain from sexual activity for seven days after receiving the single dose antibiotic or until completion of the seven day course of antibiotics.

If left untreated, chlamydia vaginitis can cause "pelvic inflammatory disease" (PID) which can become very serious and lead to infertility and/or an ectopic pregnancy. An ectopic pregnancy is when the embryo implants in the fallopian tube instead of the uterus, and can be life threatening!

Gonorrhea

Gonorrhea is the second most common bacterial sexually transmitted disease in the U.S. and frequently occurs occurs along with chlamydia.

Causes

Neisseria gonorrhoeae is a gram negative bacteria that causes a gonorrheal infection, also referred to as "the clap, drip or GC". This organism, when introduced through the vagina, infects the urethra, cervix and upper reproductive organs in women. Gonorrhea can also infect the rectum and throat.

Symptoms

Most women commonly DO NOT experience symptoms with this infection. You must be screened for this if you are sexually active, especially if you have multiple partners.

Some women may experience a yellow creamy vaginal discharge and/or an increase in pain and frequency of urination. These symptoms can be very mild and often times may be mistaken for a bladder or vaginal infection.

Screening Recommendations: You should be screened for gonorrhea annually if you are sexually active and are:

• 25 years of age and younger

• 25 years of age or older and at increased risk with a new partner or multiple partners.

NOTE: Chlamydia and gonorrhea both have similar screening and treatment procedures.

Treatment

If you have been diagnosed with either gonorrhea or chlamydia, it is recommended that you be treated for both infections.

Dual therapy is now recommended for the treatment of gonorrhea. An antibiotic injection may be given along with a different single dose antibiotic given by mouth on the same day due to the recent emergence of antimicrobial resistant strains.

You should refrain from sexual intercourse for seven days after receiving treatment and until your sexual partner or all partners have been treated for the same seven day period.

Gonorrhea can also cause "pelvic inflammatory disease" (PID) which can lead to possible infertility and/or an ectopic pregnancy.

NOTE: A pregnant woman may pass this infection to her newborn during delivery resulting in serious harm to the baby.

Fungal Infections

Candida Infection

Candida infection, also known as a *yeast infection,* is very common in women of all ages. Yeast is normally found in your mouth, digestive tract and vagina, but when it grows out of control, an infection can occur.

Causes

A yeast infection occurs from an overgrowth of *Candida albicans* and when your body is out of balance. This infection is facilitated under certain conditions such as when you are:

• Taking antibiotics

• Pregnant or taking the birth control pill

• Menstruating

• Experiencing a hormonal imbalance

• Experiencing a weakened immune system

• Taking a steroid medication

• Being treated for a thyroid condition, diabetes and/or any other metabolic condition

Symptoms

This fungal condition typically presents itself as a thick white curdy (cottage cheese) type of vaginal discharge or as a thin watery discharge. Sometimes there is an odor, intense vulvar itching, swelling and redness.

Treatment

There are many over-the-counter vaginal creams, prescription suppositories and a pill that you take only once.

It is important for you to consult with your clinician, especially if over-the-counter preparations are ineffective.

Parasitic Infections

Trichomoniasis

Trichomoniasis, sometimes referred to as "trich" (pronounced trick) is a common cause of vaginitis. Trichomoniasis is primarily an infection of the urogenital tract and the most common sites of infection are the urethra and vagina in women.

Causes

Trichomoniasis is usually a sexually transmitted infection caused by a single celled flagellated protozoan called *Trichomonas vaginalis.*

Symptoms

This infection usually presents with a yellow-green bubbly or frothy malodorous discharge. The cervix can appear spotted with red dots, referred to as a "strawberry cervix". Some women may not have any symptoms at all.

Trichomoniasis can also cause itching and soreness of the genitalia, a burning sensation during urination and intercourse can become painful.

Symptoms can be more apparent after your period and during pregnancy.

Treatment

This infection responds well to oral medications that can be given in a single dose and both you and your partner or partners need to be treated.

Viral Infections

Genital Herpes

Genital herpes is a sexually transmitted disease which causes grouped painful blisters or ulcerated lesions of the genitalia.

Causes

Two types of the *herpes simplex virus* (HSV) can cause this incurable and recurrent genital herpes infection.

- Type 1 (HSV-1): This is the type that usually causes cold sores or fever blisters on or around the facial lips, although it can be spread to your genital area during oral sex.

• Type 2 (HSV-2): This is the type that commonly causes genital herpes, affecting areas below the waist. The virus spreads through sexual contact and skin-to-skin contact. HSV-2 is very common and highly contagious, whether or not you have an open sore. HSV is the most common cause of a genital ulcer disease in the US.

NOTE: This virus dies quickly outside the body so it is nearly impossible to get the infection through contact with toilet seats, towels or any other objects used by an infected individual.

Symptoms

A woman may experience the following symptoms with the initial outbreak:

• Feeling sick, flu like illness

• Swollen lymph glands (nodes in groin region)

• Intense pain

• Burning with urination, depending on the location of the outbreak

• Watery discharge if the outbreak is on the cervix

Recurrent outbreaks are usually less severe and can happen within the first year of infection. Many things can trigger an outbreak including:

• Stress (emotional)

• Hormonal changes/menstruation

• Decreased immune response

• Ultraviolet light exposure/sunburn

• Vigorous sexual activity

Many times a woman will feel a tingling or burning sensation in the area of the lesion before the sore actual appears.

NOTE: You can pass the Herpes virus to your partner without having an outbreak! Consistent use of a condom reduces the chance of getting or spreading herpes.

Treatment

There is no cure for herpes, although antiviral medications can help reduce viral shedding, the frequency of outbreaks, transmission to partners and to newborns from pregnant women.

An initial outbreak is treated for seven to ten days with antiviral medications.

If you have six or more outbreaks within one year, antiviral medications can be taken daily or twice daily to reduce the number of outbreaks.

Human Papilloma Virus, (HPV)

The Human Papilloma Virus (HPV) is the most common sexually transmitted disease seen in the U.S.

Causes

This infection is caused by the *Human Papilloma* virus. There are several types of HPV. Some types can cause genital warts and other types have been found to cause cancer of the cervix and vulva.

Genital Warts: These warts are caused by *condylomata Acuminata* and they grow on the genitalia, groin and/or anal areas. HPV types 6 and 11 are associated with these genital warts. Anorectal warts caused by condylomata acuminata can also be associated with cancer.

Types 16, 18, 31, 33 and 35 are associated with the development of cervical cancer. These lesions appear as flat warts which are not easily visible without using special procedures to locate them.

HPV types 16 and 18 can also cause vaginal, vulvar, penile, anal and head/neck cancers.

It is also possible to develop HPV of the vocal cords as a result of engaging in oral sex. This can cause permanent hoarseness and result in multiple painful surgeries to remove the stubborn and recurrent HPV lesions. This is not very common but can seriously impact your quality of life.

NOTE: This virus can spontaneously resolve or seem to leave the body (especially in younger women) with a healthy immune system, although it doesn't always clear.

Symptoms

- Painful warts that have a cauliflower-like appearance.
- Increased vaginal moisture and itching in the areas where the warts are present.
- Abnormal vaginal discharge and/or vaginal bleeding (not associated with a menstrual period).
- Some individuals do not have any symptoms.

Diagnosis

- Be sure to have a routine pap smear, which also screens for HPV and other sexually transmitted diseases. (Please see Chapter 19 for routine screening recommendations).
- When a woman becomes infected with one of these types of HPV, and the virus doesn't go away on its own, abnormal cells can develop in the lining of the cervix. If these cells are not found early, changes can occur, leading to cancer. In some cases a female may not even know she has contracted this virus until a pap test is abnormal.

Treatment

Genital warts should be treated by a medical professional. Do not use over-the-counter remedies intended to treat other types of warts.

Your clinician may:

- Apply a skin treatment in the office
- Prescribe a medication that you apply several times per week at home
- Recommend a surgical treatment: cryosurgery (freezing), electro cauterization (burning), laser therapy or just cutting them out.

Prevention

Practice safe sex.

Gardasil is a vaccine available to help prevent the development of the human papillomavirus (HPV) in those not previously exposed. This vaccine provides protection against many strains that are responsible for causing cervical cancer and genital warts.

• *Gardasil* was approved in May 2006 and is recommended for females and males, ages 9 through 26 years and helps protect against HPV types 6, 11, 16 and 18.

This vaccine is administered by injection. If the series is started before the individual's 15th birthday, two doses will be given at least 6 months apart. If started at 15-26 years of age, three doses of the vaccine will be needed. This vaccine should NOT be given during pregnancy.

Side effects of this vaccine include pain, swelling, itching, bruising and redness at the injection site. Headache, fever, nausea, vomiting and dizziness can also occur.

Recent reports have associated neurologic complications such as seizures, paralysis and speech problems as being possibly linked to the Gardasil vaccine.

If you have already contracted the human papilloma virus you may still benefit from receiving the vaccine because it offers protection against many different types of the virus.

Current studies are under way for women and men over 26 years of age.

Human Immunodeficiency Virus (HIV)

HIV is sexually transmitted. HIV is a retrovirus that attacks the immune system, the body's natural defense system. White blood cells are an important part of the immune system. HIV invades and destroys certain white blood cells called CD4 T-cells. The body can no longer defend itself against infection if too many CD4 T-cells are destroyed. Once your immune system becomes weak, you are then susceptible to life threatening illnesses, such as infections and cancers.

The progression of HIV to the advanced stage of the disease is called "AIDS" (acquired immunodeficiency syndrome). Having HIV does not mean that you have AIDS. It can take a long time for HIV to progress to AIDS, sometimes up to 10 to 12 years, even without treatment.

If HIV is diagnosed before progressing to AIDS, there are medications that can help slow or even stop the damage to the immune system for a period of time.

Many individuals receiving treatment for HIV can live long active lives.

Causes

HIV is caused by the human immunodeficiency virus. If you are sexually active and are not using a male latex condom, you can get HIV/AIDS from having sex with someone who is infected with the virus.

The HIV virus passes from the infected person to another through exchange of body fluids such as blood, semen and vaginal fluid.

HIV can enter a woman's body during intercourse through mucous membranes or any opening, such as a tear or cut in the lining of the vagina, vulva, rectum or mouth. The same is true for men with the virus entering the body through the penis, rectum or mouth.

Another common way of acquiring the virus is by sharing drug needles with an individual who is infected with HIV.

The virus can also be passed from a mother to her baby during pregnancy, birth or breast-feeding.

NOTE: There are no known cases of HIV being transmitted through kissing or sharing drinking glasses, because it does not survive well outside the body.

Symptoms

Many individuals DO NOT even know that they have been infected early on because they may NOT have symptoms, aside from a mild to moderate flu like symptoms, referred to as "Acute HIV Syndrome".

Common early symptoms can be:

• Fever

• Sore throat

• Headache

• Muscle aches and joint pain

• Swollen glands

• Skin rash

It can take just a few days to several weeks for flu-like symptoms to manifest after an individual is first infected. These early symptoms usually go away within 2-3 weeks. After these early symptoms go away, an infected individual may not experience anything for several years before developing more serious signs of HIV, referred to as "Symptomatic (Advanced) HIV infection".

Without treatment, the virus continues to grow in the body and attacks the immune system.

Symptoms that can reappear and persist over time include:

• Swollen glands

• Extreme tiredness (fatigue)

• Weight loss

• Fever

• Night sweats

Diagnosis

Once you have been exposed to HIV, your immune system then makes antibodies in an attempt to destroy the virus, which can be detected by a blood test.

Screening tests are now available that can detect the HIV antibodies in urine or fluid from your mouth and blood.

If the urine or fluid from your mouth tests positive for HIV you will need a blood test called a Western blot (WB) to confirm the results.

NOTE: Did you know that menopausal women are also at risk for developing HIV infection?

Within the past seven years, the number of new HIV cases in sexually active individuals 50 years of age and older has nearly doubled. Two thirds of the women contracted the virus from infected sexual partners. Another third of the women contracted the virus from sharing needles. Of all the women ages 50 and above who developed AIDS, 70% were Hispanic and Black.

The Possible Connection between HIV/AIDS and Women in Menopause

• There is no longer a fear of getting pregnant and a condom is not being used to practice safe sex.

- Vaginal dryness is common, increasing the likelihood of small tears or abrasions occurring during intercourse, thus increasing the risk of contracting HIV.

- These women may have less of an understanding of how this virus is spread.

- Women typically live longer than men and with the increase in divorce rate more women are now dating and having sex.

It is so important to communicate with your clinician and request an HIV test. It may take as long as six months for the HIV antibodies to show up in a blood test.

If you think you've been exposed to HIV and your test is negative:

- Get re-tested in six months to be sure you are not infected.

- Continue to use precautions to prevent the spread of the virus.

NOTE: If you are infected, you can pass HIV to another individual during this time period.

Treatment

There are many medicines called highly active antiretroviral therapy (HAART) that when used in combination can help slow down the rate at which the virus multiplies.

The earlier you are diagnosed, the better the prognosis, life expectancy and quality of life.

Practice Prevention

- Get to know your partner well and talk about previous partner exposure prior to engaging in intercourse for the first time.

- Find out if he or she is at risk for HIV and get tested before you engage in sexual intercourse! You both should be tested initially and again in 6 months.

- Practice safe sex and use a condom.

- Do not have multiple sex partners.

- Do not drink alcohol or use drugs, which can alter your decision to practice safe sex.

- Do not share personal items, such as toothbrushes or razors.

- Never share needles or syringes with anyone.
- Be sure to have regular check-ups and ask to be tested for HIV if you are at risk.

NOTE: A new monthly vaginal ring that releases a continual dose of dapivirine (an antiretroviral medication) has been reported to reduce the risk of HIV-1 infection by 61% among women 25 years of age and older according to research published online in the New England Journal of Medicine.

Websites for further information on:

Acquired Immune Deficiency Syndrome (AIDS)
HIV/AIDS Basics: **https://www.aids.gov/hiv-aids-basics/**

AIDS information-HIV/AIDS Treatment, Prevention and Research: **https://www.aidsinfo.nih.gov/**

Female reproductive system
Female Reproduction System: Organs, Function: **http://www.webmd.com/sex-relationships/guide/your-guide-female-reproductive-system#1**

Human papillomavirus (HPV) vaccines
Gardasil (Human Papillomavirus Quadrivalent): **https://www.aidsinfo.nih.gov/**

U.S. Food and Drug Administration-Safety Information and Adverse Event Reporting Program: **https://www.fda.gov/Safety/MedWatch/default.htm**

Sexually transmitted and vaginal infections
Centers for Disease Control and Prevention-Sexually Transmitted Diseases: **https://www.cdc.gov/std/healthcomm/fact_sheets.htm**

Centers for Disease Control and Prevention-Sexually Transmitted Diseases Facts-Trichomoniasis: **https://www.cdc.gov/std/trichomonas/stdfact-Trichomoniasis.htm**

Herpes Facts-Herpes Virus: **http://www.herpes.com/**

Chapter 2

UNDERSTANDING HORMONES

Definition Of A Hormone

Hormones are "chemical substances" produced in the body by an organ, or cells of a certain organ, which have a specific regulatory effect on the activity of another organ in the body. In plain English, they are chemical messengers.

Hormones are typically released from a gland and travel through the body in the bloodstream until they reach the "target" cell. The target cell has a specific receptor (like a door lock) that allows the specific hormone to enter.

We have many different hormones circulating in our body, although for the understanding of female hormones in this chapter, we will focus on the sex steroid hormones.

These natural hormones known as sex steroids are made from cholesterol. Our bodies do need healthy nutrients and enzymes to create these hormones.

Most of us think that cholesterol is all bad but it is actually a very important player in our sex life.

Sex Steroid Hormones

Estrogens

The three most common estrogens found circulating in the female human body are:

- **Estradiol:** This is the most active and powerful form of estrogen produced in the ovaries and is considered "the work horse" hormone during your reproductive years.

- **Estrone:** This is the inactive form of estrogen which is also produced in the ovaries during the reproductive years and in fat cells after menopause. Estrone has the ability to change into estradiol (the strong form of estrogen), but is the most common form found in postmenopausal women.

- **Estriol:** This is the weakest form of estrogen and is produced in large amounts by pregnant women. Women who are not pregnant have lower levels circulating in their bodies. This hormone helps neutralize active estradiol and estrone by competing for the same receptor sites. Some researchers think estriol can protect against breast cancer.

Scientists have discovered that estrogen is a powerful antioxidant, which can protect the body from damage by free radicals. Free radicals are unstable compounds that can attack and damage healthy cells/tissues and antioxidants help prevent this process from occurring.

Women have estrogen receptors throughout their body, located in the brain, heart, blood vessels, bones, skin, intestines, respiratory system and urinary tract.

Estrogen affects a woman in many ways, ranging from how her skin looks to how her heart beats. Isn't that amazing?

Progesterone

Progesterone is produced in the ovaries and the adrenal glands, which are seated on top of the kidneys. Progesterone is another main player in the female reproductive cycle. The word progesterone means for gestation, which is for a pregnancy. This hormone prepares the womb and maintains a pregnancy.

It also signals the uterine lining to shed if a pregnancy is not achieved.

Progesterone is also known as "the feel good hormone" because of its ability to enhance mood and provide a sense of calm and well-being. When progesterone is metabolized, it binds with gamma-aminobutyric acid (GABA) receptors in the brain, producing a calming effect.

Some studies show that progesterone can stimulate the bone building cells called osteoblasts, which can help maintain strong bones.

Progesterone in excess can promote breast tenderness and somnolence. Progesterone replacement is usually given at bedtime.

Testosterone
Testosterone is an androgen (male) hormone and is produced in both the adrenal glands and the ovaries of a woman, even after menopause.

Testosterone is referred to as "the hormone of desire" because of its enhancing effect on a woman's libido (sexual desire). Recent studies suggest that testosterone may play a role in bone growth, which may help prevent osteoporosis.

If the level of estrogen in your brain is low, the circulating testosterone can turn into estrogen. These two hormones work together to make sure you can think clearly and maintain a healthy libido.

During perimenopause and menopause as the level of estrogen begins to decline, the balance of testosterone and estrogen can be altered, resulting in a higher level of circulating testosterone.

This higher level of testosterone may influence the body in the following ways:
• Fat tends to migrate toward your waist.
• Hair can disappear from your head and appear on your chin and upper lip.
• Blood pressure and cholesterol levels can become elevated.

DHEA (Dehydroepiandrosterone)
Dehydroepiandrosterone (DHEA) is also an androgen hormone and the building block for testosterone. This is the most abundantly produced sex steroid.

DHEA:
• Is produced in the adrenal glands and is converted into testosterone during the reproductive years. Your ovaries must be functioning for this process to occur.

- Is also produced in the skin and brain.
- Works with other sex steroid hormones to maintain hormonal balance.
- Can convert into both testosterone and estrogen, especially when these levels are fluctuating or declining, which is commonly seen during perimenopause.

Research suggests that DHEA may also promote bone growth, similar to testosterone and help prevent osteoporosis.

You need estradiol to be present to achieve the benefits of DHEA and testosterone. Be careful with over-the-counter DHEA (as with any other supplement) without the advice of a medical professional because hormones should be in balance and you could end up making things worse! In addition, the dosages vary widely and it is difficult to know for certain just exactly what you are taking in an over-the-counter supplement.

Cortisol
Cortisol is not technically a "sex steroid" hormone, although it behaves similarly and intimately interacts with them. It belongs to the glucocorticoid group and is produced in the adrenal glands.

Cortisol, commonly known as "the stress hormone" helps you cope with stress.

Cortisol also determines how proteins, carbohydrates and fats from your diet are used to help build your immune system and provide energy.

Negatives of excess cortisol production:
Too much cortisol production over long periods of time due to increased stress may cause damage to your body. The following are a few problems that may occur:
- Blood sugar problems
- Fat accumulation
- Bone loss
- Exhaustion
- Heart disease

Your brain can override the message to stop cortisol production if it perceives ongoing stress. Your level stays high because your brain thinks your body needs it to cope with the stress, which is not good.

DHEA and cortisol work together. Under normal conditions, when the body perceives stress, cortisol is produced to give you energy. Once the stress is over, DHEA helps you to recover. This is one way your body handles stress.

How Hormones Create A Menstrual Cycle

Women are born with two ovaries, which contain many tiny sacs called follicles where the eggs are stored. Once a female reaches puberty a new egg ripens every month. The ovaries receive a message from the **Follicle Stimulating Hormone (FSH)** which regulates egg production. Estrogen along with FSH, signal the ovaries that it is time to prepare the eggs to be fertilized. Several eggs begin to mature in the sac (follicle) but ordinarily only one will move to the outer surface of the ovary. The follicle then ruptures and releases the egg into the fallopian tube and it begins its journey toward the uterus. It is here that the egg can become fertilized. At the same time, the uterus is preparing to receive the fertilized egg, known as a zygote.

Estrogen is the hormone responsible for building up the uterine lining and stimulating the follicles to develop eggs in the first two weeks of the cycle, referred to as proliferative or follicular phase.

Ovulation (the release of an egg) occurs in the middle of your cycle in response to the secretion of *luteinizing hormone (LH),* which regulates egg maturation and release. The ruptured follicle (the sac which contained the egg) then undergoes a name change becoming the *corpus luteum,* which then begins to produce progesterone. Your body temperature goes up about one degree at the time of ovulation.

Progesterone is responsible for the change in vaginal mucus (resembling egg whites), making it sperm friendly. Estrogen and progesterone direct the uterine lining (endometrium) to become thickened with blood and nutrients, ready for the fertilized egg to implant and grow in to an embryo. If a pregnancy does not occur within 10-12 days after ovulation, estrogen and progesterone levels fall suddenly, triggering the shedding of the uterine lining. This shedding of the lining is well known as your period. This second half of the menstrual cycle is referred to as the *luteal* or *secretory* phase.

Table 2.1

Hormone	*Functions*
Estrogens	• These female hormones are responsible for breast development, menstrual cycles, ovulation and fertility. • Increase tolerance for pain. • Help with sleep, mental alertness, focus, memory, communication, coordination and mood. • Help raise the levels of endorphins, serotonin and dopamine • Help with sensory function (vision, hearing, taste, touch and smell). • Help with digestion, sex drive and skin tone. • Can help relieve menopausal symptoms. • May help protect against osteoporosis, heart disease, colon cancer, urinary incontinence and tooth decay.
Progesterone	• Improves mood and has a calming effect. • Is necessary for fertility, prepares the womb and helps maintain a pregnancy. • Increases energy and improves libido (sex drive). • Helps balance blood sugar, improves thyroid function and regulates mineral and fluid balance. • May help relieve menopausal symptoms. • Helps decrease the risk of developing endometrial (uterine) cancer and may reduce the risk of breast cancer, fibrocystic breast disease and osteoporosis.
Testosterone	• Helps improve sense of well-being. • Helps increase energy and improves libido (sex drive). • Builds muscles and promotes muscle tone. • Helps to strengthen bones.
DHEA	• Can enhance energy level, libido, memory and immune system. • Protects against the effects of stress. • Helps to prevent wrinkles and dry eyes. • May help protect against diseases such as heart disease, osteoporosis, diabetes, cancer, dementia, lupus and rheumatoid arthritis. • May help promote weight loss.
Cortisol	• Helps you respond and cope with stress. • Increases energy and metabolism. • Can help to keep blood vessels healthy and regulate blood pressure. • Reduces allergic and inflammatory response.

The normal menstrual cycle is about 26-28 days in duration and is due to the balance of these four hormones:

• Estrogen

• Progesterone

• FSH (follicle stimulating hormone)

• LH (luteinizing hormone)

If your periods become irregular, these hormones are no longer in balance.

During perimenopause your hormone levels are unpredictable and you could still periodically ovulate and guess what? Yes, have a "change of life" baby! Even if you are skipping periods (referred to as amenorrhea) you should continue whatever birth control method you have been using if you wish to prevent a pregnancy.

Contraception & Birth Control

In review, during your reproductive years from menarche (your first menstrual cycle) until menopause, an egg is usually released each month from one or both of your ovaries and then travels down through the fallopian tube to the uterus. If the egg is fertilized, it will implant in the lining of the uterus, which is called the endometrium. When the egg is not fertilized, the endometrium, which has built up in preparation for a pregnancy, is then shed. This tissue and the unfertilized egg leave the uterus through the cervix and exit the body through the vagina, also known as your menstrual period.

I will now outline the different birth control method options and how they work to prevent pregnancy. Remember, you can still become pregnant during midlife, so it is important to understand how the different methods work to help prevent a pregnancy.

Definition Of Contraception
Contraception is the use of any method, device or medication used to prevent pregnancy by interfering with ovulation, fertilization and/or implantation. Contraception is commonly referred to as birth control.

If you have intercourse without using birth control, there is a chance that you could become pregnant. Yes, you could possibly become pregnant even if you haven't started having periods or if you are in perimenopause. The risk of pregnancy increases starting five days prior to the day of ovulation, peaks on the day of ovulation and then rapidly decreases to zero the day after ovulation. The only way to be sure you won't become pregnant is to refrain from having sex!

When choosing a contraceptive method, many factors need to be considered including:

• Age

• Hormone levels

• Health

• Lifestyle

• Sexual habits

It is important to review your personal and family history with your clinician to identify any risk factors before making your contraceptive choice.

Barrier Methods
Diaphragm, Cervical Cap, Sponge and Condoms

The diaphragm, cervical cap, sponge and condom are all classified as barrier methods and block the sperm from entering the uterus. You must be fitted for a diaphragm and a cervical cap by your clinician.

Barrier methods must be used correctly every time you have intercourse.

Positives of choosing a barrier method:

• Condoms, if used along with a spermicide, can offer protection against sexually transmitted diseases, which is a real plus!

Negatives of choosing a barrier method:

• You may be allergic to latex or nonoxynol-9 products, which are used in spermicides. Be sure to check with your clinician before using any of these methods if you have an allergy to avocados, chestnuts and/or bananas.

• Use of spermicidal products containing nonoxynol-9 may cause irritation and this irritation can increase your risk for contracting a sexually transmitted disease.

• Use of the sponge is not recommended if you have had an abnormal pap smear.

• Condoms do not provide protection against infections transmitted skin-to-skin, like herpes and HPV (human papilloma virus).

- Diaphragms and cervical caps need to be refitted with a weight gain or loss of 10-15 lbs or more. The use of these devices may increase your risk of developing:

  - *Yeast infections:* An infection can develop from leaving the sponge or diaphragm in the vagina for longer than the recommended time period.

  - *Urinary tract infection:* This type of infection can also occur from over extended use of these devices and/or from using unclean hands.

  - *Toxic Shock Syndrome:* This is a bacterial infection known to be caused from the use of tampons or the introduction of other foreign objects into the vaginal canal. It can present similar to a severe flu with fever and chills and overall illness. This condition is rare but very serious and usually requires hospitalization for treatment with intravenous antibiotics.

Spermicides

Spermicides can be used alone or along with barrier methods and they kill sperm on contact.

Using a spermicide along with a barrier method gives you the best possible barrier method protection.

These methods work by preventing sperm from entering the cervix and are not as effective in preventing a pregnancy as the hormonal methods and IUDs.

Hormonal Birth Control Methods

Birth Control Pill

The birth control pill is one of the most common methods used in the US and works by preventing ovulation (release of an egg from the ovary). There are many different brand names for combination pills with both estrogen and progestin. There is also a pill with progestin only, commonly referred to as the mini pill. Some of the newer pills can reduce your menstrual cycles to only four a year.

Positives associated with taking the pill:

- May decrease the risk of developing ovarian and endometrial cancer.

- May help improve acne and skin conditions.
- May help reduce cyst formation in the breasts and ovaries.
- May help reduce heavy bleeding, cramping and regulate menstrual cycles.

Negatives associated with taking the pill:
- May aggravate migraine headaches
- May raise blood pressure
- May decrease the effectiveness of antibiotics and certain other medications.
- May promote the formation of gallstones.
- Offers no protection against sexually transmitted diseases.
- May be less effective if you weigh more than 180 lbs.
- May mask menstrual changes that signal the approach of menopause.
- May increase the incidence of developing a deep vein blood clot, stroke or heart attack

NOTE: Taking vitamin B supplements have been reported to interfere with the absorption of the birth control pill!

Do not take the pill if you have:
- High blood pressure, heart disease or have had a stroke
- Diabetes more than 20 years
- History of blood clots
- History of breast or uterine cancer
- History of liver and gallbladder disease
- A smoking habit and are over 35 years old

Your clinician will look at your individual "risk to benefit ratio" and then decide which pill you can take. The progesterone only pill "Mini Pill" may be a choice for breastfeeding women. The level of hormone in a birth control pill is much higher than in hormone replacement therapy medications. I tend to be very conservative and do not recommend the birth control pill as treatment if you are over age 45.

If you do elect to take the pill during perimenopause, choose a low dose pill such as: Loestrin 1/20 or Loestrin 1.5. These low dose pills have fewer side effects. You should preferably take the lowest effective dose.

Emergency Contraception

This method is referred to as the "morning-after" pill. This pill is to be used within 72 hours of having unprotected intercourse, known or suspected failure of contraception (condom breaks) or rape.

There are typically two types of hormones used with this method, similar to using the birth control pill:

• A pill containing the hormone progestin. Brand names are Plan B, Plan B One-Step, and Next Choice.

• A pill containing both hormones, estrogen and progestin. Brand name is Preven.

There are many other brands of the birth control pill that can also be used for this purpose.

Insertion of a Paragard IUD within 5 days after intercourse can also be used, so check in with your clinician.

Chemical Abortion Pill

A medical abortion is the use of medicines to end a pregnancy. A medical abortion may be done up to nine weeks of pregnancy. This method is referred as "the abortion pill" and RU-486 (Mifeprex) is the most common pill used. This pill blocks the effects of the hormone progesterone, stops the placenta from growing, softens the cervix and promotes labor.

NOTE: Many women may confuse Plan B with Mifeprex. Plan B does not cause abortions.

Contraceptive Skin Patch

Ortho Evra is the brand name of the estrogen and progestin patch, which releases hormones much like birth control pills do.

You place the patch on your upper arm, buttocks, stomach or chest once a week for three weeks and then wait a week until it is time to start over again.

Your menstrual period should begin during the week that you are not wearing the patch.

Use of the contraceptive patch during perimenopause can be associated with higher levels of circulating estrogen due to the sustained-release of this trans-dermal delivery system. This higher level of circulating hormone may increase the risk that side effects will occur, especially blood clots. Side effects for using this device are similar to the pill.

Implant Devices "Implanon" and "Nexplanon"

These devices are placed underneath the skin (sub-dermal) on the inside of your upper arm. The implant is a single, thin flexible rod, about the size of a match stick and releases the hormone progesterone for up to three years to prevent pregnancy. You must have a trained clinician to insert and remove this device.

Injections

There are two brand names of this type of contraception given by injection that provides protection for about 12 weeks. These injections work by suppressing ovulation, fertilization and implantation. (An injection is given every three months.)

Depo-Provera is the brand name for (DMPA), depomedroxy-progesterone acetate. There is also a low dose shot available called **Depo-sub Q Provera 104.**

Lunelle is the brand name for the combination estrogen and progesterone injection.

Positives associated with using injections:

• Good choice if you have trouble remembering to take the pill daily or to use your birth control method correctly each time you have sex.

• May lighten menstrual bleeding or even stop your periods.

Negatives associated with using injections:

• May increase the risk of developing breast cancer, blood clots, stroke, heart attack, high cholesterol, high blood pressure and major depression.

• May increase incidence of migraine headaches.

• May aggravate diabetes.

• May cause irregular heavy menstrual bleeding or completely stop your periods.

• May possibly delay fertility up to 18 months after discontinuation.

- May increase facial hair growth, breast tenderness and your weight.
- May promote bone loss. Bone loss associated with the low dose Depo-provera injection may be reversible.
- This form of contraception is not recommended if you have:
  - A history of depression.
  - Osteoporosis or are at risk for developing osteoporosis.
  - A heightened sensitivity to hormones.

Vaginal Contraceptive Ring

The **Nuva Ring** is the brand name for the vaginal contraceptive ring which releases both estrogen and progestin to prevent pregnancy.

It is a circular flexible ring that is inserted into the vagina for three weeks and then removed for one week. Your period should start the week the ring is out and then you insert a new ring for another three week cycle.

NOTE: This device delivers a constant low dose of hormones and seems to preserve vaginal moisture, unlike the birth control pill. The side effects for using this device are the same as the pill.

Intrauterine Device (IUD)

This device must be inserted into your uterus by a gynecologist or clinician.

IUDs have a string attached at one end which hangs down into the vagina. The string helps a woman check to make sure the IUD is still in place and helps the clinician locate it when it is time for removal.

The IUD works by altering the endometrium (uterine lining) and prevents implantation. It also changes the cervical mucus affecting sperm motility and preventing fertilization.

This method of contraception is very effective at preventing pregnancy.

Intrauterine Device With Hormone

Liletta, Mirena and Skyla are the brand names for the IUDs that contain levonorgestrel which is a progestin hormone and lasts for up to five years.

Positives associated with using this device:

- These devices may help decrease menstrual cramping, bleeding and shrink uterine fibroids.

Negatives associated with using this device:

- This method carries an increased risk for developing an ectopic pregnancy (a fertilized egg grows outside the uterus).
- Increased risk of developing pelvic inflammatory disease in the first three weeks after the IUD is inserted.
- This is not the best method if you have multiple partners because it does not provide protection against sexually transmitted diseases.

Intrauterine Devices (IUD) Without Hormone
Paragard is the brand name for the IUD which contains copper and may be left in place for up to ten years.

Positives associated with using this device:

- Good choice if you have trouble remembering to take the pill or using a birth control method correctly each time you have sex.
- Does not introduce hormones into your system.

Negatives associated with using this device:

- Increases the risk for developing a pelvic infection, which may cause sterility.
- Increases risk for developing an ectopic pregnancy (outside of the uterus).
- May cause spotting between periods, cramping and heavier menstrual bleeding.
- Does not provide protection against sexually transmitted infections.

Natural Family Planning
This is referred to as fertility awareness, when couples abstain from having intercourse on days when a woman might become pregnant.

This method also works when couples are trying to conceive a baby.

A woman must have regular menstrual cycles for this technique to be effective.

This technique requires couples to be trained in identifying cervical mucus changes, basal body temperature rise during ovulation and tracking the menstrual cycle by using the calendar method.

You need to use a special thermometer to identify the first morning basal body temperature, which falls just prior to ovulation and rises immediately following ovulation.

Couples may choose to use a barrier method during the days when a woman is considered to be fertile.

Permanent Birth Control (Female Sterilization)
These methods give you lasting protection against pregnancy and are not reversible. They are a good choice if you and your partner are certain that you don't want to have any more children.

Non-Surgical
Essure is relatively new way of achieving sterilization without having surgery. A small metallic spring-like device is placed in each fallopian tube, causing scar tissue to form over the implant. The scar tissue blocks the egg from traveling down the tube to meet sperm and fertilization is prevented.

Negatives associated with this device:
- Pelvic pain, vaginal bleeding and in some individuals hemorrhaging has been reported.
- Headaches and weight gain.
- Allergic reaction to the nickel.
- Higher incidence of possible ectopic pregnancy should you become pregnant.
- This device is currently under investigation by the FDA to determine if it should remain on the market.

Surgical
A woman may elect to have her fallopian tubes tied, which is called a tubal ligation. This procedure is an abdominal operation performed under general anesthesia.

Surgical risks can be:
- Damage to the bowel, bladder and major blood vessels.
- Adverse reaction to the anesthesia
- Complications with wound healing and possible infection, especially if you are a diabetic
- Persistent pelvic and/or abdominal pain

NOTE: Be sure to discuss your individual contraceptive needs with your clinician!

Common Premenopausal Conditions Associated with Hormonal Imbalance

Estrogen Dominance (Too Much Estrogen)

The balance of estrogen to progesterone is changed by excess estrogen or inadequate progesterone.

Symptoms

- Weight gain
- Bloating
- Mood swings
- Irritability
- Breast tenderness
- Headaches
- Fatigue (feeling tired)
- Depression
- Hypoglycemia (low blood sugar)

Estrogen Dominance can be associated with the following conditions:

- Uterine fibroids
- Endometriosis
- Thyroid dysfunction (too much estrogen impairs thyroid hormone activity and promotes weight gain)
- Fibrocystic breasts
- Breast cancer
- Ovarian cancer
- Uterine cancer

PMS (Premenstrual Syndrome)

Yes, it is real and you are not going crazy! PMS is described as, "the physical and emotional changes a female experiences every month because of her hormonal cycle." PMS is cyclic and you will notice these changes at the same time each month. The prevalence is greatest during the fourth and fifth decades. Seventy percent of women have some premenstrual symptoms.

Symptoms which can occur seven to ten days before your period begins each month are:

- Bloating and swelling of hands and feet
- Weight gain
- Headaches and backaches
- Breast swelling and tenderness
- Irritability and feeling anxious
- Depressed mood (crying for no apparent reason) and decreased ability to concentrate
- Feeling tired with decreased energy and insomnia
- Cravings for sweets, especially chocolate

You may experience any combination of these symptoms at varying degrees from mild to severe. Every system of the body can be affected; immune, digestive, circulatory, nervous, endocrine, and dermatologic (skin).

We don't know what causes PMS, although most authorities on PMS agree that it's related to the hormone progesterone, which is produced in the second half of the menstrual cycle.

Recommendations For Relieving PMS Symptoms

Dietary Changes

- Decreasing salt, your body's cells absorb sodium more readily before your menses.
- Increase fiber to bind excess estrogen.
- Decrease consumption of processed foods and red meats with xenoestrogens (environmental estrogens).
- Eat six small meals throughout the day.
- Consume vinegar which can act like a natural diuretic.
- It is ok to eat chocolate with 72% or greater cocoa. Limit to two small pieces.
- Eat your fruits and vegetables.
- Avoid alcohol and caffeine, because they stimulate the central nervous system initially and then depress it.

Supplements

- Calcium with vitamin D in divided doses.
- Vitamin B complex for decreasing stress (be careful not to take

too much B6 which can cause peripheral neuritis).

- A good one-a-day vitamin/mineral supplement with magnesium.
- Vitamin E helps restore ovarian health and reduces symptoms of PMS.

Herbs

- Evening Primrose oil, valerian and melatonin. Melatonin is considered the sleep hormone and decreases just before ovulation.
- Don Quai can help with irritability and sleep.
- Chaste Tree can help with mood changes and headaches.

CAUTION: Use caution when taking herbs, you should consult with a herbologist or your clinician to determine the proper dosage for you to take. Please see the vitamin and supplement section in Chapter 3 for further detail.

Medications

- **Natural Progesterone Cream:** given in the second half of your cycle may help relieve anxiety, enhance sleep and balance blood sugar. Progesterone can block many unwanted side effects of too much estrogen.
- **Anti-prostaglandins** such as ibuprofen or naproxen sodium may be helpful. They should be taken with food. Consult your clinician if you have bleeding problems or a history of stomach ulcers.
- **Diuretics** such as spironolactone may be prescribed by your clinician for persistent fluid retention.

NOTE: If you experience persistent anxiety and depression that interfere with your ability to perform daily activities, talk with your clinician about possible prescription medications that can help.

If you experience severe PMS that interferes with your ability to function, you may have *premenstrual dysphoric disorder* (PMDD) and this can be very serious. This disorder is associated with a decreased level of serotonin, (the "feel good" hormone) and can lead to severe depression. PMDD should be treated by your clinician as soon as possible.

Counseling (psychological), hypnotherapy and acupuncture may reduce symptoms of PMS and help you feel better.

I will close this section with a question that one of my male patients at the age of eleven asked me many years ago when I was examining his mother. He asked if "PMS" means "Pissed Mommy Syndrome?" We all just looked at each other and began to laugh.

Endometriosis

This condition occurs when tiny pieces of endometrium (cells which line the uterus), become misplaced throughout the pelvic region. These pieces are found:

• On fallopian tubes

• Within the uterine musculature, called *adenomyosis*

• On the outer surface of the uterus

• On the colon

• On the bladder

• Along the sides of the pelvic cavity

Once a month these pieces of misplaced endometrium respond to ovarian hormones exactly like the endometrium cells inside the uterus. They swell with blood and then bleed into the nearby tissues during your menstrual period. This bleeding causes inflammation which can be very painful.

The symptoms begin one to two weeks before menstruation and progress up through menstruation. Sexual intercourse or even having a bowel movement can be extremely painful.

Symptoms

• Menstrual cramps which increase in intensity with each cycle

• Pain when ovulating (mid-cycle) called "Mittelschmerz"

• Painful intercourse

• Inability to get pregnant (infertility)

• Bladder infections (tests for bacteria often are negative)

• Severe pelvic pain before and during you period

• A history of bleeding ovarian cysts which may rupture

• Bumps that can be felt on the uterus during a pelvic exam

NOTE: These symptoms also can be associated with other conditions and it is important to have regular check-ups with your clinician to monitor any changes.

Diagnosis

- Endometriosis can be a challenge to diagnose because we do not have any tests that can identify these endometrial pieces.

- Laparoscopy (looking into the abdomen through a scope) is the method used to ***diagnose*** endometriosis.

Treatment

- Natural progesterone cream has been reported to afford relief, when used for three weeks a month, beginning around the first week of the cycle. It can take up to six months before relief is noted.

- Male hormone injections can be used for a short period of time to relieve symptoms. Lupron is commonly used.

- Pregnancy helps slow the progression of endometriosis, although it may be challenging to achieve a pregnancy.

- Menopause is the cure for endometriosis.

Uterine Fibroids

Uterine Fibroids are the most common growth within the uterus. Uterine fibroids can range in size from a chicken egg to a grapefruit. These growths occur during the years before menopause and shrink (shrivel up) after menopause.

Estrogen makes fibroids grow! (So don't take estrogen, including birth control pills.)

Diagnosis

Uterine fibroids are diagnosed and followed with an ultrasound.

Treatment

- Male hormone injections, like Lupron, can be used for a short period of time to counteract excess estrogen, shrinking uterine fibroids. (Some larger uterine fibroids can make estrogen within the fibroid itself.)

- Progesterone cream may provide some benefit, if used during the second half of your cycle. Progesterone may help reduce the size of these growths by decreasing excess estrogen and restoring a normal hormone balance.

- RU 486 - This is an anti-progesterone medication. Some fibroids contain growth factors that can be stimulated by progesterone. Be sure to consult with your clinician.

- <u>Surgery</u> may be recommended for the treatment of uterine fibroids. You can choose to have a procedure that uses a laparoscope (looking through a scope into the abdomen) or to have a hysterectomy (removal of the uterus.) Many women choose to have a hysterectomy for treatment of uterine fibroids.

Benign Breast Disease

Mastodynia (Mastalgia, or Breast Tenderness)
This condition is quite common, often cyclical and increases in women taking the birth control pill or hormone replacement therapy.

Symptoms
Typically one week before your menstrual cycle begins you may experience a fullness of your breasts and they can become very sensitive to touch. This can also occur when you first begin taking the birth control pill or hormone replacement therapy and may last for several months and then resolves.

Fibroadenomas
This is the most common benign breast tumor and is typically found in young women less than 30 years of age. Fibroadenomas are described as round, firm, smooth, discrete, mobile and usually non-tender to touch. These growths tend to appear suddenly and are more commonly found in black women.

Fibrocystic Changes
This is a common breast condition seen in women 30 to 50 years of age and is referred to as *benign breast disease*. Lumps and cysts (abnormal tissue growth) can develop in your breasts.

Symptoms
These lumps and cysts can become painful usually one week before your period. Some women do not experience pain.

This condition can be aggravated by caffeine use.

Many women with estrogen dominance (relatively more estrogen than progesterone) have fibrocystic breast disease.

NOTE: Make sure you do your monthly breast self-exam about a week after your period and do it at the same time each month if you no longer are having periods.

Treatment

- Avoid trauma and wear a supportive bra.
- NSAIDs like ibuprofen (Advil) and naproxen sodium (Aleve), as well as acetaminophen may help reduce pain.
- Natural progesterone cream has been reported to help correct the hormonal imbalance with good results.
- Prescription male hormone injections such as Lupron may be recommended.
- Vitamin E and Evening Primrose oil have been reported to help relieve breast discomfort.
- Chaste Tree has been reported to help balance estrogen and progesterone levels.
- Decreasing caffeine intake may help reduce fibrocystic changes that are found in women with fibrocystic disease.
- Birth control pill users report having fewer cysts in their breasts than non-users.

(Please read Chapter 7 for information on Breast Cancer)

Websites for further information on:

Breast Health
National Breast Cancer Foundation-Breast Health Education:
http://www.nationalbreastcancer.org/breast-health-education

Contraception
Centers for Disease Control and Prevention-Contraceptive Use:
https://www.cdc.gov/nchs/fastats/contraceptive.htm

Endometriosis
WebMD Endometriosis Health Center:
http://www.webmd.com/women/endometriosis/

Estrogen Dominance
Christiane Northrup, M.D.-Estrogen Dominance:
http://www.drnorthrup.com/estrogen-dominance/

Premenstrual Syndrome (PMS)
Women's Health, US Department of Health and Human Services-
Premenstrual Syndrome Fact Sheet:
**https://www.womenshealth.gov/a-z-topics/premenstrual-
syndrome**

The Female Menstrual cycle
Mayo Clinic Women's Health-Menstrual cycle:
**http://www.mayoclinic.org/healthy-lifestyle/womens-health/
in-depth/menstrual-cycle/art-20047186**

Uterine Fibroids
Women's Health, US Department of Health and Human Services-
Uterine Fibroids:
https://www.womenshealth.gov/a-z-topics/uterine-fibroids

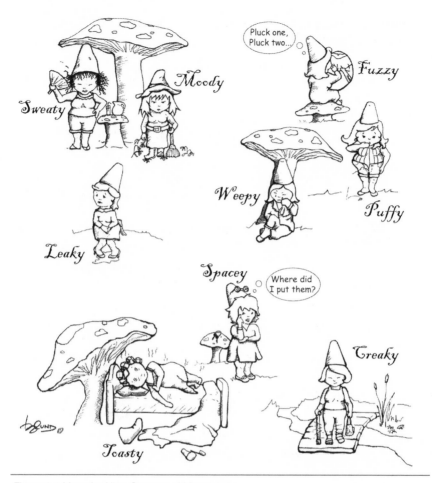

Figure 3.1 Meet the Nine Gnomes of Menopause

Chapter 3

CHAMPIONING THE CHANGE: UNDERSTANDING MENOPAUSE

Are you menopausal? You are not alone! There are about 35 million women in the United States who are over age 50. Many women find themselves in their menopausal years without any knowledge of what to expect, when the process might begin and how long it may last. I believe the more you know, the better you can plan for this transition and pursue treatment options, if needed. Understanding this process can help alleviate the stress and fear associated with the unknown.

The Stages Of Menopause

Menopause is the end of menstrual cycling and its associated fertility (a woman's ability to have a child). The word "menopause" means the last menses and the "climacteric" is the aging process when a woman moves from her reproductive years to her non-reproductive years.

This is a gradual natural midlife transition and is divided into three stages:

- Perimenopause
- Menopause
- Postmenopause

Perimenopause

Perimenopause is the first stage of the transition and the term is used to describe the years leading up to menopause, which also includes the first full year after your last menstrual period. The ovaries, where your eggs are produced and stored, begin transformation between the ages of 35 and 50. The ovaries actually shrink in size and egg production slows down along with declining estrogen and progesterone levels, which leads to a hormonal imbalance. Ovulation (release of an egg) becomes less regular and your menstrual cycles begin to change. These are referred to as "anovulatory" cycles. When the ovaries are no longer releasing an egg, progesterone is *not* produced. This leads to a lower level of circulating progesterone, although you can still be having periods.

Symptoms of Perimenopause

Mental clarity can be affected. This transition has peaks and valleys which can cause annoying mental symptoms such as lack of focus and memory. Mood changes often occur and many women can experience a depressed mood, increased irritability and stress due to low levels of estrogen mixed with high surges. You just don't feel like yourself. This can be misdiagnosed as depression or worse.

Physical symptoms can occur due to these surges of high mixed with low levels of estrogen.

Common symptoms you may experience with **high levels of estrogen,** termed *Estrogen Dominance* are:

- Weight gain, especially in your tummy (body fat shifts to your waist)
- Breast tenderness
- Water retention
- Fatigue (feeling tired)
- Heavy bleeding and cramping (seek medical attention if bleeding is severe or persistent)
- Worsening premenstrual symptoms "PMS"

Common symptoms you may experience with *low levels of estrogen* are:

- Hot Flashes, Flushes or the Toasties (a warm sensation throughout the body)
- Insomnia (unable to sleep well)
- Vaginal dryness
- Urinary Incontinence (leakage)
- Decreased libido (sex drive/desire)

Menstrual changes you may experience can vary from individual to individual but may include:

- Lighter or heavier bleeding
- Bleeding for fewer or more days than usual
- Shorter or longer cycles than usual (length of time between periods), irregular menstrual patterns or even skipped periods

Most women will experience menstrual changes 4 to 8 years before reaching menopause.

NOTE: Some evidence points to the fact that the mental and emotional symptoms are actually worse during perimenopause than during menopause due to hormonal fluctuations. We can ask our partners their opinion. Or maybe we should not- Ha! Ha!

Menopause
Menopause is the second stage of transition described as a natural biologic process that is part of every woman's life and occurs as a woman ages.

Menopause can also result from having surgery, radiation, chemotherapy, illness or any other condition or procedure that can adversely affect the hormonal axis.

Definition

Menopause occurs with your final menstrual period and is confirmed by twelve months in a row without having a period. Unfortunately, there is not a test to determine exactly when you will experience menopause.

Natural Menopause

Natural menopause is the time of a women's life when the ovaries naturally stop functioning. There is a gradual decline in the production of estrogen and progesterone during the perimenopausal years, which then accelerates as menopause approaches. Women often ovulate less and less until they no longer ovulate and the monthly periods with their associated fertility come to an end. Changes begin to occur in the tissues which respond to estrogen, such as the vagina, bladder and your bones.

Surgical Menopause

Surgical menopause occurs when the ovaries are surgically removed. This is most commonly done while having your uterus removed and is referred to as a complete hysterectomy. When you have your ovaries removed, menopause occurs immediately, because of the abrupt decline of estrogen. If you are premenopausal, this can be a real shock to your body. I describe it as, "a high speed train loaded with hormones headed for a brick wall and once it hits, everything is gone." It would be a smoother ride if the body could prepare by slowing down and bracing for the impact at a much slower speed. This is what happens with natural menopause when your ovaries are in place, as they gradually produce less and less hormone over time.

This could also be accomplished by taking hormone replacement therapy if your ovaries must be removed. Hormone replacement therapy can sometimes have risks which I discuss later in this chapter.

If you have not had your ovaries removed during a hysterectomy, you will not have periods but you will experience menopause naturally because your ovaries will still produce hormones.

Onset Of Menopause

The onset of menopause can vary from woman to woman. Menopause occurs for most women between the ages of 45 and 55, although it can happen earlier or later. I have seen women in my practice experience menopause as early as the age of 35 and as late as the age of 58! The average age is 51.5 years. Premature menopause is the term used when your period stops before age 40.

The severity of symptoms can be different for each woman. Some women may experience minor or very few symptoms, while other women have severe symptoms that can interfere with daily living.

Symptoms Of Menopause

Hot Flashes, Or Flushes, And Night Sweats

Hot flashes are sudden feelings of heat and intense sweating, often accompanied by an increase in heart rate and sometimes followed by chills.

Some hot flashes can be mild and pass quickly and other times they can be intense, very embarrassing and interfere with life. It seems like a catch 22, the more embarrassed you become, the more intense the hot flash. Frustration tends to promote a hot flash- just when you need it most. Not!

Hot flashes have been reported to affect approximately 50%-90% of postmenopausal women. These hot flashes can begin early in perimenopause and can continue through postmenopause.

The flushing symptoms seem to be more associated with the drop in estrogen level rather than the level of estrogen in your body.

Estrogen has many functions. One of them is controlling the dilation and constriction of blood vessels. When your estrogen level is dropping, as in perimenopause or menopause, one of the control monitors that limit vessel dilation is lost and your blood vessels can dilate at will, hence a "hot flash!" It's like "when the cat's away, the mice will play." The estrogen is the cat and those naughty blood vessels are the mice. When blood vessels dilate, they bring warm red blood to the surface of the skin, thus you feel hot and you turn red.

Sound familiar?

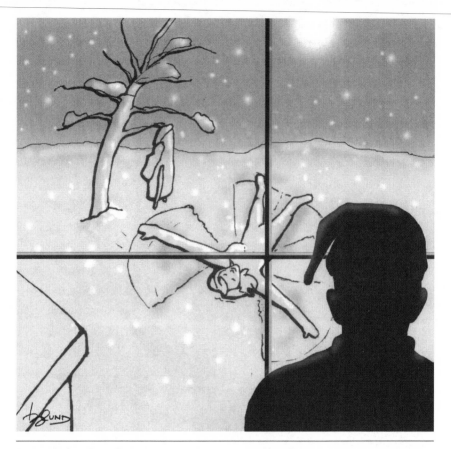

Figure 3.2 Hot Flash Snow Angel — *Where did my wife go?*

Night Sweats are hot flashes combined with intense sweating that occur at night. These can definitely interfere with a good night's sleep. These sleep disturbances can lead to daytime tiredness. This can begin early in perimenopause and continue through the post-menopausal period. Sometimes they can recur even after menopause seems to be well in the past.

Vaginal Changes

Low estrogen levels lead to thinning of the tissues of the vagina and can be associated with decreased vaginal lubrication. The vaginal tissue can actually shrink and dry out over time. These changes can cause uncomfortable symptoms such as itching, burning, irritation and painful intercourse.

Urinary Frequency And Incontinence

Low estrogen levels lead to thinning of the tissues of the urethra as well. The urethra is the opening where urine passes through, exiting the body. These changes can contribute to the inability to hold urine. The tissues become dry and thinner and muscles lose their tone leading to urinary leakage.

(Please read Chapter 9 for more detailed information on urinary incontinence.)

Skin Changes

Estrogen keeps skin moist and preserves its elasticity. Lower estrogen levels can lead to thinning of the skin throughout the body, sometimes escalating the formation of wrinkles and sagging skin. Yikes!

Mental Changes

Lower estrogen levels can lead to a decrease in serotonin which is referred to as "the feel good hormone" because it helps regulate sleep and mood. Lower serotonin levels may cause:

- Changes in memory and may increase forgetfulness.
- Fogginess and lack of focus due to decreased communication between the nerve cells in the brain.

Heart Palpitations (a pounding heart)

Lower estrogen levels can signal the brain to send out adrenaline in an attempt to trigger estrogen production so your heart beats faster.

NOTE: Palpitations can also indicate a possible heart problem. See your clinician as soon as possible if you should develop this symptom.

Hair Changes

Lower estrogen levels can lead to:

- Thinning of hair and hair loss
- Dry and brittle hair
- Frizzy and wiry hair, especially if you color it regularly.

Bone Changes

Lower estrogen levels can lead to bone loss and eventually osteoporosis, which is thinning of the bones and could possibly put you at risk for a fracture from minimal trauma.

Women may experience rapid bone loss, approximately 20% in the first few years after menopause, due to the decline in estrogen.

Bone loss does eventually level off within five to ten years after entering menopause.

(Please read Chapter 6 for further information on bone health.)

Weight Changes

Lower estrogen levels allow weight to shift to the center of the body, namely, your waist. I refer to this as the "menopausal dresser" as illustrated on page 51. I can relate, can you? Having a sense of humor helps you survive ... right?

NOTE: Any of the menopausal symptoms listed above can also be caused by other medical conditions, therefore medical advice should be sought if they are sudden, severe or persistent.

Postmenopause

Postmenopause is the last stage of the menopause transition. When you entered puberty your hormones claimed center stage and in perimenopause they rode the roller coaster with fluctuating levels. During postmenopause your hormones have now taken their final bow. In a similar manner, as in puberty, your hormone levels eventually calm down after menopause and your body adapts to this new phase of life. Many women find this stage of menopause to be liberating, claiming freedom from years of premenstrual symptoms, menstruation and fertility concerns.

Definition

Postmenopause is the period of a woman's life after she has gone through menopause. A woman is assured that she is postmenopausal when she has gone twelve months without a period.

During postmenopause, hormone levels drop dramatically and these markedly lower levels are maintained, unlike the perimenopause phase.

During postmenopause the sites where hormones are produced change as well. Prior to menopause the primary site where estrogen is produced is the ovary. After menopause the secondary sites, like fat and muscle, produce an estrogen called estrone at markedly lower levels. During postmenopause, ovarian production of estrogen declines dramatically and this much weaker form of estrogen is produced.

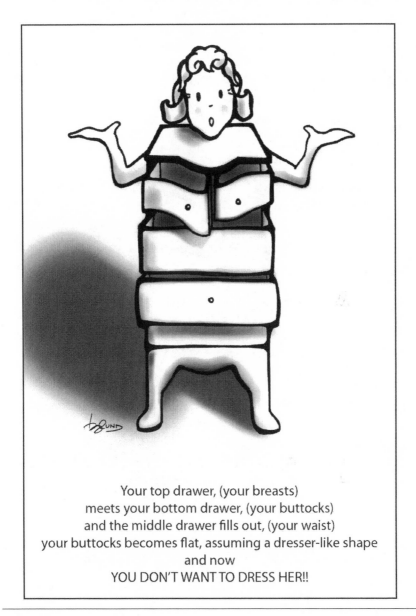

Your top drawer, (your breasts)
meets your bottom drawer, (your buttocks)
and the middle drawer fills out, (your waist)
your buttocks becomes flat, assuming a dresser-like shape
and now
YOU DON'T WANT TO DRESS HER!!

Figure 3.3

Symptoms Of Postmenopause

During postmenopause some women continue to experience uncomfortable menopausal symptoms such as:

• Hot Flashes

• Urinary incontinence

- Decreased libido

- Insomnia

Some women experience almost complete relief from menopausal symptoms during the postmenopausal period.

Hormones play an essential role in many areas of the body. When hormone levels reach permanently low levels as in postmenopause, the health implications can be significant.

As women begin to notice the symptoms of hormone deficiency, they may want to consider taking steps to stabilize their hormone production.

NOTE: Postmenopausal women are at a much higher risk for developing health conditions related to low hormonal levels. (Please refer to part 2 of this book for further details on these conditions.)

Minimizing Menopausal Symptoms

Today there are different options to help balance hormonal levels:
- Lifestyle changes
- Alternative medicine remedies using herbs and supplements
- Vitamins and minerals
- Non-hormonal prescription medications
- Non-hormonal vaginal creams and lubricants
- Traditional Hormone Replacement Therapy
- Selective Estrogen Receptor Modulators (SERMs)
- Natural Hormone Replacement Therapy

Life Style Changes
This is an especially important time in your life when you must first look at your present diet and lifestyle. Improper diet and lifestyle can worsen symptoms of hormonal imbalance and in some people, even cause them! Proper diet and lifestyle can improve the symptoms and may possibly help to avoid these symptoms altogether.

Consider making changes which can help improve your health and make you feel better. It is a must to make healthy lifestyle changes to help restore hormonal balance! Taking care of yourself should be your number one priority for getting started on the right path.

Health risks associated with being overweight increase as you approach perimenopause and menopause. This is definitely the time to get serious about a lifestyle change to promote a healthy weight. Change your thinking from dieting, to getting healthy. Take control, watch your diet, consume less sugar and processed carbohydrates to help maintain a healthy weight.

Understanding Food Groups And A Healthy Diet

A proper diet is essential to maintaining "balance" in midlife. A woman's nutritional needs change as she approaches midlife.

Estrogen production and your metabolism slow down and fat migrates to your waist.

Your body is less forgiving and you just cannot eat what you used to without gaining weight.

"No fudge because your weight won't budge" and "the butt goes and the gut grows" is true. Bummer!

If you think eating healthy means giving up foods you like, think again. It is actually about eating more basic foods like fruits and vegetables and easing up on less healthy snacks (processed sugars and carbohydrates).

The reality is that two thirds of us are overweight. There are currently 300,000 deaths a year in the US from cancer, diabetes and heart disease. These deaths can be related to being overweight and could possibly have been prevented.

Healthy eating is a personal choice. What works for one, may not necessarily work for another, so try making small changes that will fit into your lifestyle. Make gradual changes and integrate one or two new habits at a time to ensure long term success.

Many women become "carbohydrate intolerant" as they journey into midlife, so it's best to avoid refined sugars and starches in order to lose weight.

Combine food groups that help lower the insulin response and promote weight loss which is called "food pairing." When you eat carbohydrate rich foods it stimulates your pancreas to release insulin and a high level of insulin promotes fat storage and weight gain. An example of food pairing is eating a serving of lean protein with vegetables along with a small portion of a good fat such as an avocado, olive oil, olives or almonds. Eat a small portion of food every three hours and that works out to be about six times a day. Have your fresh fruit as a snack three hours after eating protein.

Eating a nutritious diet can help to minimize hot flashes. Did you know that alcohol, processed sugars, carbohydrates and caffeine can all promote hot flashes and weight gain?

NOTE: According to Dr. Alison Huang, an assistant professor of Obstetrics and Gynecology at UCSF, there is now good scientific evidence that losing weight can reduce hot flashes.

A healthy diet can also lower your risk of developing diabetes, heart disease and even some cancers.

(Again, I discuss in greater detail the effects menopause can have on your health in part two of this book.)

Here are some questions to ask yourself:

• Why do you want to eat healthier?

• Do you eat when you're not hungry?

• When and why do you eat?

• Are you an emotional eater? Does food comfort you?

• What is your idea of a perfect meal? Can you make it healthier with a few small changes?

• How did your family feel about food? Are other family members overweight? If you have children, what have you taught them about food? Do you sit down together as a family when eating a meal?

• How much time do you spend weekly planning meals versus eating out or picking up fast food?

A few small but consistent changes that can make a big difference are:

• Drink more water daily and eliminate sodas with high fructose corn syrup.

• Eat only when you are sure that you are hungry.

• Eat only foods with nutritional value.

- Eat small amounts of food every two to three hours.
- Decrease consumption of sugar, refined carbohydrates and starches.
- Food pairing to include a protein, vegetables and a small portion of the good fats as discussed above.

It is ok to have that once a week small piece of cake, cookie or brownie, if you balance it with nutritious snacks throughout the week. The key is to make sure you eat only a small amount, just enough to satisfy the craving.

Learn how to reward yourself with something other than food. Try treating yourself to a manicure, pedicure or a massage.

Think of how great you will feel once you have achieved your weight loss goal. You are now able to fit into your jeans with room to move in them—yeah!

The goal is to make these choices for life and restore a *healthy internal balance.* This means your mind and internal organs are in complete *harmony.*

Once you restore balance, your body is able to make essential hormones and enzymes needed to function properly.

When your body is functioning properly, all systems are a go and you feel great and will lose weight.

Weight Maintenance

Body Mass Index

The body mass index is a good tool for determining if you are at a healthy weight. If you fall in the overweight or obese range, your risk can be increased for developing certain diseases. Scientists have devised a formula for assessing risk using height and body weight measurements. They refer to this as the **Body Mass Index (BMI).** The higher the BMI, the greater the risk of certain diseases, including high blood pressure, heart disease, stroke, insulin resistance, type 2 diabetes, osteoarthritis and some cancers. *(See Table 3.1, page 56)*

The National Institutes of Health defines obesity and overweight using the BMI as follows:

Table 3.1: Look for your height and weight on the BMI chart and you will find your body mass index.

Body weight (pounds)

BMI / Height (inches)	19	20	21	22	23	24	25	26	27	28	29	30	31	32	33	34	35	36	37	38	39	40	41	42	43	44	45	46	47	48	49	50	51	52	53	54
58	91	96	100	105	110	115	119	124	129	134	138	143	148	153	158	162	167	172	177	181	186	191	196	201	205	210	215	220	224	229	234	239	244	248	253	258
59	94	99	104	109	114	119	124	128	133	138	143	148	153	158	163	168	173	178	183	188	193	198	203	208	212	217	222	227	232	237	242	247	252	257	262	267
60	97	102	107	112	118	123	128	133	138	143	148	153	158	163	168	174	179	184	189	194	199	204	209	215	220	225	230	235	240	245	250	255	261	266	271	276
61	100	106	111	116	122	127	132	137	143	148	153	158	164	169	174	180	185	190	195	201	206	211	217	222	227	232	238	243	248	254	259	264	269	275	280	285
62	104	109	115	120	126	131	136	142	147	153	158	164	169	175	180	186	191	196	202	207	213	218	224	229	235	240	246	251	256	262	267	273	278	284	289	295
63	107	113	118	124	130	135	141	146	152	158	163	169	175	180	186	191	197	203	208	214	220	225	231	237	242	248	254	259	265	270	278	282	287	293	299	304
64	110	116	122	128	134	140	145	151	157	163	169	174	180	186	192	197	204	209	215	221	227	232	238	244	250	256	262	267	273	279	285	291	296	302	308	314
65	114	120	126	132	138	144	150	156	162	168	174	180	186	192	198	204	210	216	222	228	234	240	246	252	258	264	270	276	282	288	294	300	306	312	318	324
66	118	124	130	136	142	148	155	161	167	173	179	186	192	198	204	210	216	223	229	235	241	247	253	260	266	272	278	284	291	297	303	309	315	322	328	334
67	121	127	134	140	146	153	159	166	172	178	185	191	198	204	211	217	223	230	236	242	249	255	261	268	274	280	287	293	299	306	312	319	325	331	338	344
68	125	131	138	144	151	158	164	171	177	184	190	197	203	210	216	223	230	236	243	249	256	262	269	276	282	289	295	302	308	315	322	328	335	341	348	354
69	128	135	142	149	155	162	169	176	182	189	196	203	209	216	223	230	236	243	250	257	263	270	277	284	291	297	304	311	318	324	331	338	345	351	358	365
70	132	139	146	153	160	167	174	181	188	195	202	209	216	222	229	236	243	250	257	264	271	278	285	292	299	306	313	320	327	334	341	348	355	362	369	376
71	136	143	150	157	165	172	179	186	193	200	208	215	222	229	236	243	250	257	265	272	279	286	293	301	308	315	322	329	338	343	351	358	365	372	379	386
72	140	147	154	162	169	177	184	191	199	206	213	221	228	235	242	250	258	265	272	279	287	294	302	309	316	324	331	338	346	353	361	368	375	383	390	397
73	144	151	159	166	174	182	189	197	204	212	219	227	235	242	250	257	265	272	280	288	295	302	310	318	325	333	340	348	355	363	371	378	386	393	401	408
74	148	155	163	171	179	186	194	202	210	218	225	233	241	249	256	264	272	280	287	295	303	311	319	326	334	342	350	358	365	373	381	389	396	404	412	420
75	152	160	168	176	184	192	200	208	216	224	232	240	248	256	264	272	279	287	295	303	311	319	327	335	343	351	359	367	375	383	391	399	407	415	423	431
76	156	164	172	180	189	197	205	213	221	230	238	246	254	263	271	279	287	295	304	312	320	328	336	344	353	361	369	377	385	394	402	410	418	426	435	443

Normal   Overweight   Obese   Extreme Obesity

- Less than 18.5 would be *underweight.* (Consult your clinician about maintaining a healthy weight.)
- 18.5-24.9 is a *healthy weight.* (Maintaining a healthy weight minimizes health risks.)
- 25-29.9 is *overweight.* (The unhealthy weight is in the waist, therefore reducing the waist size will reduce health risks.)
- 30 or higher is *obese, very high to extremely high risk.* (Even a 10% reduction in weight can provide significant health benefits.)

Exercise

Exercise is essential for good health and a healthier lifestyle. Research has shown that exercise can have a positive impact on achieving and maintaining hormonal balance.

If you do not exercise, begin today. Exercise helps you lose and maintain your weight by burning fat and increasing muscle tissue.

Benefits Of Exercise

- Increases your metabolic rate and energy
- Improves digestion and sleep
- Lowers blood pressure
- Improves cholesterol levels
- Increases mental alertness
- Strengthens muscles and bones helping to keep them strong
- Increases flexibility and stamina
- Helps improve mood and depression
- Helps decrease stress and hot flashes
- Improves self-esteem
- You can, on average, lose about 14 pounds per year just by exercising

Muscle strength declines dramatically as we age. Unless you do resistance exercise and strength training with weights or elastic bands, you may lose up to six pounds of muscle mass in a decade.

Loss Of Muscle And Increased Body Fat Can:

- Put extra strain on the heart

- Alter sugar metabolism (increasing the risk for developing insulin resistance and diabetes)
- Lower healthy lipids (HDL cholesterol) which can lead to having a heart attack or stroke

Follow These Recommendations:

- Exercise 20 to 30 minutes a day, at least 3 to 4 times a week.
- Be sure to vary your workout to include weight bearing exercise, strength training, aerobics, stretching and core strengthening exercise such as Yoga, Pilates or Tai Chi.

Weight Bearing Exercise

This includes walking, hiking, dancing and low impact aerobics. Benefits include:

- Improved sleep
- Improved mood
- Improved balance
- Improved bone density
- Can help to balance testosterone levels
- Can help decrease stress and hot flashes

Strength Training Exercise

A complete strength training program consists of:

- Lifting free weights
- Weight machines
- Isometrics (pulling/pushing resistance exercises)
- Swimming

The duration should be for 20 minutes, two to three times a week.

Do slow reps with a low weight to the count of 10 (ten seconds to lift and ten seconds to lower the weights). You will continue this until you are unable to lift anymore. This is called, "lift to failure". Your muscles will probably be shaking after you finish.

You will definitely feel that you have worked out even after only 20 minutes. It is hard work, but you can do it and it works.

Be sure to vary the type of exercise on alternate days. This has a dual benefit in that it gives your body needed rest from one type of activity while increasing your body's response by challenging different muscle groups. After you reach 45 years of age, your metabolism may slow down and you have to wake it up.

Doing these exercises for 20 minutes a day, two to three times a week for ten to twelve weeks can:

• Rebuild three pounds of muscle and increase your metabolism by 7%, which can burn fat and calories.

• Enhance oxygen rich blood flow to the brain and vital organs, possibly decreasing your risk of developing dementia (Alzheimer's disease).

• May extend the length and quality of your life.

Remember, these exercises make your body work against gravity. Strength training builds muscle tone, endurance, bone density and also speeds up your metabolism which burns fat.

Stretching And Core Strengthening

Yoga, Pilates and Tai Chi are examples of this type of exercise. These forms of exercise are excellent for increasing strength, flexibility and promoting relaxation.

These exercises can help preserve balance and reduce stress. Certain poses force your muscles to hold your body weight and this is great for resistance training.

Yoga gently moves joints, stretches and tones muscles and encourages deeper breathing. When you concentrate on your breathing and posture, you can relax and de-stress.

Breathing, bending and twisting help to stimulate and cleanse the many systems of the body and eliminate toxins.

You can gain great benefit from a five minute workout doing just the *sun salutation*. Go to *www.verywell.com (https://www.verywell. com/illustrated-stepbystep-sun-salutation-3567187)* and print out the sun-salutation steps to follow.

NOTE: Always breathe through exercises and never hold your breath.

Exercise Pearls

Always warm up and cool down. This puts your muscles and cardiovascular system on alert that they are about to work.

Studies show that just 30 minutes of moderate exercise a day can have a tremendous impact on every cell in your body.

Warm up with some gentle walking or cycling. As you get started with your exercise routine, begin with five minutes a day and add a minute each day until you reach 20 to 30 minutes. Within a month you will have achieved your goal of exercising for a 30 minute session. The "Wii" is a great way to exercise at home, especially if you live in a cold climate and are unable to go outdoors.

Exercise can:

• Increase blood flow to vital organs
• Reverse the natural decrease in oxygen efficiency and muscle mass due to aging
• Reduce inflammation.
• Reduce your risk of heart disease by 50%
• Reduce your risk of developing high blood pressure, diabetes and colon cancer by 30%
• Slow down your resting heart rate, decreasing the overall amount of oxygen needed
• Reduce the rate at which you create harmful free radicals which can damage cells

Aerobic exercise:

• Burns fat
• Increases circulation
• Increases endurance
• Increases good cholesterol (HDL) and lowers triglycerides, total and bad cholesterol (LDL)
• Can help lower blood pressure
• Can help decrease anxiety and emotional stress
• Can help improve mood, sleep and depression

Exercise Tips:

• Choose a partner and try to exercise at the same time of day.
• Drink cold water on an empty stomach (it burns more calories) and warm water after a meal, which can promote proper digestion.

- Start slow and warm up to prevent injuries.
- Stretch after each workout and never bounce to avoid injury.
- Check your heart rate for ten seconds and then multiply that number by six. To calculate your "target heart rate" zone, you must first determine your average maximum heart rate. The maximum heart rate calculation should be 220 minus your age. Your heart rate during exercise should range between 50 to 85 percent of your average maximum heart rate. Exercising with a goal of 80% will be: If you are 50 years of age, 220 minus 50 equals 170, then multiply 170 x .80 which equals 136 and this is your target heart rate.
- Vary your workout for greater results and to keep it interesting.
- Make sure your changes are gradual and permanent. Do not start anything today that you will not be able to continue for a life time.
- You can walk for ten minutes three times a day and that counts as a 30 minute workout.
- Don't forget to reward yourself and schedule a massage or a pedicure!

NOTE: Be careful, over exercising can actually lower estrogen levels!

Designing An Exercise Plan

- Determine how strenuously you would like to exercise (intensity) and check it by the exertion effort (walk-talk-test). If you can still talk while you are working out, you are doing just fine.
- Determine how many times a week you want to exercise (frequency) with the goal of achieving 30 minute sessions up to five times a week.
- Determine how long each exercise session should last (duration).

Example of an Exercise Plan

- *Day 1:* Warm-up for five minutes, then do 30 minutes of aerobic exercise followed by 20 minutes of strength training.
- *Day 2:* Yoga or Pilates for 55 minutes

- *Day 3* Swim for 30 minutes
- *Day 4:* Off
- *Day 5:* Same as day one for 55 minutes
- *Day 6:* Your choice for 30 minutes: yoga, swimming, walking, hiking, etc.
- *Day 7:* Rest and enjoy the day!

The American Heart Association recommends moderate exercise for 150 minutes and rigorous exercise for 75 minutes per week which breaks down to:

- Three days a week of rigorous exercise for 25 minutes and 30 minutes of moderate exercise five days a week.
- You can combine your workout and on three days a week exercise for 55 minutes. Then workout for 30 minutes doing moderate exercise on the other two days of the week. ***You can do it!***

Now that I have finished writing this section, I will go for a 30 minute walk with my daughter and our golden retriever named Kuddles. Kuddles is a heartworm survivor and she filmed a public service announcement with LaDainian Tomlinson (L.T.), former star running back for the San Diego Chargers, to increase the awareness of heartworm disease.

Recent Study Update
August 27, 2012, research from investigators at Utah Southwestern Medical Center and The Cooper Institute found:

Being physically fit during your 30's, 40's and 50's not only helps extend your lifespan, but also increases the chances of aging healthily, free from chronic illness. "We've determined that being fit is not just delaying the inevitable, but is actually lowering the onset of chronic disease in the final years of life," said Dr. Jarett Berry, assistant professor of internal medicine and senior author of the study, available online in the *Archives of Internal Medicine.*

"Aerobic activities such as walking, jogging or running translates not only into more years of life but also into higher quality years, compressing the burden of chronic illness into a shorter amount of time at the end of life," Dr. Berry said.

Stress And Stress Reduction

Conquering stress can greatly reduce menopausal symptoms. Stress is one of the most common triggers for a hot flash.

Approximately ninety percent (90%) of adults report suffering from major stress at some point in their life. Seventy-five percent (75%) of all health care visits are related to stress.

Stress is how we react physically, mentally and emotionally to various conditions, changes and demands in our lives. Stress is the opposite of peace, described as one or more imbalances in the body and mind.

When your body is under stress, it produces the hormone *Cortisol,* commonly referred to as the *stress hormone.* This hormone helps your body ramp-up to meet the demands of external stressors.

Cortisol also determines how proteins, carbohydrates and fats from your diet are used to build your immune system and provide energy.

Prolonged cortisol production in the body (as in response to chronic stress) can cause physical damage to your body.

Your brain can override the message to stop cortisol production if it perceives ongoing stress. Your cortisol level then remains high because your brain thinks your body requires it to cope with the stress.

Elevated cortisol for a long period of time can cause:

Blood sugar regulation problems: This can lead to insulin resistance which I discuss further in Chapter 10.

Fat accumulation: The fat deposits primarily around your waist.

Fatigue, and prolonged fatigue can lead to exhaustion.

Possible heart disease

Bone loss: Calcium from your bones ends up being excreted in the urine. When you are under continued stress, your body will eliminate the calcium you need for bone formation and this can eventually lead to osteoporosis.

(I discuss bone health in Chapter 6)

DHEA and Cortisol work together under normal conditions when the body perceives stress and cortisol is made to give you energy. Once the stress is over, DHEA helps you to recover.

Tips For Managing A Stressful Life

- Identify your stressors and confront them if possible.

- Reduce caffeine intake. Studies show that caffeine can increase stress hormone levels which can last up to several hours.

- Try substituting your morning coffee with half decaffeinated and gradually decrease the caffeinated portion until the desired affect is achieved.

- Don't take multiple over-the-counter medications.

- Do not take unfamiliar supplements.

- Inform your clinician about any supplements, drugs and herbs that you are taking. You might consider bringing all your pills, including vitamins, to your appointments.

- If you are experiencing anxiety or stress, do not ignore any physical symptoms. You could possibly prevent the onset of a serious illness.

- Drink six to eight glasses of water or half your body weight, in ounces, per day. (The body is made up of approximately 70% water.) This also helps you feel full so you will be less apt to snack. Stress can lead to a desire to snack.

- Make sure to get enough sleep. Try to get a minimum of six hours a night and make it a goal to achieve eight to nine hours a night. Your body recovers from the stress of the day during sleep and reduces the level of the stress hormone cortisol. The body needs to rest, relax and repair.

- Get moving. Your body is designed to move. This generates endorphin production in the brain. Endorphins help to minimize stressful feelings and can promote many other positive benefits for both the mind and body.

- Have a trusted social support system. Be honest with yourself and discuss your feelings and problems with friends and/or family as needed. *No woman is an island!*

- Make time for yourself and go have a massage, pedicure or manicure. You deserve it.

- Adopt a pet. The research is in. Petting your pet as little as ten minutes a day may help lower your blood pressure, cholesterol and stress.

- Listen to your favorite music. Music therapy promotes mental and physical health.
- Try aromatherapy, hypnotherapy or acupuncture with Chinese herbs. These can be very effective for reducing stress.
- Try Meditation, Yoga, Pilates or Tai Chi for relaxation and exercise. Exercise releases 'feel good' hormones called *endorphins*. Take a class and learn how to do the different positions correctly and prevent injuries.
- Have fun! Enjoy the outdoors or your favorite activity with friends. Maintaining ongoing friendships is important. Try to surround yourself with happy people, but don't write off people who are not happy. Some individuals can have a change in mood if you take the time to let them know you care. It also makes you feel good that you have helped someone feel better.
- A UCLA study on "Friendship Among Women" (updated February 27, 2012) concluded that the more friends a woman has, the less likely she will develop physical ailments. When women are under stress they release the hormone named oxytocin, which is called the "cuddle" hormone. This hormone encourages women to "tend and befriend" - producing a calming effect.
- Oxytocin is a pro-social calm inducing hormone that affects the brain as a result of its interaction with gonadal steroid hormones like estrogen and progesterone. Oxytocin is the same hormone responsible for promoting uterine contractions and allows the breasts to let down milk in pregnant and lactating women. It is also released during a sexual orgasm. Men do not release oxytocin because testosterone suppresses its release.
- Go ahead and laugh! A study at the University of Maryland, School of Medicine found that laughter causes the tissue that forms the inner lining of blood cells to expand, increasing blood flow to the heart and other organs. When you laugh, your brain releases endorphins which create feelings of joy and euphoria. There are actually laugh therapy classes available.

NOTE: Having a sense of humor is key to creating balance in your life!

Short term stress can be a good thing. Stress is a positive experience if there is a feeling of control and satisfaction. This kind of stress is referred to as eustress, such as excitement over something positive.

Long term stress, the kind you cannot control or resolve can be harmful. A study at UCSF showed that chronic stress appears to shorten telomeres, (the caps at the end of our chromosomes). This can lead to premature aging of our cells. Another study at John Hopkins University showed that increased levels of stress hormones can lead to decreased functioning of the part of the brain called the hippocampus, which is associated with memory. Yikes-we certainly don't need that to happen!

"B-R-A-I-N" – Tips to use when you feel stressed:

- ***Breathe*** deeply as soon as you start to feel stressed. Slow deep breaths will help calm the mind. (Exhale slowly to the count of ten.)
- ***Relax*** while you breathe deeply. Saying the word "relax," calmly, will help soothe muscle tension.
- ***Ask*** yourself how you would rather be feeling? A positive question will promote a feeling of calm. Remember, "You are what you think!"
- ***Imagine*** feeling calm, powerful, content and in control. You can envision a time when you felt that way and your body will respond to those feelings with a sense of calm.
- ***Notice*** the change. If you practice these simple thought exercises, you can help prevent future stress.

You can also try these A, B, C and D's

- ***Accept*** the anxiety and don't fight it.
- ***Breathe*** slowly and relax your body (exhale to the count of ten).
- ***Calm*** yourself with relaxing thoughts.
- ***Distract*** yourself with some other activity.

NOTE: Remember to reward yourself! See your clinician for routine check-ups. Refer to the promoting health guide in Chapter 19. Prevention is the best cure!

Quit Smoking

If you smoke, you probably already know that quitting will help reduce your risk of developing a blood clot, heart disease, cancer and/ or a stroke.

Smoking also increases your risk of developing:

- Osteoporosis (thinning of the bones): This will increase your chance of having a bone fracture with slow healing
- Lung infections, lung conditions such as asthma, COPD, emphysema and lung cancers
- Stomach irritation and inflammation, which can lead to an ulcer
- Several other cancers such as mouth, tongue, pharynx, larynx, esophagus, pancreas, cervix, kidney and bladder
- Vitamin D deficiency: This can also affect calcium absorption and weaken your bones. (I discuss bone health further in Chapter 6)
- Low estrogen levels

Women who smoke are at even greater risk for developing some of the above conditions, especially if they are also taking hormone replacement therapy. Lung cancer kills more women every year than any other cancer. Call 1-800-no-butts today to help you quit and their services are free. Consult your clinician today for treatment options.

Treatment Options For Menopausal Symptoms

Non-Hormonal Treatments

Cooling Products

Menopause is not a disease and some women will elect not to treat the symptoms, which is perfectly fine. Some women do not become uncomfortable at all during menopause but many women do experience bothersome symptoms that can affect their quality of life. It is interesting to note that in some cultures menopausal symptoms are not experienced at all, begging the question: What role do cultural influences play in the way that women experience "the change". Certainly diet, lifestyle and the cultures beliefs, customs and attitudes toward aging come into play. In the North American culture there are many products available to help keep you cool when a hot flash strikes without taking hormones or medications. These products may sound a bit silly, but don't knock 'em till you've tried 'em!

Chillow Pillow: This soft comfort device, placed around the neck, can help relieve hot flashes and night sweats. You can also sleep directly on it and it acts like memory foam without the heat. This can enable you to get a good night's sleep and it doesn't require refrigeration. It comes in three sizes, Original Chillow, Chillow Plus and the Chillow Mini.

Cool Downz Neck Cooling Wraps: Place this product in cool water for about 30 minutes and it will swell up to form a soft comfortable gel roll. Tie this around your neck like a scarf and it will keep you cool. Cool Downz can also help soothe neck pain due to arthritis. Google Cool Downz cooling bandana and they have many cooling products available to choose from.

Mini fans: You can carry these battery operated fans in your purse.

Personal cooling system, Coolware: Fill this device with a few ounces of water, place it around your neck and a tiny fan creates evaporative cooling.

Bed fan device: This device keeps cool air circulating under the sheets during the night.

Cooling mattress pad, sheets, pillow cases, blanket and comforter: Gilligan & Ferneman, LLC Cooling bedding was featured on the Dr. Oz show. The Wicking sheets and cooling blanket were promoted as the "night sweats solution!" Google coolingmattress. com to check out these items.

NOTE: I have no affiliation with these products and I am sure there are similar products that achieve the same results.

Alternative Medicine Remedies Using Herbs And Supplements
Alternative treatments for menopause have gained popularity over recent years due to the unfavorable press that hormone replacement therapy has received.

It is very important that you check in with your clinician or registered naturopath prior to taking any herbal regimens, due to possible interactions with your prescription medications and to identify any possible unwanted side effects or reactions.

There are two types of herbs commonly used to help relieve menopausal symptoms: *Phytoestrogenic Herbs* and *Non-estrogenic Herbs.*

Phytoestrogenic Herbs

These are plant compounds that contain *phytoestrogens* with chemical structures similar to human estrogen, allowing them to become a perfect fit for some of the body's estrogen receptor sites.

Phytoestrogens are much weaker than human estrogen, about 1/400 to 1/1000 weaker in strength. They work by either stimulating or suppressing the effects of estrogen, depending on how much natural estrogen is present in the body.

During menopause when estrogen levels are low, *phytoestrogens* can stimulate the receptor sites, relieving hot flashes and vaginal dryness.

When estrogen levels are high, *phytoestrogens* can occupy the same receptor sites, blocking out the stronger estrogen in an attempt to maintain hormonal balance.

There are six common types of phytoestrogens found in fruits, vegetables and grains:

- *Flavones* are found in cereals.
- *Flavonols* are found in onions, kale, broccoli, lettuce, tomatoes, apples, grapes, berries, tea and red wine.
- *Lignans* are found in flaxseed, whole grains, some fruits and vegetables.
- *Chalcones* are found in the tomato peel.
- *Flavonones,* (bioflavonoids) are found in the pulp and pith of citrus fruits, cranberries and grape seeds.
- *Isoflavones* are found only in legumes, such as soybeans and red clover.

The flavones and isoflavones are thought to be the most potent and tend to provide more relief from menopausal symptoms such as:

- Hot flashes
- Menstrual irregularities
- Mood disturbances

Non-Estrogenic Herbs

These herbs do not contain estrogen like components. These herbs work by stimulating your own glands to produce hormones more efficiently, helping to restore balance.

The following is an alphabetical list of the most commonly used herbs and supplements:

Amberen Supplement (Non-Estrogenic)

This supplement has recently gained popularity in helping to provide relief from:

- Hot flashes and night sweats
- Mood swings and irritability
- Weight gain
- Difficulty concentrating
- Low energy
- Sleeplessness

Black Cohosh (Estrogenic Herb)

This herb promotes some estrogen activity by stimulating estrogen receptor sites in the body. Black Cohosh has become very popular for treating:

- Hot flashes
- Night sweats
- PMS/mood disturbances/ irritability
- Insomnia
- Vaginal dryness

Some studies claim it can help reduce your cholesterol and blood pressure too.

The American College of Obstetricians and Gynecologists supports short term use of Black Cohosh, 20 mg twice daily for up to six months for treating menopausal symptoms. Treatment is required for at least eight weeks to alleviate symptoms.

You may recognize these two over the counter preparations which contain Black Cohosh - Remifemin and Estroven.

Caution: *Do not use this herb if you:*

- *Have a liver disorder. This herb can be toxic to your liver.*

• *Have a history of breast cancer.*

• *Have an allergy to aspirin.*

• *Are taking birth control pills or hormone replacement therapy.*

Chasteberry (Non-Estrogenic Herb)

The Chasteberry has been used to help balance hormones by stimulating the pituitary gland to make more LH (luteinizing hormone), which increases progesterone production and reduces prolactin production. Prolactin is the hormone which aides in milk production. Chasteberry also acts like a mild sedative and antispasmodic, (reducing spasms). Chasteberry may help reduce:

• Acne

• PMS, menstrual cramping, menstrual cycle irregularities and breast tenderness

• Headaches

• Anxiety and depressed mood

Caution: Do not take Chasteberry if you have ever been diagnosed with cancer.

Cranberry (Non-Estrogenic Herb)

This herb helps to prevent urinary tract infections by not allowing the bacteria to adhere to the walls of the bladder and urethra. However, if you do develop an infection you will need to take antibiotics to kill the bacteria.

Try to drink at least one 8-10 ounce glass of cranberry juice daily or one tablespoonful of Cystex liquid, the equivalent of up to twelve glasses of cranberry juice, without the sugar or calories.

Cranberry extract is also available in pill form, which is equivalent to drinking 8-10 ounces of the juice.

D-Mannose is a natural occurring simple sugar that is related to glucose and also helps to decrease the occurrence of bladder infections. It works by coating the bacteria, preventing it from attaching to the inner walls of the bladder and urinary tract. D-Mannose is now available in a tablet that also contains cranberry extract.

(See Chapter 9 for further information on urinary conditions.)

Dandelion (Non-Estrogenic Herb)

Dandelion is a rich source of potassium and vitamin A.

This herb may help:

• Regulate hormone production
• Reduce PMS symptoms
• Reduce incidents of bladder infections
• Improve liver function and digestion
• Reduce fluid retention

Dong Quai (Estrogenic Herb)

Dong Quai is sometimes referred to as "women's ginseng". The roots of this herb contain naturally occurring estrogens which are called phytosterols. Dong Quai may help:

• Reduce hot flashes
• Reduce vaginal dryness
• Improve menstrual irregularities
• Improve sleep disturbances

NOTE: In Chinese medicine Dong Quai is given along with other herbs.

Caution:

• *Dong Quai can act as a blood thinner and increase your risk of bleeding.*
• *Do not take this herb if you are taking a blood thinner, such as Aspirin, Ibuprofen or Warfarin (Coumadin).*
• *Dong Quai may elevate your blood sugar.*
• *Do not take this herb if you have a history of breast cancer.*
• *Be careful with sun exposure and use a sun screen.*

Evening Primrose Oil (Non-Estrogenic Herb)

This herb contains gamma-linoleic acid (GLA), which is an Omega-6 essential fatty acid and may help reduce:

• Hot flashes
• Irritability and mood swings
• Breast and joint pain
• Insomnia

Flaxseed And Linseed (Non-Estrogenic)

Flaxseed is a good source of soluble fiber and Omega-3 fatty acids. One to two tablespoons or 10 to 20 grams of ground flaxseed daily may help moderate estrogen and progesterone levels, reducing:

• Hot flashes

• Vaginal dryness

• Dry skin

• Breast tenderness

• Excessive menstrual bleeding

• Constipation

• LDL (bad) cholesterol

Fish Oil/Omega-3 Fatty Acids (Non-Estrogenic)

Fish oil may help reduce:

• Triglyceride levels

• Painful menses

• Blood pressure (Although in some individuals it may cause a slight increase.) Be sure to monitor your blood pressure while taking this supplement.

• Joint inflammation

NOTE: Fish oil may also help improve brain function and decrease inflammation, relieving joint pain. It may also cause a slight elevation of LDL cholesterol.

Ginkgo (Non-Estrogenic)

Ginkgo is thought to improve blood flow to tissues and organs which can help enhance:

• Libido

• Brain function and memory

• Sleep

Caution: Do not take this herb if you are taking:

• *A blood thinner, such as Aspirin or Warfarin*

• *An anti-depressant medication*

Ginseng (Non-Estrogenic)

This herb is thought to boost your immune system and sexual performance. Ginseng may help reduce:

• Fatigue

• Stress

• Memory lapses

• Hot flashes

Caution: Do not take Ginseng if you have a history of breast cancer.

Kava (Non-Estrogenic)

This herb may help:

• Reduce anxiety and irritability

• Reduce painful joints and muscle tension

• Promote sleep

Caution: This herb can cause liver dysfunction.

Licorice (Non-Estrogenic)

This herb may aide in:

• Calming down estrogen fluctuations

• Balancing hormone levels

Caution: This herb may deplete the body's potassium level and raise blood pressure.

Macafem (Non-Estrogenic)

This herb may help stimulate your hormonal glands to work more efficiently, helping to restore hormone balance. This herb has been used to help relieve:

• Hot flashes

• Night sweats

• Vaginal dryness

• Mood swings and irritability

• Breast tenderness

Melatonin (Non-Estrogenic)

The pineal gland, located in the brain, produces this hormone. Melatonin is stimulated by darkness and suppressed by sunlight.

Recent studies have shown that melatonin supplementation during perimenopause may help:

- Enhance thyroid function
- Improve mood
- Improve sleep

Be sure to have your melatonin blood level checked before beginning this supplement. Melatonin is much more effective when exposure to light is limited for at least one hour before bedtime (this includes computer and TV use). It can take up to six weeks to become effective. A sublingual (under the tongue) form is now available and may begin working within 20 minutes.

Red Clover (Estrogenic Herb)
A common supplement name you may recognize is Promensil.

This herb may help:

- Reduce hot flashes and night sweats
- Reduce mood swings, depression and anxiety
- Reduce ovarian cysts
- Increase good cholesterol (HDL)
- Reduce bone loss by compensating for estrogen loss

Caution: Do not take this herb:

- *If you have a history of breast or uterine cancer, stroke, liver disease or high blood pressure.*
- *If you have an aspirin allergy.*
- *With birth control pills or hormone replacement therapy.*

Sage (Non-Estrogenic)
This herb can help reduce:

- Hot flashes
- Night sweats
- Mood swings
- Headaches

Soy (Estrogenic)
The phytoestrogens (plant estrogens) found in soy are similar to human estrogens, although very weak compared to the estrogens

produced by the human body. The ***isoflavones*** found in soy are one type of plant hormone, (about 1/400 to 1/1000 as potent as human estrogen). These *isoflavones* resemble human estrogens just enough that the cell receptor allows them to bind to the cell surface membrane to exert their effect. (Our intestinal bacteria can turn the digested soy into a substance similar to human estrogen.) Soy contains the *isoflavones genistein* and *daidzein,* which are two powerful phytoestrogens commonly found in:

• Whole soybeans

• Textured soy protein

• Soy flour and milk

• Tofu and tempeh

You can also take a daily soy supplement, which is typically a soy extract containing 50mg of isoflavones.

One over the counter product is called *Soy Care Menopause,* which contains 25mg of isoflavones per capsule.

Soy is also a good source of protein (amino acids), B vitamins, calcium, zinc, iron and potassium. Soy when compared to other

Table 3.2

Isoflavone Content Of Some Selected Foods

Food	Isoflavone (mg/100g food)
Soybeans, green, raw	151.17
Soy flour	148.61
Soy protein isolates	97.43
Soy protein concentrate (Alcohol extracted)	12.47
Miso soup, dry	60.39
Tofu (Mori-Nu), silken, firm	31.32
Tofu (Azumaya), Extra firm, steamed	22.70
Tofu yogurt	16.30
Soymilk	9.65
Vegetable burgers, prepared (Green Giant Harvest Burgers)	8.22
Soy sauce (from hydrolyzed Vegetable protein)	0.10

Source: United States Department of Agriculture, Iowa State University, 1999.

legumes, contains more protein, is higher in essential fatty acids, lower in carbohydrates and a good source of fiber.

Soy may help reduce:

• Hot flashes and night sweats

• Vaginal dryness

Taking soy for a period of time may provide certain benefits such as possibly:

• Reducing the risk of postmenopausal osteoporosis

• Reducing your cholesterol, which can help reduce the risk for heart disease

• Improving insulin regulation and weight control

There are two camps regarding the use of soy:

• Some experts believe that soy may carry some risk for developing cancer due to its estrogen like qualities.

• Some studies report that soy may have a protective effect.

An interesting fact is that Asian women, living outside of the United States, have a much lower incidence of menopausal symptoms than Americans. Studies estimate that less than 25% of Japanese women and 18% of Chinese women complain of hot flashes. These observations have led researchers to consider the possible benefits of an Asian diet on menopausal symptoms, which includes more soy food consumption.

Be sure to consult with your clinician before adding soy to your diet.

Valerian (Non-Estrogenic)
This herb may help:

• Promote sleep

• Decrease anxiety

Wild Yam (Estrogenic)
Wild Yam is a hormone like substance found in some yams. You would have to eat large amounts to achieve a level that would help your symptoms. However, Wild Yam preparations placed onto the skin may help relieve:

• Vaginal dryness

• Hot flashes

Be sure to reference the U.S. Pharmacopeia (USP). The USP is a program that helps to inform and protect consumers who use dietary supplements. The USP sets strict standards concerning the quantity and strength of the ingredients stated and the product purity. Look for the USP certification on the label.

Vitamin And Mineral Supplements

B-Complex

B-Complex contains Thiamine (B1), Riboflavin (B2), Niacin (B3), Pantothenic Acid (B5), Pyridoxine (B6), Folic Acid (B9), Cyano-cobalamin (B12) and Biotin. These B vitamins work in harmony to help support your liver, brain and glucose (sugar) metabolism.

B-complex can help alleviate: Emotional stress, fatigue, insomnia and depression associated with menopause.

Vitamin B6 Can Help:

• Reduce uncomfortable bloating due to water retention and breast tenderness.

• Rid the body of excess homocysteine and make collagen for strong bones.

Homocysteine is a byproduct of protein metabolism and increased levels can be linked to developing osteoporosis and heart disease. Premenopausal women are better able to rid the body of excess homocysteine. (Please refer to Chapter 5 for further information on homocysteine and heart disease.)

Vitamin B9 (Folic Acid)

Supplementation with folic acid has been shown to help lower levels of homocysteine in postmenopausal women.

Food Sources of Vitamin B

• **Vitamin B3** is found in meat, poultry, fish, beans and whole wheat bread.

• **Vitamin B6** is found in meat, poultry, fish, bananas, dairy products and wholegrain cereals.

• **Vitamin B12** is found in poultry, fish, eggs, milk and B12 fortified foods. Vitamin B12 is absorbed through your stomach.

Be sure to have your B12 blood level checked before starting a supplement.

Individuals with thyroid disease are more prone to developing a B12 deficiency.

Taking daily antacids and acid-blockers, like Prilosec for heartburn can be associated with developing a Vitamin B12 deficiency. Vitamin B12 deficiency is called Pernicious Anemia. Ask your clinician to check your vitamin B12 blood level.

Vitamin C
Vitamin C may help:

- Promote estrogen production

- Maintain collagen, which can help your bones, connective tissue and reduce wrinkles

- Keep vaginal tissues moist, therefore preventing bladder and vaginal infections. These infections tend to increase during menopausal years since the tissues become thin, allowing bacteria to permeate.

- Support the adrenal glands and immune system, which is especially important during our menopausal years

- Reduce cholesterol levels

NOTE: Check with your clinician before taking Vitamin C if you are on a "statin" drug like Simvastatin (Zocor) or Atorvastatin (Lipitor) to help lower your cholesterol. Combined use of a Vitamin C supplement and a statin medication may reduce the effectiveness of both substances intended to improve your cholesterol levels. Interactions can also occur between grapefruit products and certain statins, resulting in an increased level of the statin medication in the blood.

Food Sources for Vitamin C

- Fortified breakfast cereals
- Citrus fruits
- Cantaloupe and honeydew
- Vegetables such as Brussels sprouts, broccoli, cauliflower and cabbage

- Dark green leafy vegetables such as kale, spinach and collard greens
- Red, green and yellow peppers

Taking Vitamin C along with Vitamin B6 may help reduce bloating, anxiety and insomnia. Vitamin B complex taken along with Vitamin C and plant estrogens may help reduce stress and hot flashes.

Vitamin D

As we age our Vitamin D level can decrease. There are two forms found to be important in humans:

- Vitamin D2, which is made by plants
- Vitamin D3, which is made by humans. The sun can stimulate vitamin D production through the skin if you are not wearing sunscreen. Vitamin D has to be converted in our bodies to a more active form. This process requires both magnesium and the trace mineral boron to be present.

Vitamin D helps:

- Maintain normal blood levels of calcium and phosphorus
- Our bodies absorb calcium to build and maintain strong bones, decreasing the risk for developing osteoporosis

New research suggests that Vitamin D may help provide protection from:

- Osteoporosis
- Hypertension (high blood pressure)
- Cancer
- Autoimmune diseases (including diabetes)

NOTE: If you have a history of kidney stones, check with your clinician before taking a vitamin D supplement. Ask if you should have your vitamin D level checked. See Chapter 6 for more information on bone health and vitamin D.

Food Sources for Vitamin D

Vitamin D is found in fish (canned tuna and salmon), eggs, fortified milk and cod liver oil.

Vitamin E

This vitamin has been termed the "menopause vitamin" due to its chemical actions which are similar to estrogen. Vitamin E may help:

- Fight infection and boost the immune system due to its powerful antioxidant activity
- Keep thyroid function in check
- Reduce breast tenderness and PMS symptoms due to hormonal fluctuations
- Relieve hot flashes
- Reduce vaginal dryness: You may insert a gel capsule into the vagina and use it as a suppository.

Food Sources for Vitamin E

Vitamin E is found in eggs, green leafy vegetables, cereals, nuts (almonds, peanuts and walnuts), dried legumes, wheat germ, whole grains and vegetable oils (i.e., corn and safflower).

Boron

Boron is a trace mineral which may help activate vitamin D and estrogen. Boron is found in soybeans. Eating a diet rich in soy can provide you with the little amount of boron your body needs.

NOTE: Researchers have found that a small amount of boron can help reduce urinary excretion of calcium and magnesium, which helps keep your bones healthy.

Calcium

Calcium taken with vitamin D can help:

- Reduce the risk of osteoporosis
- Possibly lower blood pressure
- Possibly lower risk of colon cancer

Food Sources for Calcium

Calcium is found in dairy products, dark green leafy vegetables, seeds, nuts and fish with bones. Canned salmon and sardines have a higher calcium content because the canning process softens the bones and they are easily digested.

(I discuss calcium and bone health in greater detail in Chapter 6.)

Magnesium

Magnesium is also important for bone health. It is a component of the enzyme that helps crystallize calcium into bone and helps convert vitamin D into its active form.

Magnesium may help:

- Increase bone strength, when taken with calcium and vitamin D
- Reduce fatigue and boost energy
- Reduce migraine headaches
- Reduce heart palpitations
- Reduce breast tenderness
- Reduce cramping
- Relieve constipation

Food Sources for Magnesium

Magnesium is found in whole grains, dark green leafy vegetables, nuts, dairy products, meat, fish, dried and cooked beans like soy beans.

NOTE: Magnesium may cause loose stools when taken as a supplement. There is a chelated form called magnesium glycinate, which is better tolerated and less likely to cause loose stools.

Selenium

This mineral may help:

- Improve mood
- Promote cardiac health
- Improve thyroid health: Selenium is a cofactor involved in converting inactive T4 into the active T3. (I discuss thyroid conditions in Chapter 8.)
- Maintain hormonal balance/function

Zinc

Zinc is an important mineral which may help:

- Control blood sugar
- Prevent infections and promote wound healing

Non Hormonal Vaginal Creams And Lubricants

Lower levels of estrogen during your menopausal years can cause a decrease in blood supply to the vagina. This decrease in blood flow can certainly affect vaginal lubrication, resulting in vaginal dryness and discomfort with intercourse.

All Natural Preparations

Vitamin E Vaginal Suppositories: Use a natural source vitamin E product and insert into the vagina at night to help alleviate vaginal dryness.

Natural Oils: Grape seed, almond, sunflower or apricot oil can be quite soothing for use during intercourse.

Sylk: This lubricant is made from the extract of the kiwi fruit vine. Sylk vaginal lubricant is 100% natural without any parabens or propylene glycol. *"Sensation"* vaginal lubricant is a natural warming product with cinnamon extract added, which is also made from kiwi fruit extract.

Synthetic Preparations

Albolene: This lubricant is marketed as a moisturizing cleanser and works well to afford relief from vaginal discomfort during intercourse due to dryness. This product contains mineral oil, petrolatum, paraffin, ceresin and beta carotene. It should not be used with condoms or a diaphragm since petroleum jelly degrades latex.

Astroglide: This lubricant has been quite popular for years helping to reduce the discomfort during intercourse, due to vaginal dryness. You can buy a formulation that is glycerin-free and paraben-free.

Replens Vaginal Moisturizer: This vaginal moisturizer has been recommended by gynecologists for years and contains purified water, glycerin, mineral oil, polycarbophil, carbomer 934P, hydrogenated palm oil glyceride, sorbic acid, methyparaben and sodium hydroxide.

Femlube: This lubricant contains wild yam, rose essential oil, neroli essential oil, Lady's mantle, aloe and vitamin E. This product is in a gel base which contains glycerin and propylene glycol.

NOTE: You may need to try several products until you find the one that works well for you.

Prescription Non-Hormone Therapies

Antidepressants

Scientific evidence shows that postmenopausal women taking certain antidepressants in doses lower than those used for the treatment of depression may experience some relief from hot flashes. The antidepressants commonly used are from two different classes:

(NSRIs) Norepinephrine/Serotonin reuptake inhibitors:

• Venlafaxine (Effexor)

• Desvenlafaxine (Pristiq) and Duloxetine HCL (Cymbalta), are two newer medications

(SSRIs) Selective serotonin reuptake inhibitors:

• Paroxetine (Paxil)

• Fluoxetine (Prozac)

• Citalopram (Celexa)

• Escitalopram (Lexapro)

• Sertraline (Zoloft)

All the above medications have been reported to help reduce hot flashes. I typically will start a patient on half the recommended dosage to help alleviate these menopausal vasomotor symptoms.

Paroxetine mesylate (7.5 mg) is currently recommended by the American College of Obstetricians and Gynecologists and is the only FDA approved non-hormonal formulation recommended for the treatment of vasomotor symptoms. This is a much lower dosage of Paroxetine (Paxil) than regimens typically used to treat psychiatric conditions.

Talk with your clinician to determine which treatment would be best for you.

Gabapentin (Neurontin): is a medication used for treating seizures and chronic nerve pain. Some studies have shown this medication to be moderately effective in reducing hot-flashes. *Drowsiness* is a side effect of this medication and that could be a plus, if you are unable to sleep.

Clonidine: is a medication used to treat high blood pressure and has been found to be effective in reducing hot flashes. It is available in a pill or patch form and may also make you feel drowsy.

NOTE: Dizziness, constipation and dry mouth can occur while taking this medication, so check in with your clinician and make sure you have your blood pressure monitored.

Hormonal Therapies

Definition of Hormone Replacement Therapy

Hormone replacement therapy (HRT) is the practice of taking supplemental hormones to replace those that your body is no longer producing. These hormones are given to relieve symptoms of hormonal imbalances, which occur most commonly during midlife.

History behind Hormone Replacement Therapy

For the past fifty plus years, HRT referred to only synthetic hormones, which have been given to women to help relieve menopausal symptoms and make them feel better. More recently, non-traditional hormone therapies are available referred to as "natural or bio-identical" hormones.

Traditional Hormone Therapy

These hormones are referred to as "synthetic hormones" and are made in a lab, creating a molecule that looks similar to a natural estrogen although different from an estrogen found in nature. A conjugated horse (equine) estrogen was the first replacement hormone used in the United States, which contained only conjugated estrogens. (Conjugated estrogens are a mixture of estrogen hormones used to treat symptoms of menopause.) Women began to develop uterine cancer after taking this medication because the uterus requires progesterone to balance the effects of estrogen or uterine cancer can develop. The pharmaceutical industry then recognized the need to add a synthetic progesterone called *"Progestin"*.

Progestin was similarly created in a lab to mimic natural progesterone. Years later a combination drug called *Prempro* was formulated which contained both estrogen and progestin.

Today there are many different forms, dosages and brand names available to choose from when considering HRT. *(See table 3.3 on page 90.)*

Non-Traditional Hormone Therapy

These hormones are referred to as *"bio-identical"* hormone replacement or Natural Hormone Replacement, NHR. These natural hormones are derived from a plant source such as wild yams and soybeans. These compounds are then modified in a lab to mimic the hormone molecules found naturally circulating in the female body. *See the end of this chapter for further information and how to locate a compounding pharmacy.*

When To Consider Hormone Replacement Therapy

If you are experiencing moderate to severe menopausal symptoms that interfere with your daily living, such as:

• Hot flashes

• Night sweats

• Vaginal dryness

If you are at high risk for developing osteoporosis
If your "quality of life" is incompatible with daily living
If your mood is depressed and/or you feel extremely anxious
If you are unable to sleep
If you are unable to focus/concentrate or remember things

NOTE: There are also prescription treatments available that can treat each of these symptoms individually without hormones. (See previous section on non-hormonal prescription therapies.)

Benefits And Risks Of Hormone Replacement Therapy

Possible Benefits of Choosing HRT

There is no individual treatment or therapy, other than HRT, that can treat and minimize all of the menopausal symptoms. HRT is indeed the panacea for what ails the menopausal woman but may come with a price.

Short term use of HRT (less than five years) may help improve:

• Memory

• Mood

- Sleep
- Vaginal and urinary tract dryness and incontinence
- Hot flashes/flushes

Long term use (greater than five years) may:

- Help increase bone density
- Help decrease hip and spine fractures
- Decrease colon cancer risk

Possible Risks of Choosing HRT

- Increased risk of developing breast cancer
- Increased risk for developing gallbladder disease
- Increased risk for developing heart disease or a heart attack
- Increased risk of developing a stroke
- Increased risk of developing a deep vein clot

NOTE: Please refer to the final section in this chapter for further details about the Women's Health Initiative Study and its implications for hormone replacement therapy.

Types Of Hormone Replacement Therapy

Synthetic (Traditional) HRT

Synthetic hormonal therapy is referred to as "HRT". Medical practitioners refer to it as "traditional" because it was the earliest form of HRT used. HRT is the most effective medication approved by the Food and Drug Administration (FDA) that has been proven to treat moderate to severe menopausal symptoms and to help prevent bone loss.

HRT is indicated for the prevention of postmenopausal osteoporosis and can help:

- Protect against bone loss
- Build bone in the hips and spine
- Reduce the risk of hip and vertebral (spine) fractures

There are two types of synthetic hormone therapy:

- *Estrogen-plus-progestin therapy* (which is for women with a uterus.) Estrogen helps relieve your menopausal symptoms and the progestin helps protect the uterine lining. If you take only estrogen and you still have your uterus, the lining can become too thick (endometrial hyperplasia) and this could lead to endometrial cancer, which is cancer of the uterus.

• *Estrogen-alone therapy,* which is for women who have had their uterus removed (undergone a hysterectomy). This is referred to as unopposed estrogen replacement therapy.

Non Prescription Hormone Therapies
The most common hormone imbalance during perimenopause is too little progesterone due to an-ovulatory cycles (not releasing an egg), which can lead to an overall decreased level of progesterone.

There are non-prescription progesterone creams available that are much weaker than prescription pharmaceutical grade progesterone cream. These progesterone creams are about a fourth less potent and are well absorbed through the skin.

Pharmaceutical grade progesterone has been shown to reduce hot flashes. It is thought that progesterone reduces hot flashes by possibly being converted into estrogen in the body.

Many perimenopausal women do well with a small amount of progesterone cream applied directly to the skin.

When estrogen is not properly balanced with progesterone, your thyroid function can be affected causing you to feel tired with some weight gain.

Progesterone may help balance the excess estrogen and improve thyroid function.

Low dose estriol (1 mg) is the only non-prescription estrogen product available and can be found in a cream form or vaginal suppository.

Supplements such as soy and other products that contain phytoestrogens are thought to act like estrogen in the body but are not actually estrogen.

NOTE: Discuss the use of the above named treatments with your clinician!

Prescription Hormone Therapy Products
There are a number of ways to take hormone therapy and many prod-

ucts are available in varying doses. (See table 3.3 on page 90 for a listing of some prescription hormone therapy products.)

These hormone preparations can be given as "estrogen alone' therapy or in combination with a progesterone or progestin.

The tablet form is the most commonly prescribed.

The patch is quite popular and is applied to your skin usually once or twice a week. The patch delivers estrogen to the body through the skin, avoiding the liver and provides a steady level of hormone therapy.

The cream and gel preparations can be applied directly to the skin or inserted into the vagina. You can also apply cream inside the vagina if you are experiencing mainly vaginal symptoms such as dryness, itching and discomfort. The vaginal creams can also be helpful in relieving urinary symptoms, such as leakage and irritation due to dryness.

Estrogen preparations are also available in a lotion and spray which are applied directly to the skin.

Vaginal suppositories and a ring that can be inserted into the vagina are available as well. (See Table 3.3 on page 90.)

NOTE: You and your clinician can discuss which dose and form would be appropriate for you.

Selective Estrogen Receptor Modulators (SERMs)

SERMs are used as an option to provide the beneficial effects of estrogen therapy, without the increased risk of heart attack, breast cancer and stroke. These drugs are unique in that they act like estrogen on some cells in the body and in other cells can block the action of estrogen. These drugs work well for preventing breast cancers and recurrences that need estrogen to grow.

(See Chapters 7 and 16 for more information on cancer.)

The three SERMs typically used are:

• *Arimidex* (chemical name: anastrozole): This medication *may promote* bone loss, increasing the risk for developing osteoporosis.

• *Nolvadex* (chemical name: Tamoxifen): This medication *may promote* bone loss, increasing the risk for developing osteoporosis.

- *Evista* (chemical name: raloxifene): This medication is unique and sometimes referred to as the first "designer" estrogen. Evista is used to help *improve bone density,* decreasing the risk for developing osteoporosis.

Table 3.3

Prescription Hormone Therapy Products

Generic Name	Product Name
Oral estrogens	
Estradiol	Estrace
Esterified estrogens	Estratab, Menest
Conjugated equine estrogen	Premarin, Cenestin
Estropipate	Ogen and Ortho-Est
Oral combination Estrogen and Progestin	
Conjugated equine estrogen/MPA	Prempro
Estradiol/ Norethindrone Acetate	Activella
Estrogen skin patches	
Estradiol	Alora, Climara, FemPatch, Vivelle dot and Menostar
Combination Estrogen and Progestin skin patch	
Estradiol/norethindrone acetate	CombiPatch
Estradiol/Levonorgestrel	Climara Pro
Estrogen Creams	
Conjugated equine estrogen creams	Premarin and Estrace vaginal
Estrogen Gels	
Estradiol vaginal gels	Divigel, Estrogel and Elestrin
Estrogen Lotion	
Estradiol topical emulsion	Estrasorb
Estrogen Rings	
Estradiol (90 day delivery system)	Estring and Femring vaginal rings
Estrogen Spray	
Estradiol transdermal spray	Evamist
Estrogen Suppository	
Estradiol	Vagifem
Progestins	
Medroxyprogesterone acetate (MPA)	Amen, Cycrin and Provera
Progesterone	
Oral micronized progesterone	Prometrium

The most common side effects of SERMs are:

- Hot flashes and night sweats: What a catch 22!
- Vaginal discharge and bleeding
- Mood swings
- Water retention
- Nausea

SERMs are typically used as treatment to increase bone density or to prevent a breast cancer recurrence in breast cancer survivors and may also cause some serious side effects such as:

- Increased risk of blood clots forming in the legs and lungs
- Increased risk of high blood pressure leading to a stroke
- Increased blood cholesterol levels
- Increase in tumor size or development of new tumors
- *Tamoxifen* can increase the risk of developing uterine cancer.

Natural Hormone Replacement Therapy (NHR)

If diet and other lifestyle changes have not helped to alleviate your symptoms of perimenopause and menopause and you have decided to try natural HRT, maybe "bio-identical" hormone replacement would be right for you.

Natural replacement hormones are derived from a plant source, such as wild yams and soybeans. These compounds are then modified in a lab to become like the hormone molecules found naturally circulating in the female body.

The sex steroid hormones that your female body produces are all *"natural"* hormones, which are made from cholesterol. Isn't that amazing? The word, "natural" when describing natural hormones refers to the chemical structure of the molecule, *not* where it originates. These hormones are called *"bio-identical"* hormones and are referred to as Natural Hormone Replacement, "NHR". These identical hormones can be replaced in similar proportions that your body produced during your reproductive years.

The three most common estrogens found circulating in the human body of a premenopausal female are:

- Estradiol, which is the *active* and *strongest* form produced in the ovaries.

- Estrone, which is the *inactive* form produced in the ovaries during your reproductive years and in the fat cells in postmenopausal women.
- Estriol, which is the weakest form and is produced in large amounts during pregnancy.

These three hormones are the predominant estrogens that circulate during the child bearing years. They naturally occur roughly in the following percentages: 80% estradiol, 10% estrone, and 10% estriol.

The two most common formulations used when replacing natural estrogens are:

- **Tri-est** is approximately 10-20% estradiol, 10-20% estrone and 60-80% estriol.
- **Bi-est** is approximately 10-20% estradiol and 80% estriol.

These formulations attempt to mimic the naturally occurring hormone ratio.

Replacement estrogen therapy is typically considered after your menstrual periods have ended.

Natural progesterone should be added if you still have a uterus and in some cases testosterone or DHEA may be needed as well.

Natural hormones can be formulated in pill form, or a gel, lotion, cream, oil or drops. You will need a prescription from your clinician and you will fill that prescription at a compounding pharmacy near you.

The body can easily recognize these bio-identical hormones and often lower doses can be used with fewer side effects. The dosage can be titrated up or down depending on your individual replacement needs. It is important to alert the compounding pharmacy if you have any allergies.

Natural estrogens are lower in strength than synthetic estrogens. You can replace hormones in "physiologic doses" (only what your body needs) and give just the right amount to provide balance and alleviate the unpleasant symptoms of menopause.

Remember, natural hormone replacement prescriptions are custom compounded to meet your body's unique hormonal needs.

NOTE: It is important to make sure the compounding pharmacy is accredited through "The Pharmacy Compounding Accreditation Board" to ensure the quality and consistency of the products made.

Getting Started With Natural Hormone Replacement Therapy

When you schedule your initial appointment to discuss hormone replacement with your clinician, you should request enough time to fully address this issue. This initial encounter is important as it guides your clinician toward the best approach for your unique treatment plan.

You the patient, provide the most valuable information about your body, because *you* live in it every day. This also provides an opportunity to review any environmental concerns that could influence the treatment plan.

I highly recommend that every patient receive a complete physical, which includes blood work, a pap smear and a mammogram. This serves a dual purpose by providing baseline information for comparison in the future and can identify any medical condition that could present with similar symptoms. In my practice, I am a stickler for "screening your ticker" for heart disease and you know what the number one killer of women is? *Yes, it is heart disease!*

I would encourage you to learn as much as you can, so that you will be informed when making these health care decisions. You and your clinician together can proceed in formulating a treatment plan that is right for you. Yes, the old saying is still true, *"Everybody is different!"*

How To Identify Your Hormone Levels

Every woman's hormone profile is different. Hormone levels can change daily, weekly and even monthly. Hormone replacement can be challenging due to the variability of an individual's response. To achieve the best results, you need to be tested initially to identify which hormones you might need.

The typical initial hormone panel that we may order includes the following blood tests: FSH, LH, total estrogen, estradiol, progesterone, testosterone and/or DHEA.

Hormone level testing can be done through urine, blood and saliva.

Urine testing measures how much hormone you have used (metabolized) and is the most accurate. Unfortunately, many labs do not offer this method of testing due to its high cost.

Saliva testing is commonly done and you can take a simple saliva test in the privacy of your own home and then mail it to the lab. Saliva testing measures the amount of free hormone circulating in your body tissues. Relax, this will require a little patience on your part, because you will need to collect a fair amount of saliva from your mouth and place it into a little tube. Yes, you can do it! Try chewing some gum or sucking on a lemon drop, which can help create more saliva.

Your clinician will be notified of the results from the lab and then they can instruct the compounding pharmacy to customize your individual prescription. Once you have begun therapy, your hormone levels may be retested to determine how well you are responding and the dosage can be adjusted if necessary.

Many times your symptoms can be the best indicator of how well you are responding to therapy. The goal is to achieve symptom relief with the lowest possible dosage.

Natural low dose estrogen cream, *estriol* can be given alone or in combination with other hormones to help relieve vaginal dryness and urinary symptoms.

NOTE: Remember when estriol cream is inserted into the vagina there is minimal estrogen absorption.

Several clinician authors have reported the following benefits for patients taking NHR:

• Prevention of osteoporosis and improved bone strength

• Reduced hot flashes, vaginal dryness and thinning of tissue

• Progesterone can help balance excess estrogen and improve thyroid function. (When estrogen is not properly balanced with progesterone, your thyroid function can be reduced causing fatigue and weight gain.)

• Improved maintenance of muscle mass and strength

• Possible protection against heart disease and stroke

- Improved cholesterol levels
- Reduced risk of endometrial cancer
- Improved sleep, mood, concentration and memory
- Prevention of dementia and Alzheimer's disease
- Improved libido (sex drive)

Many traditional practitioners are NOT comfortable or willing to prescribe compounded hormone replacement therapy, because they are NOT approved by the FDA! Bio-identical hormones are manufactured in a lab to have a similar molecular structure as those circulating in your body. Synthetic hormones are made differently and can be patented, studied and approved by the FDA. Pharmaceutical companies are unable to patent a "bio-identical" compound, hence NO studies to be done and NO approval by the FDA. A natural occurring compound cannot be patented.

The FDA has approved many bio-identical based products from pharmaceutical companies commonly referred to as "natural" HRT, which include estradiol (estrogen) and Prometrium (progesterone).

Estradiol products are available by prescription in different forms:
- *Cream:* Estrace
- *Gels:* Divigel, EstraGel and Elestrin
- *Lotion:* Estrasorb
- *Patches:* Alora, Climara, Menostar & Vivelle dot
- *Spray:* Evamist
- *Vaginal ring:* Estring and Femring (90 day delivery system)
- *Suppositories:* Vagifem and Bezwecken
  (Vaginal suppositories (1mg of estriol) are available without a prescription.)

Prescription progesterone is available in a capsule called Prometrium (micronized progesterone in peanut oil).

NOTE: Trans-dermal delivery (through the skin) via patch, cream or spray avoid going through your liver and may decrease the risk of stroke. Oral forms can stimulate the liver to make more clotting factors, which can increase your risk of stroke.

It's important to achieve balance and never take more hormones than you need. The purpose of hormone replacement therapy is to bring your hormones into a healthy balance. You can talk with your clinician and revisit your decision periodically.

Remember, what is normal at 25 is not normal at 55!

You do have treatment options! And, yes Virginia, there is life after menopause!

How To Find A Compounding Pharmacy
If you have made the decision to use natural hormone therapy you may want to find a compounding pharmacy near your home. If you cannot locate a nearby pharmacy your prescription can be sent via fax or transmitted electronically (if your clinician uses electronic health records) to a compounding pharmacy. The pharmacy will compound your hormone prescription and then mail it to your home.

The best way to locate a compounding pharmacy is to contact the International Academy of Compounding Pharmacists (IACP) or try the Professional Compounding Centers of America Incorporated (PCCA). The PCCA can provide a list of compounding pharmacies located in your area.
• Telephone: (800) 331-2498
• Fax: (800) 874-5760
• Website: www.thecompounders.com

The address for the IACP is PO Box 1365, Sugar Land, Texas, 77487. Telephone: (800) 927-4227, Fax: (281) 495-0602.

You can call any compounding pharmacy and ask for a list of local clinicians in your area that prescribe compounded hormone replacement therapy.

Risks Associated With HRT

The Women's Health Initiative Study
Many women began having concerns about taking synthetic HRT after hearing about the results of a study called the "Woman's Health Initiative," referred to as the "WHI" in July of 2002.

The WHI was initiated by the U.S. National Institutes of Health

(NIH) in 1991. The study was intended to look at strategies that could potentially reduce the incidence of major health problems such as heart disease, breast cancer, colorectal cancer and fractures in postmenopausal women.

The WHI enrolled more than 160,000 postmenopausal participants into a set of clinical trials between 1993 and 1998, with an age range between 50 to 79 years (mean age of 63.5 years at the time of enrollment). The study was divided into two parts:

• A randomized clinical trial.

• An observational study.

The clinical trial had three components:

• Hormone therapy trial: Estrogen alone or estrogen and progesterone versus placebo were given and then studied to determine the incidence of coronary heart disease, osteoporotic fractures and risk for developing breast cancer in these women.

• Calcium with Vitamin D trial: Calcium and vitamin D versus placebo, given to look at the incidence of osteoporotic fractures and colorectal cancer.

• Dietary modification trial: A low fat, high fruit/vegetable and grain diet versus a regular diet, given to look at the incidence of coronary heart disease, breast and colorectal cancer.

The Observational Study (WHI-OS)
This study observed 93,000 women from the same clinical coordinating centers.

Estrogen-Progestin versus Placebo
This phase studied estrogen, specifically conjugated equine estrogen, plus progestin (Prempro made by Wyeth Pharmaceuticals) compared to placebo (the "WHI-E+P" trial) among healthy postmenopausal women. This trial was terminated in early 2002 when researchers found that subjects experienced:

• Increased risk of stroke

• Increased risk of myocardial infarction (heart attack)

• Increased risk of breast cancer

• Increased risk of blood clots, including deep venous thrombosis (DVT) and pulmonary embolism (PE)

- Increased risk of dementia (the study included women ages 65 years and older)
- No protection against memory loss (mild cognitive impairment)

On a positive note this study showed:

- Fewer hip and vertebral (bone) fractures
- Decreased risk for developing colorectal cancer

Conjugated Estrogen versus Placebo

This phase studied estrogen, specifically conjugated equine estrogen (Premarin made by Wyeth Pharmaceuticals), alone versus placebo (the "WHI-CEE" trial) in women with a prior hysterectomy. This trial was conducted among women with a hysterectomy so that estrogen could be given without a progestin. (In women with a uterus, a progestin is needed to counteract the risk of endometrial cancer in women taking estrogen alone.)

This trial was stopped in 2004 when researchers found that subjects experienced:

- Increased risk of stroke
- Increased risk of blood clots (usually in one of the deep veins in the legs)
- No effect on risk for heart disease (heart attack called a myocardial infarction)
- No effect on risk for colorectal cancer
- An uncertain effect on breast cancer risk
- No protection against memory loss (there were more cases of dementia in those who took the therapy than those on the placebo, although not statistically significant)

On a positive note, this study showed a reduced risk of bone fractures.

NOTE: Estrogen alone or with progesterone should not be used to prevent heart disease! Women in this age group can be at increased risk for having a heart attack, especially if they have been diagnosed with high blood pressure, high cholesterol, obesity and diabetes, which can all increase the risk for developing heart disease.

Calcium and Vitamin D versus Placebo

This phase of the trial compared calcium plus vitamin D versus placebo ("WHI-CalcVitD"). This study had two primary end-points:

- Colorectal cancer endpoint: Long term daily supplementation of calcium with vitamin D had no effect on the incidence of colorectal cancer among postmenopausal women.

- Fracture endpoint: Long term daily supplementation of calcium with vitamin D resulted in a small but significant improvement in bone density, although did not significantly reduce the number of hip fractures and increased the risk of kidney stones.

NOTE: A secondary endpoint was postmenopausal weight gain. Long term daily supplementation of calcium with vitamin D resulted in a small prevention of weight gain.

Conclusions

- In some women, co-administration of MPA (medroxyprogesterone acetate, a type of progestin) with CEE (conjugated equine estrogen) was associated with a slightly higher incidence for developing breast cancer.

- Based on these studies, CEE and MPA are no longer recommended to prevent cardiovascular disease in older women. The conclusions regarding heart disease were somewhat conflicting. Unfortunately we still do not have clear data to guide us regarding HRT and a woman's cardiac health.

- Other forms of estrogen (esterified estrogens) or topical administration of estradiol may reduce the risk of blood clotting compared to that of oral CEE.

- The low fat dietary phase of the trial yielded conflicting and controversial results. This trial has been criticized by epidemiologists for its lack of validity because:

  - The desired endpoint for fat reduction in diet was not fully achieved.

  - A group of postmenopausal women is not applicable to all women.

Recent Updates On HRT

New studies now suggest that women under 60 years of age and who are within ten years of menopause may benefit from HRT with less risk than older women.

USA Today (3/7/12) Szabo reports: "For certain women, taking estrogen supplements for a few years close to menopause appears safe," as published online in the Lancet Oncology (The Lancet) medical journal.

NOTE: The average age of the women enrolled in the WHI study was 63.5 years of age. Older women in general are at higher risk for developing breast cancer, heart disease and stroke.

Heart Disease And Cholesterol

If HRT is initiated within ten years of menopause and/or a woman is less than 60 years old, she may benefit from taking HRT with a reduction in risk of coronary heart disease. Remember, the risk of heart disease goes up as you age, so it's generally best to not start estrogen treatment after age 60.

The PEPI (Postmenopausal Estrogen Progestin Intervention) trial done in 1997 suggested that women between the ages of 45 and 60 taking equine estrogen alone (Premarin) or in combination with natural progesterone had an increase in HDL, the "good" cholesterol, compared to those taking equine estrogens with a synthetic progestin (i.e."Prempro").

We now know that estrogen (estradiol) given in transdermal form, (across the skin) can help reduce the level of triglycerides in your blood.

NOTE: Estrogen given in pill form, both synthetic and bio-identical can increase C-reactive protein and triglyceride blood levels. Please refer to Chapter 5, "Heart Disease" for further information on C-reactive protein and triglycerides levels.

Blood Clots (Deep vein thromboembolism)

Estrogen taken in pill form increases your risk for developing blood clots and is a risk when taking birth control pills as well.

Low dose estrogen given as hormone replacement trans-dermally (across the skin) does not carry this risk. (In birth control doses, it can actually increase the risk.)

There is recent information that suggests the use of natural pro-gesterone may carry less risk for developing blood clots than us-ing a synthetic progestin.

Do not take HRT if you've had a blood clot during pregnancy or when taking birth control pills.

Some individuals may have inherited an increased risk for devel-oping blood clots and a simple blood test can be done to determine the risk.

Breast Health

Women who had undergone a hysterectomy, ages 50 to 59, tak-ing estrogen alone did not have an increased risk for developing breast cancer.

Women of the same age, who had not undergone a hysterectomy and had taken estrogen with synthetic progesterone, *did* show an increase risk for developing breast cancer.

Other studies show that *estrogen alone therapy* may increase your risk for developing breast cancer. If you have already had breast cancer, have a strong family history of breast cancer, or have been diagnosed with breast disease that may lead to breast cancer, es-trogen is not recommended.

It is important to consider age, symptoms and the duration of ther-apy before beginning hormone replacement. Be sure to discuss your individual risk with your clinician.

Cognitive Health

The Women's Health Initiative Memory Study (WHIMS) in 2004 suggested that women who were initiated on HRT (synthetic estro-gen alone and/or estrogen with progestin) at an older age (over 60) had a decline in cognitive function, (decrease in brain function) compared to those who began HRT at the onset of menopause. The participants in the study were between the ages of 65 and 79 years of age and there is an increased possibility that irreversible neuronal degeneration may have already been present. Also, a significant number of the participants in the study already had risk factors such as hypertension and diabetes which can increase the risk of vascular damage (i.e. dementia).

Another study looked at women between the ages of 50 and 63 years on HRT and it showed a decreased risk for developing dementia.

There is not yet a definitive answer regarding the use of estrogen for treating memory loss or cognitive impairment. There is inconsistency between the available studies and estrogen's role in memory loss. The available facts indicate there may be a window of time when HRT is most beneficial and least likely to cause health risks.

NOTE: You probably have noticed that some of these studies seem to contradict each other. The point is that obviously the research is not clearly supporting the safety or effectiveness of HRT. We need more good studies, so in the meanwhile, we need to cautiously approach the decision to treat with hormone therapy. Choosing the lowest possible effective dosage for the shortest duration of time is highly recommended when choosing HRT. Be sure to discuss your family history and individual risk with your clinician!

Recent Statement Just Released From Medical Professionals Regarding The Use Of Hormone Replacement Therapy

Over the past ten years, there has been a lot of debate and confusion based on the interpretations of the first results of the WHI study discussed above. In response to this confusion, fifteen organizations have reviewed and endorsed recommendations about the appropriate use of hormone replacement.

Fifteen top medical organizations, including the North American Menopause society, the American Society for Reproductive Medicine and the Endocrine Society have come to an agreement and have issued a statement regarding the risks and benefits for hormone replacement for women suffering from symptoms associated with menopause.

According to the consensus of the group:

• Systemic HRT is the most effective treatment used for most menopausal symptoms, including vasomotor symptoms and vaginal atrophy, however individualization is key in the decision to use HT.

- Progesterone therapy is required to prevent endometrial cancer when estrogen is used systemically in women with a uterus.

- Local estrogen therapy is effective and preferred for women whose symptoms are limited to vaginal dryness or discomfort with intercourse. Low dose vaginal estrogen cream is recommended in this setting.

- Systemic hormone replacement therapy is an acceptable option for relatively young, healthy women (up to age 59 or within 10 years of menopause) who are bothered by moderate to severe menopausal symptoms.

- When making the decision to prescribe HRT, considerations should be given to:

  - Impact of symptoms on quality of life.

  - Personal risk factors such as age and time since menopause.

  - Risk of blood clots, heart disease, stroke and breast cancer.

Conclusion

The group concluded that the leading societies devoted to the care of menopausal women agree that hormone replacement has an important role in managing some symptoms for women during the menopausal transition and in early menopause.

Chapter Summary

After reading this chapter you may be feeling a little overwhelmed as to which path you should choose.

You first need to establish a relationship with a clinician that you can trust and feel comfortable with, knowing that he or she will address you as an individual.

Treating the symptoms of perimenopause and menopause can be challenging due to the variability of symptoms and an individual's response to different treatments.

The symptoms can vary from individual to individual and can change throughout the transition from perimenopause to menopause.

You should be re-evaluated as you progress through each stage of menopause.

Some women do well with just a lifestyle change where others are unable to function without hormone replacement. It is very important to address your family history and consider your quality of life.

It is always best to use the lowest dose of hormone replacement for the shortest duration needed that provides relief of your symptoms.

You and your clinician can decide which treatment or combination of treatments will provide symptom relief and restore your quality of life.

Websites for further information on:

Diseases and Conditions associated with menopause

Menopause-Mayo Clinic: **http://www.mayoclinic.org/ diseases-conditions/menopause/basics/definition/con- 20019726?reDate=13012017**

The North American Menopause Society: www.menopause.org: **http://www.menopause.org/for-women**

Office on Women's Health, U.S. Department of Health and Human Services: **https://www.womenshealth.gov/menopause/**

National Institutes of Health. National Heart, Lung and Blood Institute. Women's Health Initiative Study: **https://www.nhlbi.nih.gov/whi/**

Women's Health-Hormone Health Network: **http://www.hormone.org/diseases-and-conditions/womens-health**

Diet, Herbs and Exercise

American Herbalist Guild: **http://ww42.americanherbalistguild.com/**

American Yoga Association: **http://www.americanyogaassociation.org/general.html**

Fit Day-Free Weight Loss and Diet Journal: **http://www.fitday.com/**

Dietary Guidelines: **https://health.gov/dietaryguidelines/**

National Center for Complementary and Integrative Health: **https://nccih.nih.gov/**

Physical Activity-American Heart Association: **http://www.heart.org/HEARTORG/HealthyLiving/PhysicalActivity/Physical-Activity_UCM_001080_SubHomePage.jsp**

Chapter 4

LIBIDO CHANGES DURING MIDLIFE

Sex Does Change After Menopause

The loss of estrogen following menopause can lead to changes in a woman's sexual drive and function. You may find it takes longer to become aroused, and may have even noticed a decrease in sensitivity to touching, which can result in less sexual desire.

The fluctuation of hormone levels during perimenopause and early menopause can certainly have an effect on your sex life.

You may even experience brief periods of a higher or lower than usual sex drive during this time period.

The most common cause of a low sex drive in women is *hormonal imbalance.*

During perimenopause, declining ovarian function leads to lower levels of the sex hormones estrogen, progesterone and testosterone, which all contribute to a healthy libido.

Estrogen keeps the vagina moist and elastic. Loss of estrogen can result in a decreased blood supply to the vagina, affecting lubrication, which can lead to dryness and thinning of the vaginal walls and intercourse can become uncomfortable to quite painful.

Progesterone is also very important in promoting a healthy sex drive and its production naturally declines during perimenopause as well.

Testosterone is primarily produced in the ovaries prior to menopause and in the adrenal glands after menopause. Testosterone certainly contributes to a healthy orgasm and sexual fantasies.

NOTE: When the level of testosterone increases in relation to the level of estrogen, some women my experience an increase in sexual desire!

Frequent intercourse has been known to help decrease vaginal atrophy (drying out) by increasing blood flow to the vaginal tissues, thus stimulating lubrication.

Women who remain sexually active during menopause and beyond may experience less discomfort with intercourse than women who are only sexually active intermittently. For example: A woman who has been married and had consistent sexual relations will have less problems with vaginal atrophy than a woman who has been asexual for several years.

Improving Libido
Consider the following to improve libido:

- *Check your attitude:* Women who enjoyed sex in their younger years often will continue to enjoy sex in their later years.
- *Be comfortable with your body image:* Accept midlife changes and you will have a stronger sense of self-esteem which can help improve sexual desire.
- *Address the fatigue:* Hormonal imbalance and poor nutrition can cause fatigue.
- *Decrease carbohydrates and caffeine:* Include more protein in your diet and decrease sugar and caffeine intake. This can help improve your energy and appetite for sex.
- *Review your medications:* Discuss possible side effects of medications you are currently taking with your clinician as there are some medications which can affect libido.

- *Address health conditions:* Chronic illness and surgery can certainly decrease sexual desire.

- *Consider incontinence:* Urinary incontinence can occur after menopause which is embarrassing and you will want to avoid having sex. *(Please read Chapter 9 for more information on urinary conditions and incontinence.)*

- *Decrease your stress:* Issues with work, family and relationships can interfere with sexual desire.

- *Check your testosterone level:* Low testosterone impairs sexual desire and fantasies. Testosterone replacement may help improve sexual function.

- *Consider your partner's health:* Health issues in your partner can be associated with sexual dysfunction.

- *Use of a vaginal lubricant:* Using a lubricant when having intercourse may help with vaginal dryness. Use water soluble lubricants such as Astroglide or K-Y Jelly. Do not use non-water soluble products like Vaseline because they can weaken latex, the material condoms are made of. Non-water soluble lubricants can also contribute to bacterial overgrowth resulting in an infection, especially if your immune system is lowered.

- *Consider hormone vaginal creams:* These preparations can help improve vaginal dryness. Lower doses can be used resulting in fewer side effects. *(Please read Chapter 3 for more information on vaginal lubricants and creams.)*

- *Consider counseling with a healthcare professional:* If you and your partner are dissatisfied with your sex life, you may want to consider seeking some counseling. Select an individual with whom you both feel comfortable and make sure he or she specializes in sexual dysfunction.

Questions To Ask Yourself

- What is causing you to be dissatisfied with your sex life?
- How long has this problem been going on?
- Is this a recent problem or is there a specific event that may have triggered it?
- What else is happening in your life now?

Age, Sex & Intimacy

Midlife Positives

- You have reached a level of maturity, which can lead to greater freedom to express yourself sexually.

- The children may have left home by now, allowing for more leisure time and opportunity for spontaneity.

- You can become more accepting of yourself and your partner, which can lead to greater intimacy.

- Many women continue to have a happy and satisfying sex life well into their seventies and eighties.

- Some women report having an increase in sex drive and better orgasms.

- Communication is key! Talk to your partner about your feelings and experiences. Tell him or her what feels good.

- Go ahead and express your sexual creativity and freedom.

Improving Sexual Intimacy After Menopause

Learn about your anatomy, sexual function and how your body changes with age. Attempt to locate the "G" spot. Understanding these changes can help decrease fear and frustration with sexual behaviors and responses.

Enhance your sexual experience with the use of appropriate materials for stimulation. Use books, videos, masturbation and don't forget about "Bob" (battery operated boyfriend). Try new sexual routines in different environments.

Use distraction techniques to increase relaxation and decrease stress. Try different types of music, videos, television, and even consider different movements which can also be a form of exercise.

Try non-coital behaviors like a sensual massage. This activity can help you relax and enhance communication between you and your partner.

Avoid any positions which cause pain. Try taking a warm bath before engaging in intercourse and be sure to use a vaginal lubricant. *(See vaginal lubricant section in Chapter 3 for further recommendations.)*

Take the time to relax and enjoy. You deserve it!

Not all intimate relationships are created equal. It is not at all unusual or abnormal for sexual intimacy to evolve into a less physical and more emotional level as we age. If you and your partner have less desire and you both are comfortable with that, don't fret! The media would have you believe that your sex life must continue with the same intensity and frequency as it did when you were 20. This is not the norm, so you can relax and enjoy a new level of intimacy!

New Medications

Recent Drug Approval From The FDA For Postmenopausal Women Experiencing Pain During Sex

On February 1, 2014 the FDA approved Osphena (ospemifene) to treat women experiencing moderate to severe dyspareunia (pain during sexual intercourse), a symptom of vulvar and vaginal atrophy (thinning of tissue) due to menopause. This medication is taken in pill form once daily with food and acts like estrogen on vaginal tissues to make them thicker and less fragile, reducing pain with intercourse. This drug is a new selective receptor modulator (SERM) which stimulates growth of the uterine lining (endometrium) and you should be followed closely by your clinician.

First Prescription Drug For Premenopausal Women With Low Sexual Desire Is Now Available

On August 18, 2015 the FDA approved Addyi (flibanserin) for the treatment of low sexual desire in premenopausal women.

Addyi is the first drug to receive approval for the treatment of generalized hypoactive sexual desire disorder (HSDD) in premenopausal women.

This new medication regulates several brain chemicals which may affect sexual desire. Flibanserin is a non-hormonal medication which comes in a 100 mg tablet and should be taken once daily. This prescription is a multifunctional serotonin agonist (MSAA) and considered to be the new "little pink pill" termed "Female Viagra."

This drug cannot be taken with alcohol and can have potential serious side effects such as: severe low blood pressure termed hypotension and loss of consciousness, termed syncope. You need to discuss all possible side effects and potential drug interactions with your clinician.

Websites for further information on:

Medication for Decreased Sexual Desire in:

Pre-menopause: Addyi (flibanserin): **https://www.drugs.com/**

Postmenopause: Osphena (ospemifene): **https://www.drugs.com/**

Menopause and decreased sexual desire (libido)

Healthline-Managing the Symptoms of Menopause: **http://www.healthline.com/health/menopause/managing-the-symptoms#overview1**

HealthyWomen: **http://www.healthywomen.org/content/article/whats-really-causing-your-low-sex-drive**

The North American Menopause Society, Decreased Desire: **http://www.menopause.org/for-women/sexual-health-menopause-online/sexual-problems-at-midlife/decreased-desire**

Sexuality in Menopause, Christiane Northrup, M.D: **http://www.drnorthrup.com/sexuality-in-menopause/**

WebMD Menopause Health Center: **http://www.webmd.com/menopause/guide/sex-menopause#1**

Chapter 5

HEART DISEASE

I begin this section of the book with heart disease because it is *the number one killer of women, causing 1 in 3 deaths among women each year! It is estimated that 43 million U.S. women have heart disease and only half of them recognize it as being the leading cause of death. One-third of women still believe breast cancer is the greatest healthcare problem among women.*

More females die from cardiovascular disease than all forms of cancer combined. Breast cancer claims the lives of 41,000 women per year compared to 215,000 lives claimed annually from coronary heart disease. The National Heart, Lung and Blood Institute reports, "One out of ten women in the US between the ages of 45 and 65 have some form of heart disease." When you reach age 65 your risk increases to one in five.

Women do have a lower rate of heart disease and stroke prior to menopause and natural estrogen may have a protective effect. In addition, heart disease rates are two to three times higher for postmenopausal women than for those women the same age who haven't reached menopause yet.

Cardiovascular Disease (CVD)

Cardiovascular disease is the term used to describe a number of conditions that affect your heart, brain and circulatory system (blood vessels).

Health statistics reveal that a woman's risk of dying from CVD is eight times greater than the combined risk of breast and ovarian cancer.

More than half of all deaths in women over age 50 are the result of CVD. Death rates for American women aged 35 to 54 are increasing; likely due to the obesity epidemic paving the path for developing hypertension (high blood pressure), high cholesterol and triglycerides as well as diabetes. Smoking also increases your risk!

Cardiovascular diseases include atherosclerosis, coronary artery disease, arrhythmia (an irregular heartbeat), heart failure, hypertension, heart valve disease (infectious disease of the heart and endocarditis), cardiomyopathy (an enlarged heart) from prolonged high blood pressure, autoimmune disease, alcohol and/or drugs, diseases of the aorta and its branches, disorders of the peripheral vascular system and congenital heart disease.

In this chapter, I will focus on the most common causes of CVD which include atherosclerosis, coronary heart disease, hypertension and peripheral vascular disease.

Coronary artery disease (CAD) also known as atherosclerotic heart disease, coronary heart disease (CHD) or (IHD) is the most common type of heart disease and the cause of heart attacks!

We now know that women with heart disease often have different symptoms than men, particularly after menopause, so I will provide great detail outlining those differences throughout this chapter.

Atherosclerosis

We will now direct our focus to the disease called atherosclerosis in which cholesterol plaque builds up on the inside of your arteries. Your body has many arteries, which are blood vessels that carry oxygen rich blood to the heart and other vital organs. Plaque is made up of fat, cholesterol, calcium, and other particles found in the blood. Plaque hardens over time and can eventually cause narrowing of the inside lining (lumen) of your arteries and is commonly referred to as "hardening of the arteries." This disease can cause serious problems like a heart attack, stroke or even death. Atherosclerosis can affect any artery in the body and symptoms typically do not occur until the artery becomes so narrowed that blood flow is impaired or even blocked completely.

Coronary Artery Disease (CAD)
This condition occurs when plaque builds up on the inside of the coronary arteries leading to the heart. Coronary artery disease causes coronary heart disease.

Coronary Heart Disease (CHD)
In coronary heart disease, *plaque typically builds up on the insides of the major arteries leading to the heart.* This condition is also referred to as obstructive coronary disease and is **more commonly found in men.** The terms CAD and CHD are often used interchangeably.

Ischemic Heart Disease (IHD)
This condition occurs when plaque builds up on the insides of the small arteries leading to the heart. This condition is also referred to as ischemic coronary disease where the heart muscle is denied oxygen and may be related to coronary atherosclerosis, vascular spasm (blood vessels constrict) or vasculitis (inflammation of the vessels). This term includes different types of heart disease: acute coronary syndrome (ACS), coronary artery disease (CAD) and stable and unstable angina. Microvascular coronary dysfunction (small vessel disease) can be the cause of ischemic heart disease and can occur without the presence of atherosclerotic disease and **is more commonly found in women. Plaque can build up on the insides of the very smallest arteries leading to the heart causing ischemic heart disease.** Significant and specific differences exist in women with ischemic heart disease when compared with men.

Symptoms and further detail on ischemic heart disease to follow later in the chapter.

Carotid Artery Disease
This condition occurs when plaque builds up in the carotid arteries, which are located in your neck and supply oxygen rich blood to your brain.

Peripheral Vascular Disease (PVD) Or Peripheral Arterial Disease (PAD)
This condition occurs when plaque builds up in the major arteries of the legs, arms and pelvis.

Risk Factors For Developing CVD

A risk factor is a condition or circumstance that makes it more likely that an individual will develop the disease.

More than 80% of middle-aged women have one or more traditional cardiac risk factors.

The presence of a single risk factor at 50 years of age is associated with a substantially increased lifetime absolute risk for developing cardio-vascular heart disease and a shorter duration of survival.

Non-Modifiable Risk Factors

Advanced Age: Postmenopausal women are at greater risk.

Gender: Women typically develop heart disease ten years later than men.

Race: African-American, Native American and Hispanic females carry a greater risk. (The highest coronary heart death rates occur in black women.)

Body Type (Apple or Pear Shape): Where you store your body fat can be a *sign of your risk for CVD*. If you have a "pear shaped" body and carry more fat in your hips and legs, you are at less risk than women who carry their fat in the abdomen (around the waist) referred to as an "apple shape." *(The shape you were born with is non-modifiable but weight loss is modifiable.)*

Family History of CVD: If your mother, father, grandmother and/ or grandfather had a heart attack or stroke you carry a greater risk.

Modifiable Risks (Habits and Lifestyle)

Obesity

Obesity is a disorder of excess fat accumulation. It is caused by an imbalance in the hormonal regulation of adipose (fat) tissue and fatty acid metabolism which is termed *adiposopathy*. More fat is being made and deposited in our tissues than metabolized and mobilized. Simply put, more fatty acids are entering and being stored rather than are leaving the cells. Insulin is the primary regulator of fat storage. When insulin levels are elevated, either chronically or after a meal, we accumulate fat.

Once this hormonal imbalance is corrected then weight loss occurs.

Obesity is prevalent in one third of women, including 7% with a body mass index of greater than 40. Body mass index (referred to as BMI) is defined in Chapter 3 on pages 55 and 56. A healthy body mass index range should be between 18.5 and 24.9.

Inactivity

It is important to exercise regularly to lower your risk of developing heart disease. A well-balanced exercise program should include aerobic exercise, strength training and stretching. Check with your clinician to discuss a program that is appropriate for you.

Too Much Alcohol

Women should not drink more than one alcoholic beverage per day. Less is even better.

Smoking

Women in the United States who smoke experience twice the amount of deaths from cardiovascular disease than from any cancer. ***Tobacco use is the leading cause of heart attacks in younger women!***

Cigarettes contain carbon monoxide, nicotine, and many other toxic chemicals that can damage the inside of the arteries. Smoking has been shown to increase blood pressure, decrease HDL cholesterol (high density lipoprotein, the good type), and increases the chances of developing a blood clot in the coronary arteries.

Women who smoke have a higher risk for stroke. The risk is even higher if you are 35 years or older and take birth control pills.

Never start smoking. However, if you do smoke, it is important to quit! This is the single best way to reduce your risk of heart disease. It is important to also limit your exposure to second-hand smoke.

The American Heart Association considers smoking to be the leading preventable risk for developing heart disease!

It can be very challenging to quit on your own, so talk to your clinician about a plan which might include use of the newer medications available. Enrolling in a smoking cessation program can improve your chances of success in quitting for life.

Yes, you can quit! If you live in California, you can call *1-800-No-*

BUTTS today and it is free! The American Cancer Society is also a great resource for programs in your area.

(See Chapter 3, page 66 and 67 for further information on smoking and your health.)

Mixed Risks (Can Be Modifiable)

Hormone-Related Metabolic Abnormalities

Insulin Resistance

When you have insulin resistance, your body's cells have a decreased ability to respond to the action of the hormone insulin. The ability of your cells to respond to insulin is called insulin sensitivity. This sensitivity can decline years before diabetes develops. Your pancreas then tries to compensate by producing more insulin to keep up with higher glucose levels. This may work for a while, but then the cells become more and more resistant and the pancreas works harder and harder until it eventually burns out.

The more overweight you are, the more resistant the cells become to insulin and the less sensitivity you have for insulin and its effects.

Today too many calories consumed in our daily diet come from processed (refined) carbohydrates, sugars such as sucrose (combination of glucose and fructose) and high fructose corn syrup that quickly enter the blood stream. These sugars are particularly harmful as glucose stimulates insulin production, and fructose can elevate triglyceride levels.

An elevated triglyceride level (fasting or after a meal) is an independent risk factor for heart disease, particularly in women.

Refined carbohydrates, starches and sugars, through their direct effect on insulin and blood sugar, are major contributors to the dietary cause of coronary heart disease, diabetes and obesity.

If you have been diagnosed with "Insulin Resistance" or "Metabolic Syndrome," your risk for developing heart disease is increased.

The hallmarks of the syndrome include:

• Central obesity, a waist circumference of greater than 35 inches for a female and greater than 40 inches for a male. Your waist measurement should equal half your height in inches. (20% of insulin resistant patients are NOT overweight and have a BMI under 26.) See chart on page 56 in Chapter 3 to find your BMI number.

- A fasting blood triglyceride level greater than or equal to 150mg/dl
- HDL cholesterol 40mg/dl or less in males and 50mg/dl or less in females
- A blood pressure reading of 130/85mmHg or higher or on medication for hypertension.
- A fasting blood sugar of 100mg/dl or greater

This syndrome is found to be more common in Hispanic and African-American females. Your overall risk of developing metabolic syndrome does increase with age, especially during your menopausal years.

NOTE: Insulin resistance is common in African Americans but they may not have high triglycerides (TG) or a low HDL-C but rather obesity, glucose issues and hypertension (high blood pressure).

Diabetes

Diabetes is a group of diseases associated with high levels of sugar circulating through your body and occurs when your body fails to keep blood sugar under control. When we eat non-glucose containing food, some of it is converted to sugar known as "glucose," our body's main source of energy. (90% of Type 2 diabetics are insulin resistant.)

Two out of every three women in the United States over age 20 are overweight or obese. Current numbers reported are: 1.9 billion men and women are overweight and 600 million are obese. Diabetes is present in over 12 million women. It is twice as common in Hispanic women versus white non-Hispanic women (12.7 versus 6.45%).

Women with type 2 diabetes are seven times more likely to develop heart disease, have a heart attack and die from it than an individual without diabetes!

(Please see Chapter 10 for further detail on metabolic syndrome and diabetes.)

Hypertension (High Blood Pressure)

Classifying Hypertension

Having a diagnosis of hypertension can greatly increase your risk of having a heart attack or stroke.

After age 65 a higher percentage of women than men have hypertension.

A blood pressure reading has two numbers; a top number called the systolic and a bottom number called the diastolic blood pressure. The systolic reading records the highest pressure in the arteries and occurs when the heart contracts. The diastolic reading records the lowest pressure in the arteries and occurs when the heart relaxes. Both are important for your cardiac and vascular health.

A systolic blood pressure reading of less than 120 and a diastolic reading of less than 80 is classified as normal in a healthy non diabetic person. Lower blood pressures are common and can also be healthy in active individuals.

Diabetics and individuals who have heart disease (CAD) need to maintain a systolic blood pressure of less than 130 mm Hg and diastolic of less than 80 mm Hg.

If your blood pressure readings average a systolic reading between **120-129** and a diastolic reading of less than **80 mm Hg** your blood pressure is considered elevated and you are at increased risk. The "pre-hypertension" classification has been eliminated and now categorized as **"elevated."**

If you have three or more blood pressure readings of **130-139/ 80-89** or higher over a two to three week time period, then you have hypertension! This is classified as **"Stage 1 Hypertension."**

If your blood pressure readings average a systolic greater than or equal to **140 mm Hg** and diastolic greater than or equal to **90 mm Hg** you have **"Stage 2 Hypertension,"** which is more severe.

Risk Factors

• *Age:* The risk for developing high blood pressure increases as you age. Women are more likely to develop high blood pressure after *menopause.*

• *Race:* High blood pressure occurs more commonly in African-Americans and typically at an earlier age than in Caucasians. The current prevalence in black women is at 44%.

Complications such as stroke and heart attack are also more common in African-Americans.

- *Family History:* High blood pressure commonly runs in families.
- *Overweight or Obese:* The more you weigh, the more blood you need to supply oxygen and nutrients to your tissues. An increased volume of blood circulating through your vessels increases the pressure on your arterial walls leading to high blood pressure.
- *Inactivity:* Individuals who are inactive tend to have higher heart rates. The higher your heart rate the harder your heart has to work which increases pressure on your arteries, leading to high blood pressure.
- *Smoking:* Smoking, inhaling second hand smoke, and chewing tobacco will raise your blood pressure for a short duration immediately after exposure. The chemicals in tobacco eventually damage the lining of your arteries causing them to narrow, increasing your blood pressure.
- *High Dietary Salt (Sodium) Intake:* Consuming too much sodium in your diet can cause your body to retain fluid, which increases blood pressure.
- *Drinking Too Much Alcohol:* Heavy consumption of alcohol can damage your heart. Drinking more than two drinks a day can raise your blood pressure.
- *Stress:* High levels of stress can raise your blood pressure.
- *Chronic Health Conditions:* Diabetes, high cholesterol, kidney disease and sleep apnea can all elevate your blood pressure.

Symptoms
Most individuals with hypertension (high blood pressure) do not have any signs or symptoms, even if blood pressure readings reach dangerously high levels. A few people with early stage hypertension may have a slight headache, feel dizzy or experience an increase in nose bleeds. These symptoms typically do not occur until hypertension has reached a serious stage.

Pregnancy and Hypertension
Pregnancy can cause hypertension in females who usually have normal blood pressure and can make pre-existing hypertension worse.

Hypertension during pregnancy carries great risk for both the mother and unborn baby.

Hypertension is one of the leading causes of illness and even death in pregnant women.

Age and Hypertension

As women age they might develop a wide pulse pressure which occurs when blood vessels lose their flexibility, causing the systolic (top number) to go high and the diastolic (bottom number) to stay the same or even go down.

Your risk for heart attack, stroke and developing congestive heart failure increases if there is a 60 point difference between the top and bottom numbers.

If your blood pressure is elevated when you have it taken at the doctor's office and normal at home, this is called "white coat hypertension." You should ask your clinician for a blood pressure monitoring device that you can use at home to determine what your overall readings are. Keep a log of your readings at different times of the day so you can discuss it at your follow up appointment.

Monitoring your blood pressure regularly can keep you aware of your cardiovascular health, so you can seek treatment early and prevent further disease.

It is also important to be aware of your salt intake and read labels. Try to consume no more than 2 grams or 2,000 milligrams of sodium per day as too much salt can increase blood pressure.

New HTN Treatment Guidelines

Clinicians use guidelines based on recent research evidence along with expert opinions from the Joint National Committee to guide them in treating high blood pressure. The American College of Cardiology (ACC) and the American Heart Association (AHA) recently lowered the definition of Hypertension. High blood pressure should now be treated earlier with lifestyle changes and in some patients with medication when your readings are at **130/80 mm Hg** rather than the previous JNC reading of **140/90 mm Hg** which allows for earlier intervention.

Summary of new guideline blood pressure categories as follows:

• Normal: Less than 120/80 mm Hg

• Elevated: Systolic between 120-129 and diastolic less than 80

- Stage 1: Systolic between 130-139 or diastolic between 80-89
- Stage 2: Systolic at least 140 or diastolic at least 90 mm Hg

Hypertensive Crisis: Systolic over 180 and/or diastolic over 120 with individuals needing immediate medication changes or hospitalization to reduce blood pressure to a normal range to prevent organ damage.

Sleep Disturbances

Sleep Deprivation (Insomnia)

Several recent studies show a shortened sleep duration (less than six hours per night) carries an increased risk of developing heart disease. One 2008 study from the University of Chicago found a link between shortened sleep and increased coronary artery calcification (calcium deposits), which is a good predictor of coronary artery disease. (This study was conducted by Diane Lauderdale, PhD, professor of epidemiology at the university's Pritzker School of Medicine.) Dr. Lauderdale's study also revealed that shorter sleep can be associated with worsening hypertension (high blood pressure).

Sleep Apnea

This is a condition in which an individual stops breathing for a short duration and may even gasp for air while they sleep. As you know, your body depends on oxygen to function properly. According to the National Heart, Lung and Blood Institute, there is an increased risk for heart disease, high blood pressure and heart failure for individuals with sleep apnea. See your clinician and ask for a sleep study if you experience the above symptoms.

Calculations To Help Predict Cardiovascular Disease Event Risk

Pooled Cohort Risk Assessment Equations (PCE)

This calculator can be found online or you can download the app to your cell phone and uses the Pooled Cohort Equations to estimate the 10 year primary risk of ASCVD (atherosclerotic cardiovascular disease) among patients without pre-existing cardiovascular disease who are between 40 and 79 years of age. Individuals are considered to be at "elevated" risk if the Pooled Cohort Equations predicted risk is > 7.5%. The risk factors used are gender, age, race, total cholesterol, HDL cholesterol, systolic blood pressure (the top number), if an individual is currently receiving treatment for high blood pressure, has diabetes and/or if they are a smoker.

Current guidelines for treating individuals with elevated cholesterol blood levels to help reduce cardiovascular risk recommend that the following four groups of patients will benefit from initiating therapy with a statin medication:

- Individuals with clinical ASCVD (Heart Disease)

- Individuals with primary elevations of LDL > 190 mg/dl

- Individuals 40 to 75 years of age diagnosed with diabetes and an LDL of 70 to 189 mg/dl

- Individuals without clinical ASCVD or diabetes who are 40 to 75 years of age with an LDL 70 to 189 mg/dl and a 10 year ASCVD risk of 7.5 % or higher

QRISK2 Calculation

QRISK2 (most recent version of QRISK) is a prediction algorithm used for calculating an individual's lifetime risk for developing cardiovascular disease (CVD).

The QRISK tool can also be found online or you can download the app and uses traditional risk factors such as: age, systolic blood pressure, smoking status and the ratio of total blood cholesterol to high-density lipoprotein cholesterol (HDL) together with body mass index, ethnicity, family history, chronic kidney disease, rheumatoid arthritis, atrial fibrillation, diabetes and high blood pressure treatment medications.

A QRISK score over 20 indicates a need to start treatment (primary prevention) with cholesterol lowering medication, such as a statin.

This 20 score translates to a 20% risk of having a CVD event over the next ten years.

In summary, among patients who do not otherwise have a compelling indication for statin therapy, the Pooled Cohort Equations (PCE) and the QRISK2 score can be used to help estimate the primary cardiovascular risk and potential benefit for primary prevention by initiating statin therapy.

The Pooled Cohort Equations (PCE) and the QRISK2 score have now become more widely used than the commonly known "Framingham risk score" that was previously used to calculate cardiovascular risk.

Lipid Abnormalities

WARNING: This section can become very technical at times, outlining further emerging risk factors for those "scientists at heart" readers. *You may also choose to skip forward at any time to the "Conditions Associated with Cardiovascular Disease" section.*

Definition

Cholesterol is a fat-like substance (lipid) found in your bloodstream and cells. Cholesterol and triglycerides are the two main lipids found in your bloodstream and when produced in appropriate levels provide important functions for the body. Cholesterol is used as a building block for cell membranes, bile acids and many other functions including production of sex hormones.

Cholesterol

What is high cholesterol? Do you know what your numbers are?

Are you aware that cholesterol can play an important role in the development of heart disease?

Where Does Cholesterol Come From?

Every cell needs cholesterol and so our body makes it. Most cholesterol is made in the peripheral cells of our body and about 20% is made in the liver. Cholesterol can then be used by other organs to make sex hormones.

When you are told that you have high cholesterol this usually means you have too much bad cholesterol in your blood stream.

Our cholesterol level is actually determined mostly by how much our body makes rather than how much we *consume* in our diet.

Cholesterol in your diet comes from foods with animal fats that contain cholesterol and numerous other food substances. Problems arise when your body makes more than it should and this can happen frequently. If you consume a diet that is high in saturated and trans fats that come from animals your liver will make more cholesterol than it would make otherwise. Usually about half the cholesterol transported in the blood is returned to the liver or gut and then reabsorbed.

How Cholesterol Is Transported Through the Body

All cholesterol and triglycerides are carried in the blood within lipoproteins. If cholesterol and triglycerides were floating freely in our blood stream they would form clumps creating blockages in our blood vessels. For this reason, these fats are enveloped in water soluble spheres (like rubber balls) called lipoproteins. Lipids are hydrophobic (hate water) and need to be coated in hydrophilic (water-loving) particles to be transported through the blood. Lipids are always bound to these lipoproteins.

Lipoproteins have one or more proteins wrapped on their surface called apolipoproteins. These proteins help determine how helpful or harmful these particles will become.

How Cholesterol Is Measured
Cholesterol is measured in milligrams per deciliter (in the US) or mols/L (rest of the world), and most individuals refer to it as "my cholesterol number."

All cholesterol measurements or calculations simply refer to the cholesterol content within all of the various types of lipoproteins.

The main cholesterol-containing lipoproteins are the low density lipoprotein (LDL), the high density lipoprotein (HDL) and the very low density lipoprotein (VLDL).

Formula For Calculating Total Cholesterol
The total cholesterol lipoproteins calculations are reported as "cholesterol content," designated as "C." Total cholesterol (TC) is the amount of cholesterol carried inside all of the lipoproteins that exist in a specific volume of plasma (blood): mg/deciliter (dl) or liter (L).

- **LDL-C** is the amount of cholesterol carried within **all of the IDL and LDL particles** per deciliter of plasma (more about IDL particles to follow).

- **HDL-C** is the amount of cholesterol carried within **all of the HDL particles** per deciliter.

- **VLDL-C** is the amount of cholesterol carried within **all of the VLDL particles.** (VLDL is calculated by multiplying your triglyceride level by 0.20.)

- **TC** (total cholesterol) = **LDL-C + VLDL-C + HDL-C.**

Understanding Blood Cholesterol Numbers
The low density lipids, LDL-cholesterol referred to as (LDL-C) is known as the bad cholesterol. About 50% of the LDL-C finds

its way to atherosclerotic plaques. An optimal LDL-C cholesterol level is < 100 mg/dl but the desirable level (goal of therapy) depends upon one's cardiovascular disease (CVD) risk.

The goal for:
• Low risk individuals is 160 mg/dl or less
• Moderate risk individuals 130 mg/dl or less
• High risk individuals < 100 mg/dl or less
• Very high risk individuals < 70 mg/dl or less.

It is recommended that the LDL-C level be < 70mg/dL for those individuals at very high risk for cardiovascular disease, and for those who have already been diagnosed with cardiovascular disease (CAD). Diabetics with known CAD should also maintain a LDL-C level <70 mg/dl. Lower is even better.

Individuals with CAD may have:
• Had a heart attack (myocardial infarction abbreviated as an MI)
• Symptomatic angina, carotid disease and/or peripheral artery disease
• An abdominal aortic aneurysm (weakening of the artery wall due to the formation of plaque)

The high density lipids HDL-cholesterol, referred to as (HDL-C) is known as the good cholesterol and may have cardio-protective functions. The HDL-C is thought to offer protection to the heart and blood vessels by removing excess cholesterol from cells and cholesterol-containing white blood cells (macrophages) in plaque guiding them back to the liver. The HDL-C can also carry beneficial proteins and lipids, reducing the risk of heart disease.

A desirable HDL-C level for a female is approximately 50-60 mg/dL. (A level higher than 60 is considered to be protective and lower than 40 carries increased risk for cardiovascular disease) However 20% of women with CAD have a HDL-C level between 60 and 80 mg/dl and some individuals with a low level of HDL-C cholesterol may not even develop CAD.

For the majority of individuals the current recommendation is to keep the HDL-cholesterol high and the LDL-cholesterol low.

Table 5.1

Blood Cholesterol Numbers (as per NCEP ATP-III published in 2001)

Total cholesterol:

Less than 200mg/dl	Desirable
200-239 mg/dl	Borderline High
240 mg/dl and over	High

LDL- "bad" cholesterol:

Less than 100mg/dl	Optimal
100-129 mg/dl	Desirable
130-159 mg/dl	Borderline High
160-189 mg/dl	High
190 mg/dl and above	Very high

HDL- "good" cholesterol:

50 mg/dl or higher	Normal (the higher the better)
40 mg/dl or less	Low

Triglycerides:

Less than 100 mg/dl	Optimal
100-149 mg/dl	Normal
150-199 mg/dl	Borderline High
200- 499 mg/dl	High
500 mg/dl or higher	Very High

Note: *Both the American Heart Association (AHA) and American College of Endocrinology (ACE) now state that an optimal TG (triglyceride) level is < 100 mg/dl. ACE has also added a TG category called very, very high defined as > 2000 mg/dl.*

New Light On The Subject "Lipids Are Huge"

Carbohydrate (sugar) intake appears to be associated with increased triglyceride (TC) levels in insulin resistant patients, *a known risk factor for coronary heart disease, including postmenopausal women!* Be sure to avoid high sugar beverages and foods containing high fructose corn syrup, which are associated with evidence of increased inflammation and oxidative stress in your arteries. (Oxidative stress is cell damage associated with disease and the natural aging process.)

Traditionally levels of LDL cholesterol have been the primary focus of cholesterol screening (along with HDL and triglycerides) and *about half of all heart attacks occur in individuals with normal LDL levels.* Researchers then had to look at other measurements to help identify individuals at risk for cardiovascular disease.

Lipoproteins And Other Biomarkers

We have now learned that to accurately identify those at increased risk for cardiovascular disease, particularly menopausal women, we need to look beyond just the routine lipid panel and direct our focus on *non- HDL-C (sum of LDL and VLDL), ApoB and LDL-P* levels!

If the triglyceride and non-HDL-C levels are elevated and the HDL-C level is low, we should look at a more comprehensive panel that includes lipoproteins and other biomarkers related to cardiovascular (CVD) risk. This pattern can be associated with insulin resistance and may be found in menopausal women.

Newer advanced tests can further break down the HDL and LDL particle into subtypes, reclassifying them by their size (density) and particle number.

Identifying the number of particles and the size of particles in the blood is important and current research has found that certain patterns of LDL particle sizes may indicate a greater risk for the development of heart disease. Remember, these particles are the vehicles that carry cholesterol in the blood (arteries) causing atherosclerosis (hardened plaque on the artery wall).

In Review

The main cholesterol containing-lipoproteins are reported by their cholesterol content, (total cholesterol, {TC}, high density lipoprotein, {HDL-C}, low density lipoprotein, {LDL-C} and very low density lipoproteins, {VLDL-C}).

Lipoproteins can be further categorized by their buoyancy (density) and surface protein content; apolipoproteins B (ApoB) and A-I (ApoA-I).

Particle Concentration Number

The particle concentration number is the direct measurement of both large and small lipoprotein particles present in the blood. This marker is reported as "particle number," designated as a "P" after the specific type of lipoprotein as outlined below:

- **VLDL-P** (very low-density lipoprotein particle number)

- **LDL-P** (low density lipoprotein particle number)

- **IDL-P** (intermediate density lipoprotein particle)

- **HDL-P** (high density lipoprotein particle)

NOTE: Now that I have you all confused, let's try and simplify this concept. Think of the LDL-P particle number as a way of identifying all the prisoners gathered in one area, designated as "P" (the bad guys that clog our arteries). Hope that was helpful?

Lipoproteins

As previously discussed, lipoproteins are further categorized by their buoyancy (density) and surface protein content; apo-lipoproteins B (ApoB) and A-I (ApoA-I). The individual lipoprotein particle core varies due to the amount of cholesterol and triglycerides they contain.

Surface Proteins Wrapped on Lipoprotein Particles

- **ApoB containing lipoproteins** are made up of a single molecule of ApoB which contains (VLDL-P + intermediate-density lipoprotein-P {IDL-P} + LDL-P). The ApoB molecule circulates longer in the blood (longer half-life) and as a result about 90% of ApoB particles are LDL-particles. ApoB is therefore thought of as a measure of total LDL-P.

- **Non-HDL-C** is the cholesterol carried within the ApoB particles (most of them are LDL particles). This measurement is more closely related to the LDL-P not the VLDL-P.

- **Examples of Abnormal Results:** Remember, if the triglyceride and *non-HDL-C* levels are elevated and the HDL-C level is low, we should consider further advanced testing with a more comprehensive panel that includes lipoproteins and other biomarkers related to cardiovascular (CVD) risk. This pattern can be associated with insulin resistance and may be found in menopausal women.

- In other cases if the *ApoB* and *LDL-P* results are abnormal, this finding can help identify further CVD risks.

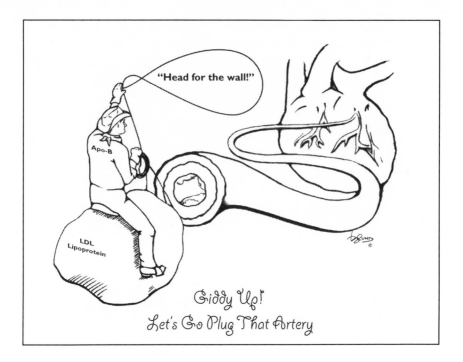

Advanced Lipid Testing

Advanced lipid testing may be considered if you are at increased risk for developing heart disease. Routine lipid screening does play an important role in identifying cardiovascular risk although it may not provide a complete picture of your heart health. Remember, nearly 50% of all heart attacks and strokes occur in patients with "normal" cholesterol levels. New detailed tests can help identify further risk and plaque buildup in your arteries.

The *NMR LipoProfile* is one of the advanced lipoprotein blood tests now available which can identify the number of LDL and HDL particles (LDL-P and HDL-P). This test also calculates the total cholesterol, triglycerides, LDL and HDL (designated LDL-C and HDL-C).

Lipoprotein markers associated with insulin resistance and diabetes risk can also be identified: Large VLDL-P, small LDL-P, large HDL-P, VLDL size, LDL size, HDL size and an insulin resistance score (LP-IR score).

Interpretation of results reported on the NMR LipoProfile test:

• **LDL-P:** This is the direct measurement of LDL particles (large and small) in a liter of plasma. This is considered the most prevalent lipoprotein particle responsible for atherogenesis and is measured as LDL-P. ***Remember, the number of LDL particles (LDL-P) is a strong and independent predictor of coronary vascular disease. (Another very important risk factor in postmenopausal women, unlike LDL-C.)***

- **HDL-P:** This is the direct measure of high density lipoprotein particles and correlates more closely with atherosclerotic risk than high density lipoprotein cholesterol (HDL-C).

- **IDL-P:** This is the direct measurement of the IDL particles in a liter of plasma.

- **LP-IR Score:** This is a lipoprotein insulin resistance test which can detect early abnormalities associated with the development of type 2 diabetes.

NOTE: Remember these newer tests can further break down the HDL and LDL particle into subtypes, reclassifying them by their size (density) and particle number. Identifying the number of particles and the size of particles in the blood is important and current research has found that certain patterns of LDL particle sizes may indicate a greater risk for the development of heart disease. These LDL particles are the vehicles that carry cholesterol around the body and into the walls of the arteries causing atherosclerosis (hardened plaque on the artery wall).

- There are other advanced lipid blood panels that can further break down the HDL and LDL particles into subtypes, reclassifying them by their size. One subclass of HDL called HDL2 (discussed below) is considered to be heart protective. These tests can also measure the amount of cholesterol within the following lipoproteins:

- **Total VLDL:** An elevated **VLDL** level corresponds to an increased risk of heart disease and diabetes.

- **VLDL-3:** This is a triglyceride-rich very low-density lipoprotein. Larger VLDL size is also a marker of insulin resistance. Studies suggest a correlation between an elevated VLDL-3 level and the development of diabetes.

- **Total ApoB100:** This is a calculated estimate of the number of apolipoprotein B containing lipoproteins in the plasma (sum of atherogenic particles). *Remember, too many apolipoprotein B-containing lipoproteins (90% of which are LDLs) help create, carry and deliver "bad cholesterol" into the arteries and are the cause of atherosclerosis. The majority of these particles, which are LDLs, are in effect the LDL particle concentration marker, LDL-P. The LDL-P marker is a strong and independent predictor of cardiovascular disease. A large particle number (LDL-P or ApoB) is associated with heart disease regardless of the cholesterol level! This measurement also helps identify the type and/or cause of high cholesterol.*

*(In contrast the **Apo A1 is the sum of anti-atherogenic lipoprotein particles** in the plasma.)*

• **Lp(a) Cholesterol or Lp(a)-C:** This is a measurement of all Apo (a) lipoproteins in a deciliter of plasma. Lp(a) is also similar to LDL and an inherited risk factor for developing atherosclerosis. ***Lp(a) is more likely to promote dangerous plaque formation than LDL. Lp(a) is considered to be more atherogenic than LDL.***

• **IDL:** These intermediate density lipoproteins are formed by degradation of the very-low-density lipoproteins (VLDLs). Once these IDL particles leave the plasma and enter the liver they are then further degraded to form LDL particles. IDL and LDL lipoproteins transport a variety of triglyceride fats and cholesterol through the bloodstream promoting plaque formation. IDL lipoprotein levels can be **elevated among individuals with a family history of diabetes.**

• Sum of Total LDL-C: The cholesterol content within all the Lp (a), IDL and all LDL particles.

• **LDL Size Pattern:** The LDL pattern A and B refers to the size of the LDL cholesterol particles in the blood. Measuring the LDL particle size pattern can also be used to identify insulin resistance. This pattern description is divided into three categories:

   • **Pattern A:** This pattern of the LDL particles are large, buoyant and less dense, making them easier for the body to remove and is associated with less likelihood of developing atherosclerosis. Individuals with LDL cholesterol pattern A are more likely to have normal blood levels of LDL cholesterol, HDL cholesterol and triglycerides.

- **Pattern B:** This pattern of LDL particles are smaller and have a higher density. These small dense LDL particles carry a four-fold greater risk of developing heart disease than those with a pattern A size. Pattern B is also used as a marker for detecting insulin resistance. Individuals with LDL cholesterol pattern B will frequently have low HDL cholesterol levels, elevated tri-glyceride levels and the tendency to develop high blood sugar levels and eventually type 2 diabetes mellitus.
- **Pattern A/B:** This pattern is a combination of light and dense molecules and is associated with intermediate risk.

- **Total non-HDL:** The sum of only LDL and VLDL levels. *A higher value indicates a higher risk for developing heart disease.*

- **HDL-2 and HDL-3:** This test further breaks down HDL cholesterol into sub classes:

HDL-2: This subclass of "good cholesterol" is considered to be protective against heart disease. *If this number is low, it is a marker of cardiovascular risk and insulin resistance.*

HDL-3: This subclass of HDL is less protective against heart disease as compared to HDL-2.

- **Sum Total Cholesterol:** The sum of HDL, LDL and VLDL levels.

Advanced Lipid Testing Summary

These advanced blood tests can identify more cholesterol abnormalities than the standard cholesterol (lipid) test and should therefore be thought of as advanced cholesterol testing for individuals at greater risk for heart disease.

The *NMR LipoProfile* test identifies the number of LDL and HDL particles (LDL-P and HDL-P) and lipoprotein markers associated with insulin resistance and diabetes risk.

Lipoprotein particles are the vehicles that carry cholesterol in plasma (blood) and potentially into the walls of the arteries, causing arteriosclerosis.

Other direct-measured cholesterol panels can identify the amount of cholesterol within the various lipoprotein sub-particles.

It is possible to have normal lipid measurements and still be at risk for developing heart disease due to dangerous particles, one of the most problematic being (apolipoprotein-B) **ApoB.**

These advanced tests can identify individuals with insulin resistance (IR) who are at risk for developing metabolic syndrome, diabetes and cardiovascular disease. If you are not on a cholesterol lowering medication and have **a pattern B LDL, a low HDL/HDL-2 and/or elevated triglycerides,** there is increased risk for developing **diabetes mellitus due to insulin resistance.** (I discuss this in further detail in Chapter 10.)

I realize this section can appear to be repetitious although I have observed through the years, the more one reads new information, the greater the understanding and retention.

NOTE: Most insurance companies view these tests as advanced lipid blood tests, NOT routine screening, so they may not pay for them to identify further risk.

Additional Important Biomarkers
Inflammation within the artery wall can now be measured with advanced biomarker testing and help determine an individual's cardiovascular risk.

C-reactive protein (CRP) is a marker which detects inflammation as discussed earlier in the chapter. *Heart disease in all humans, including women, is all about inflammation!* CRP is produced in the liver in response to substances released from inflammatory cells.

Atherosclerosis is considered to be an inflammatory condition.

Periodontal disease or any other chronic infectious or inflammatory disease can contribute to increased levels of CRP. A recent study in the Journal of Periodontology reported that inflammatory effects from periodontal disease (a chronic bacterial infection of the gums) cause oral bacteria by-products to enter the bloodstream and will trigger the liver to make proteins such as CRP that inflame arteries and promote blood clot formation. (See Chapter 18 for further information on dental health.)

We have now learned that statin medications and almost all approved lipid-lowering therapies used to treat lipoprotein disorders seem to have an anti-inflammatory effect and can help lower elevated CRP levels.

The **PLAC (Lp-PLA2)** test is the only advanced blood test cleared by the FDA to help identify increased risk for coronary heart disease and ischemic stroke associated with atherosclerosis. The PLAC test measures lipoprotein-associated phospholipase A2 (Lp-PLA2), which is a vascular-specific inflammatory marker found in association with rupture-prone plaque. *The Lp-PLA2 test helps identify cardiovascular risk in individuals that may not have been obvious from lipid and lipoprotein measurements. This test has been shown to be particularly useful in detecting cardiovascular disease and stroke risk in African American women.*

Metabolic Marker Testing

If you are at increased risk for developing CVD because of a strong personal or family history, you may want to discuss the possible need for additional testing with your clinician.

Homocysteine: This is a protein (amino acid), which makes your arteries "sticky," allowing cholesterol to adhere to the artery walls, which plays a role in plaque build-up. Homocysteine is thought to act as an oxidant, promoting oxygen free radicals. (Homocysteine can be thought of as a destructive substance.)

Consuming excessive animal protein has been shown to raise levels of homocysteine! Try eating more soy protein such as: tofu, tempeh, soy milk and soy beans, which may even help lower cholesterol levels.

Vitamin D level: Low vitamin D levels can be associated with a lowered immune system and is thought to play a role in increased risk for developing heart disease. (See Chapter 6 for further information on Vitamin D.)

Magnesium level: A low magnesium blood level has been found to be associated with an increased risk for cardiovascular disease.

Increased calcium supplement intake can lead to an imbalance of calcium to magnesium blood levels, increasing cardiovascular risk.

Supplements need to be balanced and are available in different doses. A commonly recommended dosage would contain calcium 500 mg, vitamin D 500 IU and magnesium 250 mg in one pill and should be taken twice daily for better absorption. Consult with your clinician to determine the correct dosage for you.

NOTE: *You may choose to skip forward at any time to the "conditions associated with cardiovascular disease" section if the following information is not of interest to you.*

Kidney Function Markers

Kidney disease is strongly linked to heart disease.

- **Creatinine:** Creatinine is a chemical waste molecule that is made from muscle metabolism and is transported through the blood to the kidneys. Your kidneys keep the blood creatinine in a normal range and when it becomes elevated, signifies impaired kidney function or kidney disease.

- **Cystatin-C:** This test is useful to look at kidney function when an individual is very obese, has cirrhosis (fatty liver), reduced muscle mass or is malnourished. (Auto-immune connective tissue diseases and cancer can also elevate cystatin-C levels.)

- **Urine micro-albumin or micro-albuminuria:** This test detects early signs of vascular damage, defined as albumin excretion of 30-300mg/day or 20-200mg/min. This test is considered a marker of general vascular dysfunction and is used to help predict grim outcomes for both kidney and heart patients. *Micro-albuminuria is an indicator of insulin resistance and identifies increased renal (kidney) and cardiovascular risk associated with metabolic syndrome and diabetes.*

Markers Of Cholesterol Absorption To Monitor Treatment In High Risk Individuals

Cholesterol homeostasis is maintained by a balance between absorption and production, which influences circulating cholesterol levels and development of coronary heart disease.

Your blood serum contains non-cholesterol sterols, which are reliable markers of cholesterol metabolism.

Effective lowering of LDL cholesterol by large dose statin medication is associated with a decrease in production and an increase in absorption of cholesterol.

These changes can be detected by measuring the non-cholesterol sterols in the serum and in different lipoprotein fractions.

The above-described testing can provide greater detail for the clinician and/or cardiologist to identify possible risk factors that would otherwise go undetected, guiding them in selecting the best treatment for you.

Be sure to discuss your family history with your clinician so he or she can determine which testing may be necessary.

Natural cycling estrogen is thought to delay the onset of cardiovascular disease in women, although new research suggests that estrogen replacement after menopause can possibly cause cardiovascular problems. We have learned that the pill form of synthetic estrogen used in hormone replacement therapy can raise the level of CRP in the blood. "The 2003 Women's Health Initiative" research study was stopped due to an increase in cardiac problems and cancer in its participants. The truth is, experts are divided as to whether estrogen replacement is harmful or helpful. (Please read Chapter 3 for further detail on the WHI study and hormone replacement therapy.)

Congratulations you made it through the lipid section! Are still with me? Feel free to go back and review any section, break it down at little bit at a time to help you gain a better understanding.

Conditions Associated With Cardiovascular Disease

Acute Coronary Syndrome (ACS) Or Sudden Cardiac Death
Acute coronary syndrome (ACS) refers to a group of conditions associated with decreased blood flow to the coronary arteries such that a part of the heart muscle is unable to function properly or dies. A heart attack and/or unstable angina are both considered to be "acute coronary syndromes" when the blood supplied to the heart muscle is suddenly blocked. The blockage can be sudden and complete or it can be incomplete and come and go. A clot can sometimes break open and then clog the artery again. Acute coronary syndrome symptoms are the same as those experienced when having a heart attack. It is important to take these symptoms very seriously and if not treated quickly, a heart attack can occur. When this condition occurs the heart tissue is dying, even if it is a few cells or a large section of the heart and is always considered an absolute medical emergency!

Angina
Angina is the name given to the symptoms (usually chest pain and discomfort) produced when the heart muscle is not receiving enough oxygen (ischemia). When an individual has CAD, as described earlier, the plaque narrows the lumen of the arteries and reduces the blood flow to

your heart muscle. This plaque can make your arteries sticky and blood clots are more likely to form. Blood clots, depending on their size, can partially or completely block the flow of blood to the heart and this can cause a condition called unstable angina that can be a signal of a coming heart attack.

Prinzmetal's Angina also called variant angina, can be seen more commonly in women. This condition occurs when a spasm strikes in one of the coronary arteries and usually in the smaller arteries of the heart. This is thought to be associated with endothelial dysfunction which means the inner lining of the arteries do not work normally. I discuss ischemic heart disease and endothelial dysfunction in greater detail later in the chapter. This condition may be found in women who have migraine headaches and/or Raynaud's phenomenon. I was treated for this condition at the age of 43 and am now doing well!

Signs And Symptoms
The narrowing of the blood vessels can cause the arteries to tighten up and spasm, causing chest pain, and at times, shortness of breath with exertion.

Heart Attack (Myocardial Infarction)
Heart attacks usually occur as a result of having coronary artery disease (CAD). You may not even know that you have this disease until you have a medical emergency, such as a heart attack or stroke.

A heart attack is often caused by a blockage in a coronary artery (obstructive coronary artery disease). Fatty material called plaque containing (oxidized LDL particles) bad cholesterol within white blood cells (macrophages), builds up over many years on the inside walls of the coronary arteries and is termed atherosclerosis. An area of plaque can eventually rupture and cause a blood clot to form. If this clot becomes large enough it can partially or completely block the flow of oxygenated blood to that part of the heart muscle.

New evidence supports that "young plaque" can become unstable and rupture as well. Once it occurs, time is of the essence to re-open the artery in the hospital and minimize the severity of damage to the heart.

New evidence also supports that many individuals who have had a heart attack are found to have a low magnesium level. Magnesium supplementation may play a role in prevention!

Signs And Symptoms Of Heart Attack

Be "Heart-Wise" and on the alert for signs that could indicate possible heart disease.

• Chest pain or pressure and/or pain in the shoulders, arms, neck and jaw

• Shortness of breath

• Nausea

• Prolonged fatigue (feeling tired)

• Fainting spells (lightheadedness and sweating)

• Increased abdominal discomfort with bloating and gas (indigestion)

NOTE: Shortness of breath and heartburn are frequently seen as presenting symptoms in women.

The above signs and symptoms may develop gradually or they can be present for months or years before a heart attack actually occurs.

Some women have no signs or symptoms and this is termed "silent CAD."

The symptoms can vary and may become more severe as the plaque builds up and narrows the coronary arteries.

NOTE: If any of these symptoms appear abruptly, you could be having a heart attack. Do not hesitate to call 911 immediately! Treatment is most effective when started within one hour of the onset of the symptoms!

Both women and men often delay in seeking help for heart symptoms. Denial is so common during a heart attack that it is actually considered a symptom by doctors in the emergency room. "It's not my heart, it is just indigestion," can easily be famous last words.

Minimization of symptoms is one reason why women may delay seeking care. Studies show that women tend to wait longer than men after experiencing symptoms before calling for medical help. The mean duration of delay in women seeking help ranges from 1.8 to 7.2 hours compared to 1.4 to 3.5 hours in men.

Another reason women may delay seeking care is that many women are working full-time jobs as well as performing child-care responsibilities and therefore a case of nausea would not be a major concern for them to interrupt their schedule.

Recently we have made an impact on educating women about heart disease and more women are now seeking treatment. Remember that women often have "silent" heart attacks, which makes the diagnosis even more challenging.

Facts To Remember
Heart attack is a leading killer of both women and men in the United States.

Statistics have shown that 90-95% of individuals who experience a heart attack will survive if they get to a hospital immediately.

Experts recommend:
• Calling 911 first

• Chewing an aspirin (160 mg-325 mg) immediately if you experience heart symptoms. Aspirin decreases the formation of clots in your blood vessels and chewing the aspirin makes it work faster.

• Taking a nitroglycerin pill, if your doctor has already prescribed it for you.

Do not take aspirin if you:
• Are allergic to aspirin

• Are already taking blood thinners (anticoagulants) like Coumadin (Warfarin)

• Have bleeding problems

• Have active peptic ulcer disease

Ischemic Heart Disease (IHD)
Ischemic heart disease (IHD) in women is more commonly found to be associated with the heart's smallest coronary arteries. IHD in women typically presents differently than coronary heart disease (CHD) when found in men and the symptoms can be different. Plaque tends to build up and can scatter unevenly throughout the heart's smallest arteries which can lead to blockages that limit or prevent oxygen from reaching the heart muscle.

In just the past decade researchers have learned that many women who have ongoing chest pain along with other heart disease associated symptoms have a condition called ***coronary microvascular disease (MVD),*** which affects the heart's smallest arteries. The term CHD typically refers to obstruction within the major coronary arteries and IHD or MVD refers to reduced blood flow to the smaller arteries. About 25 to 50 percent of women with heart disease do not fit the typical male CHD pattern and have IHD instead. Recent research shows that women tend to develop micro-vascular dysfunction, whereas men are more likely to have large vessel obstruction.

Women, particularly at midlife ages 45 to 65, are more likely to have abnormalities of the function of the small arteries (endothelial dysfunction). The plaque can scatter unevenly or build up evenly within the artery walls creating blockages in these tiny arteries. The tiny arteries may tighten up, causing spasms (angina), which can prevent oxygen rich blood from reaching the heart muscle. These small artery walls can become damaged over time due to cellular changes within the artery walls and surrounding muscle tissue.

Ischemic heart disease (IHD), also referred to as coronary micro-vascular disease (MVD), is thought to affect up to three million women with heart disease in the United States. IHD can be a real challenge to diagnose because the standard tests used to diagnose heart disease look for blockages in the large coronary arteries. These tests are unable to detect plaque, spasms or damage in these small arteries. Women with symptoms of heart disease are often told they have "clear arteries" and are thought to be at low risk for heart disease and they may NOT be!

Risk Factors

The rate of ischemic heart disease (IHD) mortality (death rate) increases with the number of traditional risk factors. Clustering of risk factors is common after menopause to include: obesity, hypertension (high blood pressure) and dyslipidemia (elevated triglyceride blood levels), which can potentially correlate with the metabolic changes that occur with menopause. Women typically are a decade older than men when they present with ischemic heart disease.

Death rates from heart disease have overall dropped in the past thirty years due to improved treatments. Death rates in women have not dropped as they have in men. Women overall tend to develop further complications after having a heart attack (MI) such as: a higher rate of developing heart failure than seen in men. Increased death rates among women may be related to the critical differences in how women and men present with ischemic heart disease.

The National Heart, Lung and Blood Institute's WISE study (Women's Ischemic Syndrome Evaluation) began in 1996 and looked at how heart disease develops in women. The WISE study also looked at the role of hormones in heart disease and how to improve the diagnosis of coronary micro-vascular disease (MVD). The role of hormones in heart disease is still not well understood. Further studies are currently under way to learn more about the disease, how to treat it and its outcomes.

We do know that hormonal differences and conditions distinct to women translate into altered clinical presentation, diagnostic testing and outcomes when compared to men. An increased understanding and awareness about these important differences should help guide future diagnosis and treatment strategies to help improve the quality of care for women presenting with cardiac disease.

Signs And Symptoms
The signs and symptoms of IHD and CHD may differ. **Women** with IHD may describe having chest pressure although typically present with **shortness of breath and indigestion. They may also experience neck pain, throat pain and palpitations.**

Men with CHD typically describe having chest pain and pressure.

NOTE: Ischemic pain (angina) is often precipitated by exertion, cold weather, meals or stress. The chest discomfort usually goes away within 5 to 20 minutes, although can last longer. You should seek medical attention immediately!

Cardiomyopathy
This condition is characterized by heart disease which affects the contractility of the heart muscle and potentially causes heart failure. The major causes of cardiomyopathy are ischemia (decreased oxygen to the heart), hypertension, heart valve and congenital defects.

Cardiomyopathy is classified into three types:

• Dilated cardiomyopathy is the most common type and accounts for 25% of all cases of congestive heart failure (CHF). It can be associated with alcohol abuse, toxins and infection. This condition is more commonly found in males.

- Restrictive cardiomyopathy can be associated with connective tissue disease (auto-immune disease), nutritional deficiencies and infection.
- Hypertrophic cardiomyopathy is caused by long term hypertension typically seen in the elderly and can also be associated with a genetic disorder in young athletes which can result in sudden death.

Heart Failure

If an individual has had a previous heart attack, persistent high blood pressure, a heart valve abnormality and/or an enlarged heart muscle (cardiomyopathy), heart failure can eventually develop. This condition is associated with a decreased pumping action of the heart and is commonly called congestive heart failure (CHF).

Signs And Symptoms Of Heart Failure And/Or Cardiomyopathy

- Shortness of breath with exertion and/or wheezing
- Rapid heart rate and/or palpitations (awareness of the heartbeat)
- Dizziness or feeling faint
- Swelling of lower extremities
- Fatigue and weakness

Stroke, Cerebral Vascular Accident (CVA)

Definition

Stroke is a cardiovascular emergency that occurs in your brain. Stroke symptoms which resolve within a few minutes or hours may alert you to an impending brain attack, referred to as a *TIA (transient ischemic attack).* Suffering a stroke can be even more devastating than a heart attack because survivors are often left with a serious disability.

Each year 55,000 more women than men have a stroke and a condition called *atrial fibrillation* is responsible for about 15 to 20 percent of these strokes.

Atrial Fibrillation (also called AF or AFib)
Stroke risk increases five-fold when you have been diagnosed with an irregular heart rhythm called atrial fibrillation. Atrial fibrillation is when your heart beats irregularly, allowing blood to pool and form clots, which can travel to your brain. Most blood clots form in the heart, increasing the chances of a possible stroke.

When a stroke occurs, a blood clot blocks a vessel (artery), or a blood vessel breaks open, crowding out or interrupting the flow of blood to a specific part of the brain. When this process occurs, brain cells die in the area involved. A substance is released that sets off a chain re-action called an "ischemic cascade," which affects nearby brain cells involving a larger part of the brain. Once brain cells die, you can lose function in areas that control your speech, sensation or movement of any part of your body.

NOTE: You need to seek treatment immediately!

At the onset of a stroke, medical experts have about a three hour window in which they might be able to save your life, prevent further damage and hopefully, permanent disability.

Most Common Stroke Symptoms

- A *sudden* onset of numbness of the face, arm or leg and especially if it is only on one side of the body.

- A facial droop may be present (one side of the face does not move as well as the other side). This can also occur with non-stroke conditions like Bell's palsy, but a medical professional should examine you to rule out a dangerous stroke.

- A sudden onset of confusion or difficulty with speaking or under-standing.

- A sudden loss of vision, (experiencing difficulty seeing with one or both eyes) or double vision.

- A sudden loss of the ability to walk or maintain your balance.

- A sudden onset of dizziness or a severe headache without a known cause.

- A sudden onset of nausea, vomiting or fever which could very easily be confused with the common flu.

- A sudden onset of altered consciousness (fainting, confusion, con-vulsions or even coma).

*NOTE: If you experience or witness any or all of the above symp-toms, call 911 and get to an emergency room as soon as possible! New treatments, if administered early within three hours or less, can prevent death or serious disability. **Remember, a stroke is always a 911 emergency!***

Peripheral Vascular Disease

This condition is a disease of the intima (inner lining) of the artery wall and causes narrowing of the arteries supplying blood to the upper and lower extremities. The lower extremities are most commonly involved.

Peripheral vascular disease (PVD) is highly associated with cerebro-vascular disease (stroke) and cardiovascular disease (CAD).

Signs And Symptoms

- Pain and cramping in the legs is the most common symptom and is termed "claudication," which typically can be relieved with rest.
- Fatigue and weakness with walking
- Skin appears pale and cool to touch
- Pulses are decreased in extremities
- Ulcers or sores may form and hair loss can occur.

Screening And Diagnostic Testing

Conventional Screening For Risk

Medical History And Physical Examination

You first need to schedule a complete physical exam to include a detailed medical history which can help *identify cardiac risk factors and any family history of heart disease and/or stroke.*

Pregnancy History And CVD Risk

Pregnancy can produce cardiovascular and metabolic stress on the body.

A history of preeclampsia during pregnancy can be associated with approximately double the risk for future ischemic heart disease, stroke and venous thromboembolic events (blood clots) within 5 to 15 years after pregnancy.

It is important to inform your primary care clinician in detail about your pregnancy history to include: gestational diabetes, preeclamp-sia, preterm birth or birth of an infant small for gestational age.

Close follow up with your primary care clinician after delivery is recommended so you can be monitored if a positive history has been identified.

History Of Autoimmune Diseases And CVD Risk

Autoimmune diseases such as systemic lupus erythematosus and rheumatoid arthritis may be unrecognized risk factors in women and have been associated with a significant increased risk for developing CVD.

Women with autoimmune disease should be considered at risk and screened for CVD risk factors.

Women with a history of a previous CVD event should be screened for autoimmune diseases and appropriate secondary prevention efforts should be addressed and instituted.

History Of Migraines With Aura And CVD Risk

The Women's Health Study (WHS) results suggest that women aged 45 years or older who experience migraines accompanied by transient neurologic symptoms (known as the "migraine aura") are at increased risk of developing major cardiovascular disease events, including myocardial infarction (heart attack), ischemic stroke and death due to ischemic cardiovascular disease.

This migraine study also found that women who experience migraine without aura (the most common form of migraine) were not at significantly increased risk for any cardiovascular event.

Blood Testing

A fasting chemistry test which includes: a blood sugar and kidney test and a liver function panel.

A hemoglobin A1c test which looks at more of an average blood sugar over several months to assess for insulin resistance as discussed earlier in this chapter.

A thyroid stimulating hormone test (TSH) to assess thyroid function.

Lipid testing:

• A fasting lipid panel to identify any cholesterol and triglyceride abnormalities.

• Advanced lipoprotein particle testing to look at ApoB and Lp(a) if an increased cardiac risk is suspected. Advanced blood testing can further help identify cardiac risk factors as outlined earlier in this chapter.

- A magnesium and calcium level to determine if the calcium is elevated and the magnesium low, which may contribute to an increased cardiovascular risk.

Novel Cardiac Blood Test Screening (especially for postmenopausal women)

ALERT: This is another detailed outline of further cardiac blood testing if this topic is of interest to you. You can also skip ahead to non-invasive imaging.

Inflammatory Biomarkers

C-Reactive Protein (high sensitivity)

We have now learned that women typically have greater levels of C-reactive protein (hsCRP) as compared with men. Women also have a greater frequency of inflammatory-mediated autoimmune diseases, such as rheumatoid arthritis or systemic lupus erythematosus, suggesting a prominent role for inflammation in IHD. The risk of future ischemic heart disease events increases proportionately with increasing levels of hsCRP.

An elevated CRP is also associated with conditions such as: cardio-metabolic syndrome, type 2 diabetes and heart failure. The cardio-metabolic syndrome is a clustering of risk factors, including at least 3 of the following: insulin resistance, dyslipidemia (increased triglyceride blood levels and decreased levels of HDL cholesterol), hypertension and abdominal obesity.

These conditions when found in women can also be associated with fluctuating levels of estrogens and androgens (male hormones) as seen in perimenopause and other conditions. (Please see Chapter 3 for further detail on perimenopause and other hormone related conditions.)

Lp-PLA2 inflammatory marker is used to identify rupture prone plaque as discussed earlier in this chapter.

Myeloperoxidase (MPO) is an enzyme found in white blood cells that is linked to inflammation and cardiovascular heart disease (CVD). It seems to be a marker of vulnerable plaque which refers to areas of thickening in the walls of arteries that are most likely to rupture and cause a heart attack or stroke.

Additional Markers Of Heart Function

NT-proBNP is a blood test that can help identify individuals at risk for having a heart attack, stroke or heart failure.

An elevated **Galectin-3** blood test in a patient already diagnosed with chronic heart failure can identify those patients with the progressive form and will aide in determining their prognosis. *This test is not used to diagnose patients with chronic heart failure.*

Coagulation Markers

Platelet reactivity testing can help determine which oral anti-platelet therapy to use.

Omega-3 index testing can help predict the risk of dying from coronary heart disease (CHD).

Free fatty acid testing to help determine if your levels of essential fatty acids and other beneficial fatty acids are adequate.

Non-Invasive Cardiac Screening Tests

Ankle-Brachial Index (ABI) Test

An Ankle-Brachial index test is used to look for peripheral vascular disease (PVD) in the legs. This test measures the blood pressure in your ankles and compares it to the reading in your arms. If your blood pressure is lower in your legs than the reading in your arms, it may indicate that peripheral vascular disease is present, restricting blood flow to your legs.

This test can be done after exercising on a treadmill and is called an exercise ABI test which can detect peripheral vascular disease (PVD) in women who only experience symptoms during exercise and have a normal measurement at rest.

A low ABI score indicates that you are at risk for other forms of artery disease, including coronary artery disease.

Recent studies concluded that women with an ABI of 0.90 or less were 3.5 times as likely to die of heart disease within 10 years compared with women with a normal ABI reading.

Arterial Doppler Study Of Extremities

An arterial Doppler study of the upper and lower extremities is a painless test used to look for any blockages in the arteries (arterial insufficiency or peripheral vascular disease). Sound waves create images of the blood flow through the arteries identifying areas of disease.

Calcium Score Testing (CAC)
This test is another imaging marker that may correlate with traditional risk factors for detecting heart disease. *The Multi-Ethnic Study of Atherosclerosis* found that women with a score of >300 had an increased annual ischemic heart disease (IHD) event rate. These women with IHD, a high CAC score and multiple risk factors were found to be at *10% greater risk for having an event* than men.

NOTE: Calcium scoring is of very limited use in women < 50-60 years of age because calcium does not develop in women's arteries as early as it does in men. A zero score may have limited value in some women who develop ischemic heart disease, as coronary spasm can also play a role as discussed earlier in the chapter.

CIMT TEST (Carotid Intima-Media Thickness)
This test helps detect risk for developing heart disease and stroke. This is an ultrasound procedure which measures the first two layers of the carotid artery located in the neck. This is an important site to investigate for the development of atherosclerosis. Artery wall thickening here can be the earliest physical indicator that plaque is being deposited in the neck and probably the heart and other sites in the body as well. This test provides early detection of risk for developing heart disease.

Who Should Have a CIMT Test?
Individuals with the following risk factors for vascular disease:
• A positive family history of heart disease and/or stroke
• If you are overweight or physically inactive
• If you are age 40 and older with other risk factors
• If you are a smoker
• If you have elevated lipids and consume a high fat diet
• If you have high blood pressure
• If you have metabolic syndrome, insulin resistance and/or diabetes
• If you are postmenopausal with other risk factors

Chest X-Ray

A simple chest x-ray can determine if the heart is enlarged (cardiomegaly), which could indicate heart failure or a type of cardiomyopathy.

Echocardiogram

This test uses ultrasound (sound waves to create images of your heart) to identify any heart wall tissue damage, pumping or heart valve abnormalities. This test is usually ordered when a murmur (abnormal heart sound) or arrhythmia (abnormal heart beat) is detected during an examination using a stethoscope. If you have an arrhythmia such as atrial fibrillation, an echocardiogram can detect if a blood clot is present, which could travel to the brain resulting in a stroke.

A **Stress echocardiogram** can be done while you exercise to look for areas of the heart that are not receiving enough oxygen and can evaluate the heart valves during stress. If a woman is unable to exercise, a chemical stress echocardiogram can be performed using a medication called dobutamine which can mimic the effect of exercise. (Further discussion to follow.)

Electrocardiogram (EKG)

A baseline EKG (also referred to as an ECG) is a low cost test that can be done in the office and gives a print out of the heart's electrical activity. This is typically the first test performed to evaluate an individual's risk factors for developing CAD, or who have had a prior heart attack or have an abnormal heart rhythm. The EKG is particularly helpful if the individual is experiencing symptoms while the test is being done.

Holter Monitor/Arrythmia Event Monitor

The Holter monitor is a device that is worn typically for 24 hours and records the heart's electrical activity. The Holter monitor is not a "routine test" and is ordered when there is a concern that an arrhythmia (irregular heart beat) may be present. This test can help detect any heart arrhythmias that may be missed with the standard EKG and can identify heart ischemia (decreased oxygen to the heart muscle). This test may also be ordered if the individual has symptoms such as palpitations, syncope (passing out) or dizziness.

Stress Treadmill/Exercise Electrocardiography (EKG)

A treadmill exercise stress test is performed by walking on a motorized treadmill which places stress on the heart and can show changes not seen on a resting EKG.

An exercise EKG test measures more than the heart's electrical activity. It also measures your exercise capacity and how your blood pressure and heart rate respond to exercise. Some heart problems only show up when the heart is working hard (stressed). This test looks for any areas of the heart that are not receiving enough blood and oxygen (ischemia) when under stress.

Non-Invasive Tests Used For Diagnosing Heart Disease

As opposed to screening, it becomes necessary to run special tests to investigate reported symptoms and attempt to diagnose cardiac disease in women. As previously mentioned, women can present differently than men in regard to heart disease and for this reason can be a challenge to diagnose and should be approached a bit differently.

Blood Tests

- A fasting chemistry panel to look at glucose (blood sugar), electrolytes (sodium, potassium and chloride), kidney and liver function.
- A hemoglobin A1C can provide useful information for identifying insulin resistance and diabetes.
- Heart enzymes to look for a possible heart attack (CPK, CK-MB and Troponin T and I).
- B-type Natriuretic Peptide (BNP): This level increases with age, is greater in females than in males and is typically elevated when you have congestive heart failure (CHF).
- A low baseline magnesium level may be associated with an increased risk for heart disease.

Stress Test

Chest pain experienced during exercise testing can be a sign of heart disease, particularly in women.

A positive EKG result can be less reliable in women than in men. Women are prone to false positive results (the test detects a problem which may not be present). Traditional stress testing is considered to have a lower sensitivity and specificity for detection of heart disease in women as compared with men.

Stress testing brings out abnormalities in the heart muscle and can aide in diagnosing heart disease. This procedure is performed with an exercise stress treadmill or a stress medication if you are unable to exercise. Some individuals are unable to run or even walk on a treadmill. In these individuals, nuclear scanning can be done with a stress medication mimicking exercise, bringing out cardiac abnormalities, aiding in the diagnosis.

Nuclear Exercise Stress Test

This procedure is similar to an exercise treadmill test and is a diagnostic test used to evaluate blood flow to your heart. This test is also called a stress myocardial perfusion scan and measures the amount of blood in your heart muscle at rest and during exercise. This test may be done after having had a heart attack or to identify areas of the heart that are not receiving enough oxygenated blood. It can also tell you how much heart muscle tissue has been damaged after having had a heart attack.

During this test, two sets of pictures are taken of the heart with a special camera, called a gamma camera. One set is taken during rest and the other set is taken after the heart has been stressed by exercising on a treadmill. A small amount of radioactive tracing material (thallium or technetium) is injected into a vein in your arm. This tracer travels through the blood and into the heart muscle identifying areas that have good blood flow. The tracer is not absorbed by areas of tissue which have been damaged by a heart attack. The resting images are then compared with the stress (exercise) images to determine if there is adequate blood flow to the heart during exercise versus rest.

NOTE: There are different names for a myocardial perfusion scan. This test may also be referred to as cardiac perfusion imaging (MPI), cardiac nuclear imaging and a radionuclide stress test. Based on the specific radioactive tracer that is used for the test it may be called a Thallium, Sestamibi (Cardiolite) or Myoview (tetrofosmin) scan. Sestamibi and Myoview are both types of radioactive Technetium that can be used for this test.

Pharmacological Perfusion Nuclear Stress Test (Non-Exercise)

This type of myocardial perfusion scan is used to simulate exercise for individuals unable to exercise on a treadmill.

A pharmacological nuclear stress test is a diagnostic test used to evaluate blood flow to the heart. During this test a small amount of radioactive tracer is injected into a vein and the special gamma camera detects radiation released by the tracer to create computer images of the heart. Combined with certain medications that dilate blood vessels to your heart, this test can help determine if there is adequate blood flow to the heart during activity versus rest.

Adenosine

Adenosine, dipyridamole (Persantine) and regadenoson (Lexis-can). These are medications that can be used during a pharmacological nuclear stress test that causes the coronary arteries to dilate. Arteries that are narrowed due to atherosclerosis cannot dilate as much as healthy arteries. *Adenosine should not be used in individuals with asthma or lung disease!*

Dobutamine

Dobutamine is another medication that can be used during a pharmacological nuclear stress test for individuals with a history of asthma or chronic lung disease. This medication has a similar effect as exercise in that it makes the heart beat faster and harder. This test medication can also be used when an individual has a cardiac condition that prohibits the administration of other types of stress testing.

Cardiovascular Computed Tomography (CT) Scan

A CT scan uses an X-ray machine to take detailed pictures of the heart and creates a 3-D image of the entire heart. This test helps identify coronary artery disease and other heart problems.

Cardiovascular Computerized Tomography (CT) Angiography

This non-invasive test uses the same x-ray machine as mentioned above to take three-dimensional images of the heart. A dye is injected into a vein which creates a clearer image of the coronary arteries and flow of blood through the heart, identifying any blockages.

Cardiac Magnetic Resonance Imaging (CMR Or MRI)

This procedure uses a computer, radio waves and magnets to create pictures of your heart. This procedure is also referred to as a cardiac MRI and is a non-invasive test that can assess heart function, *detect microvascular dysfunction* and structural abnormalities.

This scan can measure the amount of blood flowing into the heart muscle before and after the heart is given a drug that dilates the micro-vessels.

This test can also be used to identify birth defects of the heart, tumors, an enlarged heart (cardiomyopathy), and blockages within the arteries. This same type of imaging can be used to assess the carotid arteries in the neck (called a MRA) to look for blockages that could potentially lead to a stroke.

Positron Emission Tomography (PET) Scan

This procedure is another myocardial perfusion imaging test that uses a small amount of radioactive material that is injected into your vein and a scanner takes pictures of the heart. This test can detect whether damage has occurred to the heart wall after a heart attack. It can also determine if a prior heart attack has occurred and if there are any blockages in the arteries of the heart. PET scans produce a better quality picture of the heart than the standard nuclear stress tests, especially in women who are obese or have large breasts.

These scans are not routinely ordered due to their high cost!

NOTE: The above described myocardial perfusion imaging tests are used by doctors to find out if an individual could benefit from an invasive cardiac procedure to help restore blood flow to the heart. One of these invasive procedures would be a percutaneous coronary intervention (PCI) such as angioplasty and stenting and another would be a coronary artery bypass surgery called a CABG. More discussion about these procedures to follow later in the chapter.

Invasive Tests Used For Diagnosing Heart Disease

Cardiac Catheterization And Cardiac Angiogram

If an individual has an abnormal myocardial perfusion imaging test and persistent chest pain, a cardiac catheterization may be the next step to consider. A cardiac angiogram is a procedure that uses x-ray imaging to examine your heart's blood vessels. This invasive test is considered to be what we call "the gold standard" for looking at the vessels of the heart. A thin flexible tube (called a catheter) is inserted into your groin and a thin wire (called a guide wire) is used to guide the catheter into the different arteries of your heart. This is the most specific and sensitive test to evaluate heart function and the coronary arteries. This is one of the tests performed in a group of procedures termed cardiac catheterization discussed later in this chapter.

This procedure:

• Looks for any blockages in the arteries of your heart.

• Carries increased risk because of placing catheters in the heart chambers and openings of the coronary arteries.

• Is reserved for those individuals at high risk due to symptoms and/ or abnormal results from previous non-invasive tests.

• Is also used with coronary angioplasty to treat coronary artery disease (CAD).

Coronary Reactivity Test

The coronary reactivity test is an invasive procedure used to examine the blood vessels in the heart and how they respond to different medications. This angiography procedure is "the gold standard" for diagnosing coronary microvascular disease and endothelial wall dysfunction in women with ischemic heart disease (IHD). This test measures coronary-artery flow reserve termed coronary reactivity. An ultra-thin wire with blood-flow sensors at the tip is threaded deep into a coronary artery. Blood flow in the artery is measured before and after injections of one or more medications that should cause the micro-vessels to dilate detecting any abnormalities.

This test should be reserved for those individuals at high risk due to persistent symptoms and/or results from previous non-invasive testing which showed evidence of myocardial ischemia and no obstructive heart disease.

In review:

Remember our earlier discussion that women often experience chest symptoms differently than men? This is because women tend to have abnormalities of the smallest vessels rather than the larger ones and often are not detected with the standard testing used. We refer to this gender difference as "obstructive coronary disease in the larger arteries" in men and "ischemic heart disease in the smaller arteries" in women. (Ischemia means lack of blood flow and oxygen to an area of the heart.) Ischemia can be caused by a blockage in the artery or spasms of the tiny vessels.

Treatment

You cannot change your body type, although you can change your lifestyle!

Diet

Consume a sensible diet rich in fresh fruits and vegetables, whole grain high fiber foods and eat oily fish at least twice a week. Limit intake of saturated fat, cholesterol, alcohol, sodium, sugar and avoid trans-fatty acids. **REDUCE ADDED SUGARS AND PROCESSED FOODS** to help protect your heart!

Specific Dietary Intake Recommendations

- Fruits and vegetables: More than or equal to 4.5 cups a day or five or more servings a day can help lower your risk of coronary heart disease, heart attack and stroke. It also helps lower your blood pressure and risk of developing type 2 diabetes.

- Dietary Fiber and Whole grains: Research has shown that consuming three servings (30 grams) of whole grains a day can lower your risk of developing coronary heart disease, type 2 diabetes and even having an ischemic stroke. Consuming whole grain foods such as: oats, bran, barley, kasha and bulgur can help lower your total and LDL (bad) cholesterol levels.

- Nuts, seeds and legumes: Eat four times a week. Studies suggest that eating beans (dried, not canned) and other legumes at least four times a week can lower risk of developing coronary heart disease compared to those consuming them just once a week.

- Soluble Fiber: 10-25 grams per day. Beans have a high soluble fiber content which lowers cholesterol and they are rich in folic acid which helps lower homocysteine levels.

- Fish: At least two times a week. Try wild or cold water fish that are high in omega-3 fatty acids. Sardines and Alaskan salmon are in this category.

- Sugar Intake: Less than or equal to 5 times a week (Less than or equal to 450 kcal per week from sugar beverages). Less is even better and I personally would recommend NOT drinking any sugar beverages! Limit your sugar intake to 6 teaspoons a day for women and 9 teaspoons a day for men. One teaspoon of sugar equals 5 grams of sugar. Women should limit their total daily intake of sugar to 30 grams per day and men 45 grams a day. This limit should include all added sugars found in desserts and beverages. If you substitute artificial sweeteners for sugar, discuss the type and amount you consume with your clinician. Artificial sweeteners may not contain sugar but may contain other chemicals which can be harmful.

- Eat small servings of food every three hours throughout the day and have fresh fruit as a snack.

- Food Pairing: Combine food groups that help lower the insulin response and promote weight loss. An example would be: eat a serving of lean protein with vegetables along with a small portion of a good fat such as an avocado, olives, olive oil or almonds. This food combination lowers the amount of insulin produced; decreasing fat storage and risk for heart disease and diabetes. (See

Chapters 3 and 10 for further information on diet, food pairing, insulin resistance and diabetes.)

- Salt Intake: Try to consume 1,500 mg to 2,000 mg or less a day. High salt intake has been linked to high blood pressure and heart disease. Avoid processed meats and canned foods which have a high sodium content. Read the labels and substitute herbs and spices to flavor your foods. Garlic and chili peppers have been shown to help lower blood pressure and cholesterol levels.
- Cholesterol intake: Less than 150 mg a day
- Saturated Fat: Less than 7 % total calorie intake
- Alcohol: Less than or equal to one a day (5 ounces of wine, 12 ounces beer or 1.5 ounces of spirits)
- Trans-Fatty acids equals Trans Fat: 0

Do not eat Trans Fats because they raise low-density lipoprotein (LDL or "bad") cholesterol and reduce levels of (HDL or "good") cholesterol. If the label reads "partially hydrogenated oil," you should avoid consuming that product.

Trans Fat can be found in many margarines, processed and fast (junk) foods listed as saturated fat. These include:
- Crackers, cookies, cakes, frozen pies and other baked goods
- Snack foods (microwave popcorn)
- Frozen pizza
- Fast food
- Vegetable shortenings and stick margarines
- Coffee creamer
- Refrigerated dough products (biscuits and cinnamon rolls)
- Ready to use frostings, etc…

Weight Maintenance
Women should maintain and lose weight through an appropriate balance of physical activity, caloric intake, and formal behavioral programs when indicated, to maintain and achieve the following recommendations:
- BMI less than 25 in US women (Please read Chapter 3 for more information on body mass index, BMI)
- Waist size less than 35 inches. (Your waist measurement should equal half your height in inches.)

Exercise

Regular exercise can help lower your cholesterol, triglycerides, and blood pressure, which can help decrease your heart disease risk. *It also can help decrease inflammation and your risk of insulin resistance!*

Try to exercise for at least 30 minutes a day on most days to maintain weight and 60-90 minutes a day to lose weight. Remember, the American Heart Association recommends 150 minutes of moderate aerobic exercise and 75 minutes of vigorous activity per week to keep a healthy heart.

Studies have shown that regular exercise can lower your risk of developing cardiovascular disease by 40 percent or greater as compared to a sedentary lifestyle.

Stop Smoking

Remember, smoking is the number one preventable cause of heart disease!

Blood Pressure Control With Lifestyle Changes

An optimal blood pressure of 120/80 should be obtained and encouraged through weight control, increased physical activity, alcohol moderation, sodium restriction and consuming fruits, vegetables and low fat dairy products.

Lipid Control Through Lifestyle Approaches

Recommended optimal lipid levels:

• LDL-C less than 100 mg/dL

• HDL-C greater than 50 mg/dL

• Triglycerides less than 150 mg/dL(<100 mg/dL is even better!)

• Non-HDL-C less than 130 mg/dL

Stress

Reduce Stress: Uncontrolled stress can raise your blood pressure, cholesterol and homocysteine levels. Practice Yoga and meditation in your weekly exercise.

NOTE: You do not have to develop heart disease, although if you do not take action to control your risk factors, chances are you will.

Supplements

B-complex should be taken once daily to help the body eliminate homocysteine. Take vitamins B12 and B6 in B-complex formulation along with folic acid (B9) 400 mcg a day. Folic acid is the synthetic form of this B9 vitamin found in supplements and fortified foods. Folate is the natural occurring water soluble form found in foods like liver, spinach, lentils and garbanzo beans.

Coenzyme Q10 is an antioxidant which helps prevent the oxidation of LDL (bad) cholesterol and maintains healthy blood vessels. Normal aging along with statin therapy may potentially lower your blood level of coenzyme Q10. It is especially important to take a supplement if you are on a prescription statin drug, to promote the body's natural production of coenzyme Q10 and prevent muscle atrophy.

Fish Oil contains the omega-3 fatty acids found in fish. Fish oil supplements help lower triglyceride levels, increase HDL cholesterol levels, decrease inflammation and promote healthy blood vessels.

Magnesium Supplementation May Be Needed
Have your magnesium and calcium levels tested along with your kidney function to determine if you could benefit from taking a supplement. Be careful because magnesium supplements can worsen kidney function!

Medication Therapy
An important factor contributing to the relatively greater heart disease risk in women is less intensive use of available medical therapy.

Aspirin should be used daily for women only in the high risk category (secondary prevention for those already diagnosed with heart disease and diabetes mellitus). In primary prevention it depends on the risk for stroke, level of blood pressure control and/or the overall risk of the woman. (Some research supports that this therapy is more effective when used in men than women.)

Beta-blockers should be used for up to 12 months in women following a heart attack to reduce blood pressure and slow the heart rate, decreasing the heart's demand for oxygen. Long term therapy (greater than 12 months) may be considered for women with diagnosed cardiovascular disease. Beta blockers should not be used if you have been diagnosed with heart failure and/or a cocaine-induced heart attack.

Statin drugs should be used first and then ezetimibe, niacin and bile acid sequestrants to reduce atherogenic lipoproteins as measured by ApoB or surrogates of ApoB, (like LDL-C and non-HDL-C). All approved lipid medications aide in reducing inflammation.

Two new prescription injectable medications have been approved, Repatha (evolocumba) and Praluent (alirocumab) to be used along with diet and maximally tolerated statin therapy to help further lower high levels of LDL-C cholesterol. These injections are to be administered twice monthly for those individuals whose LDL-C levels remain high despite receiving treatment with statin drugs and in individuals with an inherited condition called heterozygous familial hypercholesterolemia. Repatha (evolocumba) released a once a month injection that is now also available by prescription. These individuals are typically already on the highest dose of a statin medication and their LDL-C cholesterol level still remains elevated, increasing their risk of heart disease.

Discuss the side effects of each medication with your clinician to assess the risk to benefit ratio. We tend to select medications with a higher benefit than side effect risk.

Fibrates and niacin are the preferred medications for lowering very high triglycerides (TG greater than 500 mg/dl), just published by the Endocrine guidelines. Niacin and fibrate therapy can be useful when the HDL-C is low (less than 50 mg/dL) or non-HDL-C is elevated (greater than 130 mg/dL) in high risk women after the LDL-C level is treated to goal.

High dose prescription Omega-3 or N-3 fatty acids (fish oil) and high dose niacin can be used to treat very high or extremely high TG levels, (TG greater than 500).

Angiotensin-converting enzymes (ACE-inhibitor or ACEi) should be used in women after having had a heart attack and those diagnosed with heart failure and/or diabetes mellitus.

Angiotensin receptor blockers (ARBs) can also be used as an alternative treatment to reduce blood pressure and help preserve kidney function.

NOTE: It is also very important to keep blood sugar levels under control with appropriate medications to reduce your risk!

Invasive Cardiac Procedures And Surgery

Coronary Angioplasty

A coronary angioplasty is performed during a cardiac catheterization. This non-surgical procedure is typically performed if you have been diagnosed with coronary artery disease and/or have had a heart attack. This procedure is commonly know as percutaneous coronary interventions (PCI) which includes percutaneous transluminal coronary angioplasty (PTCA) with or without stent placement. This procedure places special tubing with an attached deflated balloon up into the stenotic (narrowed) coronary arteries of the heart found in coronary artery disease. These stenotic segments are due to the build-up of the cholesterol-laden plaques that form due to atherosclerosis, as discussed earlier in the chapter.

An interventional cardiologist feeds the deflated balloon or another device on a catheter from the inguinal femoral artery or radial artery up through the blood vessels until they reach the site of blockage. X-ray imaging is used to guide the catheter threading and the balloon is inflated to widen blocked areas of an artery, increasing blood flow to the heart.

Cardiac Stent Placement
Bare-metal stents, BMS or drug-eluding stents DES (stents with medications) can also be used at the site of the blockage to permanently open the artery.

Peripheral Angioplasty
Peripheral Angioplasty (PA) refers to the use of a balloon to open blocked arteries outside of the heart (coronary arteries). This procedure is commonly used to open narrowed arteries in the abdomen, legs and those leading to the kidneys.

Bypass Surgery
This surgical procedure is also referred to as a CABG, pronounced "cabbage," coronary artery bypass graft and is open heart surgery.

This procedure treats blocked arteries by creating new passages for blood flow to your heart muscle. Arteries and veins are taken from other parts of your body, called grafts, which can reroute the blood supply around the heart. Think of it as a detour on the road to get to the same destination. The internal mammary artery, saphenous vein or radial artery, are graft vessels used today.

You may need more than one graft depending on how many arteries are blocked.

This procedure can help relieve chest pain by improving blood flow to the heart and reduce the risk of having a heart attack.

Prevention Recommendations

Eight Steps To Lower The Risks For Developing CVD
Eight steps recommended by the American Heart Association to help lower your risk of developing cardiovascular disease:

- Never smoke and quit if you do! (Even quitting for one year or more lowers your risk.)
- Maintain a blood pressure of 130/80 or below in men and 120/80 in women.
- Maintain a total cholesterol of 199 mg/dl or lower, HDL of 60 or higher and LDL of 100 mg/dl or lower.
- Maintain a body mass of less than 25, (see body mass index in Chapter 3) and a waist measurement less than 35 inches for women and 40 inches for men.
- Maintain a healthy diet by eating:
  - Fewer daily calories
  - More fruits and vegetables (half your plate)
  - Oily fish like salmon at least two times a week.
- Make sure you fit in 150 minutes of moderate intensity and 75 minutes of vigorous intensity exercise or a combination of both moderate and vigorous intensity aerobic physical activity per week.
- Maintain a normal blood sugar (fasting < 100 mg/dl) and prevent diabetes and insulin resistance from even developing. Limit daily sugar intake to 6 teaspoons or 30 grams a day for women and 9 teaspoons or 45 grams a day for men.
- A recent recommendation from the AHA is to reduce the intake of added sugars, which for most American women is no more than 100 calories per day and 150 calories a day for men.

Recent Prevention Study Updates

A study headed by Dr. Michelle A. Albert at Brigham and Women's hospital in Boston was presented at the American Heart Association meeting in Chicago and outlined in an article entitled, "Stressful Jobs May Raise Women's Heart Attack Risk." The study was conducted over a ten year period with more than 17,000 female health professionals with an average age of 57, looking at the effect of work-related stress on women's health. The results revealed that women with high job strain were at twice the risk for having a heart attack and 43% more likely to have to undergo a bypass procedure.

The New England Journal of Medicine, June 2010 edition, reported that Kaiser Permanente's Heart Disease prevention programs are working, resulting in a 24% decrease in heart attacks in members from 1999 to 2008.

Programs such as PHASE (Prevent Heart Attacks and Strokes Everyday) helped members reduce their risk by:

• Encouraging healthy eating and exercising

• Promoting the benefits of quitting smoking

• Evaluating the benefits of taking prescription medications such as statins, beta blockers, ACE inhibitors and aspirin when indicated

NOTE: Remember, women do not gain the same protective benefit from aspirin as men!

Researchers from Japan published the results of a recent study in the journal, *Atherosclerosis,* found that an increased intake of magnesium in the diet may reduce the risk of cardiovascular mortality by 50 percent! Scientists have found that low magnesium levels are linked with all known cardiovascular risk factors including high blood pressure, arterial plaque build-up, and calcification of soft tissues, as well as excess cholesterol levels and hardening of the arteries.

Researchers determined that decades of elevated calcium intake for bone health have not been balanced with increased magnesium intake, resulting in an imbalance of the two minerals.

Dr. Carolyn Dean, Medical Advisor of the Nutritional Magnesium Association concluded: "Heart disease is still the number one killer in America in spite of over two decades of statin use. The fact that low levels of magnesium are associated with all the risk factors and symptoms of heart disease, hypertension, diabetes, high cholesterol, heart arrhythmia, angina and heart attack can no longer be ignored: the evidence is too compelling." The authors note that nuts and legumes are an excellent, natural source of magnesium, yet many individuals avoid them due to the misconception that they are unhealthy due to the high fat content. Daily minimum requirements for magnesium are 320 mg for women and 420 mg for men.

Women are less likely to be properly treated, even when they have similar symptoms to men, according to an analysis in the Journal of American Medical Association. An article in USA Today (February 22, 2012) by Liz Szabo reports: "Women Less Likely to Get Immediate Heart Attack Treatment."

"Women having heart attacks are less likely than men to get immediate treatment and more likely to die in the hospital," says a ground breaking study that tracked more than 1.1 million patients.

Women are less likely to get immediate treatment to stop the heart attack in its tracks; clot busting drugs, balloon procedures to open arteries or bypass surgery, the study says. Partly because of such delays, 15% of female heart attack patients die in the hospital, compared with 10% of men." Delaying can be fatal. "Time is muscle," says author John Canto of the Watson Clinic and Lakeland Regional Medical Center in Florida. "And muscle is life."

A recent British study showed that adhering to a long-term treatment plan (greater than 10 years) with statin medications could prevent twice as many deaths from heart attack and stroke!

A recent study presented at the American Heart Association's annual meeting reported that blood pressure and blood sugar levels continue to rise in U.S. adults, mainly fueled by obesity.

• As weight goes up, so does the risk for heart disease.

• Obesity continues to be a major risk factor for heart disease and degenerative diseases.

• One out of three children and teens in the U.S. is now obese, according to the U.S. Centers for Disease Control and Prevention. These children are more likely to develop heart disease later in life.

A new study at the University of San Francisco showed that young adults whose cholesterol levels are even slightly higher than normal are at greater risk for developing artery-clogging calcium deposits later in life.

Chapter Conclusion

We have read how women can differ from men in the development, presentation, diagnosis and treatment of heart disease. We've also seen that the risk of heart disease increases after menopause. For this reason, new approaches to identifying risk, diagnosing and treating women are becoming more important. I realize some of the information presented in this chapter is quite technical, although it can become a valuable reference for future testing, if needed. Heart disease can interfere with your daily living, cause financial hardship and prevent you from enjoying life to its fullest.

Developing heart disease may be avoided if action is taken to control risk factors.

Moderation is the key to success for achieving a heart healthy diet. It is best to begin eating a healthy diet and exercise early in life to prevent heart disease. (I do screen all of my adolescent patients as part of their prevention physical exam.)

If you are unable to lower your cholesterol and triglyceride levels with diet and exercise, you do have many options for treatment.

Do not delay, and schedule your appointment today with your clinician.

I will pass along the advice our daughter gave her daddy when she was four years old, *"Daddy, be sure to watch your diet and don't eat salt or fat because I don't want you to have a "heart-a-choke!"*

Please read Chapter 3 for further information on nutrition and exercise.

I hope this chapter provides information you can take to "heart" to help make the changes you need to keep your heart healthy.

You will find personal written testimonies at the end of this book in Chapter 21.

Websites for further information on:

Heart Disease in Women

Centers for Disease Control and Prevention:
https://www.cdc.gov/heartdisease/facts.htm

Women & Cardiovascular Diseases-American Heart Association:
http://www.heart.org/idc/groups/heart-public/@wcm/@sop/@smd/documents/downloadable/ucm_319576.pdf

Heart disease-Mayo Clinic:
http://www.mayoclinic.org/diseases-conditions/heart-disease/basics/definition/con-20034056

How Does Heart Disease Affect Women?-National Heart, Lung, and Blood Institute. U.S. Department of Health & Human Services:
https://www.nhlbi.nih.gov/health/health-topics/topics/hdw

Recipes from American Heart Association:
https://recipes.heart.org/categories/31/delicious-decisions

Hypertension (High Blood Pressure)

American Heart Association-Hypertension: **http://www.heart. org/HEARTORG/Conditions/HighBloodPressure/High-Blood-Pressure_UCM_002020_SubHomePage.jsp**

Stroke Symptoms

Menopause and Heart Disease-American Heart Association-Stroke: **http://www.heart.org/HEARTORG/Conditions/The-Heart-and-Stroke-Encyclopedia_UCM_445688_SubHomePage.jsp#. WRtKGMm1uV4**

Heart Condition Centers-SCAI (Society for Cardiovascular Angiography and Interventions)-Seconds Count: **http://www.secondscount.org/heart-condition-centers/info-detail-2/women-stroke#.WRtKMsm1uV5**

National Stroke Association-Women and Stroke: **http://www.stroke.org/understand-stroke/impact-stroke/women-and-stroke**

Chapter 6

BONE HEALTH

Keeping Your Bones Healthy

During your teen and younger adult years, your bones are as dense as they ever will be and this is referred to as your "peak bone mass". Bone density is defined as the degree of mineralization of the bone matrix which continues to increase until you reach your third decade of life and then declines thereafter. Your body stores excess calcium until you reach your peak bone mass in your early to mid-thirties. After you reach your peak bone mass, your body is no longer able to store calcium and you may need to take calcium supplements. When your calcium stores become depleted, your bones become weak and can eventually become hollow, which leaves you vulnerable to break a bone. Think of how a woodpecker hollows out a tree trunk and it looks like a bee honey comb. This can happen to your bones.

Some facts about bone health:

• The risk of developing a bone fracture does increase with age.

• Approximately 55% of postmenopausal women have a low bone mass, (thinning of the bones) and they don't even know it. One out of every two women and one out of every four men over age 50 will have an osteoporosis-related fracture in their lifetime.

• Estrogen plays an important role in maintaining bone mass. Women may experience rapid bone loss (up to 20%) in the years immediately following menopause due to the lack of estrogen.

• A condition called osteoporosis is most common in women after menopause. This disease can lead to low bone mass, increased bone fragility and broken bones (fractures). This is because bones break down without estrogen and new bone does not build up as quickly.

• According to the National Osteoporosis Foundation (NOF), 10 million Americans are estimated to have osteoporosis, and 34 million have low bone mass. Approximately 30 million women age 50 and older have osteoporosis or low bone density which can lead to fractures. (Osteoporosis and low bone mass both refer to changes in the bones that have occurred over time.)

• Your bones are living tissue just like your liver or kidneys and are constantly making new bone and replacing old bone. As we age, our bones wear down faster than vitamin D and calcium can replace them and this can lead to osteoporosis.

• It's important to eat a healthy diet rich in vitamin D and calcium, while also exercising throughout your life, to prevent bone loss! The goal is to have plenty of bone calcium saved up for menopause, when your bones naturally start to lose some of their density.

• Remember, half of all women over age 50 will break a bone due to osteoporosis.

How Estrogen Affects Our Bones

Estrogen is the hormone that helps keep calcium in your bones by absorbing the calcium and magnesium you eat, which keeps bones strong. I use the train analogy, "Estrogen is like the engine and calcium is like the cargo."

Estrogen has a calming effect on bone destruction. After menopause the bone destroyer cells, which are called osteoclasts, become more active and the new bone being made cannot keep up.

Calcium

Calcium is responsible for many functions in your body. Some of the functions calcium performs are to:

• Keep your joints free of inflammation, which can lead to arthritis.

• Facilitate muscle contraction.

• Assist with brain communication by maintaining nervous system health.

• Help maintain a normal blood pressure.

• Decrease the risk of developing colon cancer.

• Solidify and strengthen your bones.

Osteoporosis

Osteoporosis is a disease that results in:

• The loss of bone because the cells that break down bone are working faster than the cells that make bone.

• A deterioration of bone strength, bone density and bone quality.

• A tendency for bone to fracture (break) from little or no trauma.

• Spinal or vertebral fractures can also be very serious, causing loss of height, severe back pain and deformity of the spine.

NOTE: Nearly three times as many women have osteoporosis than those that report having the disease! The most concerning fractures are those of the hip and spine. Women with a broken hip almost always need to go to the hospital and have major surgery. More than half of the women who have had a hip fracture are never able to walk again without help and one quarter of them will need long term care.

Osteoporosis

Why Osteoporosis Occurs

Normal bone is continually rebuilding new bone. The bone is absorbed or broken down by cells called osteoclasts.

Changes that occur with normal aging:

• Decreased vitamin D activity

• Decreased intestinal calcium absorption

• Decreased weight bearing exercise

• Decreased muscle mass

• Decreased estrogen

During perimenopause your bone loss rate is at about 1%.

During menopause, your bone loss rate is at about 3%. Women can gradually lose up to 20% of their bone mass in the first five to seven years following the onset of menopause.

During postmenopause, your bone loss rate usually slows back down to about 1% within seven to ten years.

The loss of bone minerals will continue for the rest of your life!

Bone Robbers
• Salt (high sodium diet) increases elimination of calcium.
• Acid, caffeine, and protein increase elimination of calcium.
• Fiber and aluminum bind with calcium in the stomach and this decreases the absorption of calcium. Many over the counter antacids contain aluminum and decrease the absorption of calcium.
• Tobacco decreases estrogen levels, which decreases the calcium level.
• Excess consumption of alcohol (more than two servings a day) decreases calcium absorption. It also increases elimination of calcium and can lead to poor dietary intake of calcium & vitamin D (one serving size equals 5 ounces of wine, 1-1/2 ounces of hard liquor or 12 ounces of beer).

Risks For Developing Osteoporosis
If you fit into any of the following categories, the risk of developing osteoporosis is higher if you:
• Have a relative with osteoporosis. If your mother was diagnosed with osteoporosis, you have an eighty percent chance of developing the disease.
• Smoke or drink in excess (more than two beverages a day). Smoking doubles your risk of having a fracture related to osteoporosis.
• Have other health problems, such as diabetes or a thyroid condition.
• A low body weight, small frame (thin).
• Sustain a broken bone after menopause.
• Are sedentary, with an inadequate calcium intake.
• Are a female.
• Take certain prescription medications such as steroids (prednisone) or have been taking thyroid replacement for more than three months.
• Have a decreased exposure to estrogen (low blood levels of estrogen).

Fracture Risk Assessment Tool (FRAX)

The FRAX tool was developed by the World Health Organization (WHO) task force in 2008 to assess an individual's risk of fracture to help guide treatment decisions. This tool can be found online and uses the bone density from the hip along with clinical risk factors listed below to calculate postmenopausal women's 10 year fracture risk, ages 40 to 90 years of age.

1. Femoral Neck Hip bone density (BMD), not in the spine.

2. Age, weight in kilograms and height in centimeters.

3. A previous fracture in adult life occurring spontaneously

4. Alcohol use (greater than 2 units a day)

5. Current Smoker

6. Use of systemic steroids

7. History of hip fracture in individual's mother or father.

8. A confirmed diagnosis of rheumatoid arthritis.

Calculate Your Fracture Risk

What is your current age?

<65	65-69	70-74	75-79	80-84	85+
0 pts	1 pt	2 pts	3 pts	4 pts	5 pts

Have you broken any bones after age 50?
Yes – 1 pt.   No / Not sure – 0 pts.

Has your mother had a hip fracture after age 50?
Yes – 1 pt.   No / Not sure – 0 pts.

Do you weigh 125 pounds or less?
Yes – 1 pt.   No – 0 pts.

Are you currently a smoker?
Yes – 1 pt.   No – 0 pts.

Do you usually need your arms to assist yourself in standing up from a chair?
Yes – 2 pts.   No–0 pts.

NOTE: If your total score is 4 or greater, you may be at high risk for developing a fracture due to osteoporosis. Early diagnosis and prevention are essential! Talk to your clinician about minimizing your risks. The earlier osteoporosis is diagnosed, the more effective the treatment can be.

Osteoporosis is often referred to as a silent disease, because many times you don't even know you have it until you break a bone or start losing height. Your bones may become so fragile they can break easily from such daily activities as bending over to pick up a bag of groceries! Once this disease progresses it can cause:

• Hip and back pain due to bone fractures
• Spine curvature which is called kyphosis
• Stooped posture
• Height loss (Keep track of your height)

NOTE: Remember, osteoporosis can also be caused by having a chronic disease and taking certain prescribed medications such as prednisone on a long term basis. Talk to your clinician about your individual risk.

Preventing Osteoporosis

Diet And Supplements
Eat a diet rich in calcium. Try to get at least 250mg of calcium from non-dairy sources and choose low fat dairy products. Please read labels for the calcium content of individual foods.

Foods that are rich in vitamin D:
• Fish and especially shell fish naturally have vitamin D.
• Milk, orange juice and many cereals are fortified with vitamin D.

Take a daily calcium supplement: calcium is the major mineral component of bone tissue and your body is unable to build new bone without it. Even if you are taking medication for osteoporosis, you still need adequate calcium intake through your diet and supplements. The elemental calcium content of any supplement is what matters most. Be sure to check the label. Try to take a total of 1,000 to 1,200 mg daily derived from your diet and supplements combined.

Dietary sources include: yogurt and skim milk, sardines and canned salmon with bones, dark green leafy vegetables and calcium fortified foods like soy milk and orange juice.

Take adequate vitamin D to absorb the calcium: Have your vitamin D blood level checked. New studies revealed that calcium given along with vitamin D can help reduce the risk of hip fractures, total overall fractures and possibly vertebral fractures.

Take a magnesium supplement: You should consider taking 500 mg of magnesium daily, in divided doses to help balance the effects of calcium on nerve and heart function. An example would be a supplement which contains calcium 500 mg, vitamin D 500 IU and magnesium 250 mg to be taken twice daily. Check with your clinician to determine the correct dosage for you.

New research has shown that many individuals who have had a heart attack were found to have had a low magnesium level.

Magnesium may help improve your sleep too.

Almonds are a rich source of magnesium.

NOTE: Consult with your clinician and/or herbalist to determine what supplement dosage would be best for you to take.

Some Advice When Taking Supplements
Take your supplements in divided dosages for better absorption.

If you take iron supplements for anemia, take your calcium two hours later.

Do not take antacids such as Maalox or Mylanta with your calcium. Calcium needs an acid environment to be absorbed.

Add another 20 mg of calcium for every 12 ounce caffeinated drink or 4 ounce cup of coffee consumed.

Calcium citrate is easily absorbed without food and is usually more expensive.

Calcium carbonate is inexpensive and comes in chewable tablets. It must be taken with food and in divided doses to be absorbed.

Take your calcium supplement close to the time of exercise. Exercise causes a negative charge on the bones which attracts the positive charge of calcium, thus better absorption in to the bones.

Vitamin K is also important for bone health and 90ug per day is the recommended dosage for women. Dietary sources include green leafy vegetables, cabbage, broccoli, Brussels sprouts and plant oils.

Be careful if you:

- Are taking blood thinners, such as Coumadin. Discuss all your medications and supplements with your clinician.
- Have had kidney stones. Ask your clinician what amount of calcium is right for you.
- Are at risk for heart disease, to determine which dose of calcium is appropriate for you.

Exercise Regularly

Weight bearing: walking, hiking, stair climbing, dancing, or tennis. This type of exercise can help build bone density.

Yoga, Pilates and Tai chi for stretching and core body strengthening. These types of exercise can also help your posture. To check your posture, stand up straight against a wall with your buttocks and heels touching the wall and then rotate your shoulders and upper back against the wall and walk away maintaining that position. It is amazing how much we tend to stoop forward throughout the day.

Weight lifting and strength training: This type of exercise can also help build bone density.

Preventing Bone Fractures

Remove environmental hazards like throw rugs and wear non-slip shoes.

Store items where you can reach them, so you don't need to use a stool or ladder.

Keep walkways well lit and free of clutter and install hand-rails when needed.

If you smoke-STOP!

Avoid excessive use of alcohol (remember, no more than one beverage daily).

Diagnosing Osteoporosis

The DEXA scan (dual energy x-ray absorptiometry) is the most accurate and a commonly used test for diagnosing osteoporosis. It is used for initial testing to establish a baseline and also useful for monitoring your bone density over time. This procedure is painless, quick and safe, because it delivers only a small amount of radiation - less than what you would receive from a chest x-ray.

A DEXA scan can measure bone density in the spine (back), hips, forearm and/or total body.

A recently developed test that measures bone quality is called a Trabecular Bone Score (TBS) and will soon be reported along with the Dexascan results. This test measures the architecture of trabecular bone in the lumbar spine, predicting further fracture risk.

You should consult with your clinician to evaluate the density of your bones if:

• You are of menopausal age or older.
• You have a family history of osteoporosis (your mother).
• You break a bone (this could mean that your bones are weakening).

Understanding Your Results

The bone density test reports your results as a "T"-score. If your result is:

• -2.5 or lower, you have osteoporosis! This is high risk for a fracture.
• -1.0 to -2.5, you have osteopenia (bone thinning). A low bone mass presents a medium risk for a fracture.
• -1.0 or higher, you have a normal bone mass. This is low risk for a fracture.

Medications Used To Treat Osteoporosis

Bisphosphonates

Bisphosphonates have been the main treatment for osteoporosis since 1996, when alendronate (Fosamax) was first introduced to the US. These medications work by decreasing the amount of bone that is being destroyed (reabsorbed) and are used for prevention and treatment, reducing spinal and hip fractures.

Today we have other bisphosphonates to choose from that can be taken in pill or liquid form daily, weekly or monthly. Common names you may recognize are: Actonel (risedronate), alendronate (Fosamax), Atelvia, a delayed-release form of risedronate and Boniva (ibandronate). A new formulation of alendronate sodium called Binosto is now available in an effervescent tablet that dissolves in water so you can drink it. Reclast (zoledronic Acid) is another treatment which is given by inserting a small needle into a vein once a year.

A relatively new type of medication called Prolia (denosumab) works by a different mechanism of action and may be considered if other treatments have been ineffective. Denosumab is a human antibody made by one type of immune cell and stops the growth of the osteo-clasts, preventing bone loss. Denosumab is given every six months and injected under the skin in the upper arm, thigh or abdomen. Prolia is used to treat postmenopausal osteoporosis in women who:

• Have an increased risk for fractures.

• Cannot use other osteoporosis medications, or other osteoporosis medications did not work for them.

NOTE: These medications can potentially cause serious side effects. Your clinician will determine which medication is right for you.

Hormone Replacement Therapy
Hormone replacement therapy works well for preventing bone loss, maintaining bone density and helps prevent fractures in the spine and hip.

Selective Estrogen Receptor Modulators
Selective estrogen receptor modulators, (SERMs) are artificial hor-mones which act like estrogen to help maintain bone density. SERMs may prevent fractures of the spine, but not the hip. Evista (Raloxi-fene) is a name you may recognize.

A new combination medication called Duavee is a pill that combines conjugated estrogens along with the SERM bazedoxifene. It is used by women with a uterus to help reduce symptoms of menopause, (hot flashes and vaginal dryness.) This medication helps preserve bone mass and reduces the risk of cancer of the uterus.

Calcitonin Hormone
Calcitonin hormone is produced in the parathyroid gland and regu-lates the amount of bone being destroyed. It is used to treat and pre-vent fractures of the spine, especially in elderly women. Miacalcin is the brand name of a medication used to prevent fractures.

Parathyroid Hormone
Forteo (teriparatide) and Tymlos (abaloparatide) are the two injec-tion medications available to treat very severe osteoporosis and work by rebuilding new bone.

NOTE: *Osteoporosis does not have to be a normal part of aging. Start treatment early and you can improve your bone health. Your clinician will discuss all the potential risks and benefits of these individual therapies. Together you can discuss which treatment will be appropriate for you and determine the length of therapy needed.*

Vitamin D Deficiency

We have known for years that taking vitamin D supplements can help prevent childhood rickets and absorb dietary calcium. Recently we have learned that vitamin D plays a role in protecting our body from different diseases such as:

- Heart disease
- Stroke
- Osteoporosis (thinning of the bones)
- Osteomalacia (softening of the bones)
- Many forms of cancer
- Depression
- Autoimmune diseases such as rheumatoid arthritis and diabetes (types 1 and 2)

Where Does Vitamin D Come From?

Vitamin D has two forms, Vitamin D2 and Vitamin D3.

Vitamin D2 is found in vegetables and supplements. It is made by exposing fungal cell membranes to ultraviolet light.

Vitamin D3 is mainly formed from your skin being exposed to ultraviolet B radiation with sunlight and tanning beds. It also comes from foods such as fatty fish and dairy foods with added vitamin D. Cod liver oil and many vitamin supplements also contain D3.

Both vitamin D2 and D3 do not become active until they pass through the liver. Calcitriol, the most active form of vitamin D, is produced in the kidney.

Why Vitamin D Is Important

Are minerals needed to stimulate new bone growth or replace aging bones? Yes, if you do not consume enough calcium, over time loss of bone density can occur. Mild bone loss is called osteopenia. Greater bone loss is called osteoporosis.

Vitamin D:

- Is needed to build healthy bones and to help prevent bone loss.
- Helps calcium travel from the intestine to the bone.
- Helps harden new bone and keeps bone from becoming soft and thin by providing the bone with adequate calcium.
- Can help muscles become stronger in those individuals with a vitamin D deficiency.

Is It Common To Have A Low Vitamin D Level?
Yes, vitamin D deficiency is becoming more common. More than half of the patients that go to see their clinician have it.

Many individuals do not have optimum vitamin D levels, which should be around 30ng /ml (nanograms per milliliter) or higher. Normal range should be between 30 ng/ml and 100 ng/ml.

About 70% of Caucasian and 95% of African American adults in the US have a vitamin D level under 30 ng/ml.

A level of 20 ng/ml to 30 ng/ml is considered to be *vitamin D insufficiency.*

A level of 10ng/ml or lower is very low and considered to be *vitamin D deficiency.*

Who Is At Risk For Vitamin D Deficiency?
It is now known that many individuals have vitamin D levels that are too low to support good health. We know that vitamin D is made when our skin is exposed to ultraviolet light from the sun. Many factors can limit sun exposure to our skin. Here are a few:

- Clothing and sunscreen
- Time of day and season
- Skin pigment. Dark-skinned individuals require much longer exposure to sunlight in order to make adequate vitamin D.
- Areas with less sun. Individuals with limited sunlight exposure have decreased vitamin D levels, especially those living at northern latitudes.
- Age. The elderly have a decreased ability to make vitamin D from ultraviolet light.

The two most common causes of low vitamin D levels are lack of sun and not enough intake of vitamin D by mouth.

Other causes of low vitamin D levels are:

• The body's inability to absorb enough Vitamin D due to intestinal disease or previous gastric surgery, which includes a gastric by-pass procedure.

• Chronic kidney disease.

• Liver failure.

• Anti-seizure medications.

• Having chronic musculoskeletal pain and/or Fibromyalgia. *(Not enough vitamin D in your system may be linked to chronic pain.)*

• Obesity. Overweight individuals store vitamin D in their fat cells, making it less available in the blood stream.

Testing For Vitamin D

Checking vitamin D blood levels is very expensive and not everyone needs to be tested.

Vitamin D screening should be a part of your annual physical examination if you are at risk. You may have a deficiency without any symptoms. The good news is, if you have a deficiency it can easily be corrected with vitamin D supplementation. Your clinician can determine which dosage is appropriate for you.

A Technical Word About Vitamin D Testing

When we check your vitamin D level, we will order a 25-hydroxy vitamin D blood test. Vitamin D production is regulated by our parathyroid gland. If you have a vitamin D deficiency, your parathyroid gland makes more parathyroid hormone which stimulates your kidneys to make more 25-dihydroxyvitamin D in attempt to correct the deficiency.

How To Prevent And Treat A Low Vitamin D Level

You can obtain vitamin D from foods you eat, such as fatty fish and dairy products. Foods fortified with vitamin D provide only a small amount, so you will usually need to take a supplement as well. One cup of fortified milk contains 100 international units (IU) of vitamin D and 300 mg of calcium.

The current Food and Nutrition Board recommends 400-600 IU daily. This amount may not be enough for many individuals and they will need to take more.

Vitamin D Supplements

Supplementing your diet with Vitamin D2 or D3 is a good choice as long as the optimum blood level of Vitamin D is achieved. Both D2 and D3 are hydroxylated in the liver to form their 25-hydroxy metabolites and are the two major forms found circulating in our blood. These are the highly active forms which bind to specific vitamin D receptors in our body.

Both forms can be taken by mouth once daily, ranging from 400 IU up to 2,000 IU. The recommended dose of vitamin D can vary based on the conditions that are being treated. Larger dosages of Vitamin D2 (Ergocalciferol) 50,000 IU is available by prescription in gel coated capsules or liquid and typically is taken once a week for eight weeks if vitamin D deficiency is diagnosed. You will probably need to continue taking a daily Vitamin D supplement ranging between 1,000 IU to 2,000 IU or higher after completing the prescription dose to maintain a therapeutic blood level.

NOTE: Take vitamin D exactly as prescribed because an overdose can cause serious or life-threatening side effects!

Most prescriptions of vitamin D, especially the high dose forms are made from D2.

It is best to take vitamin D with a meal that contains some fat. Vitamin D is a fat soluble vitamin and is more readily absorbed when ingested with fat.

Individuals with intestinal conditions, such as following a gastric bypass procedure, will need to take higher dosages.

NOTE: Your clinician will determine the appropriate dose for you to take.

NOTE: A common mistake that many of my patients have made is they forget to take the daily vitamin D supplement once the higher dose prescription is completed.

Chapter Summary

- It is very important to consume a nutritious diet and take adequate calcium, vitamin D and magnesium supplements to help strengthen your bones.
- Weight bearing exercises and daily stretching can help you maintain flexibility and preserve your bone health.
- Be aware of potential environmental safety hazards to prevent falls, which could result in sustaining an unwanted fracture.
- If you are postmenopausal you should have a Dexa scan done to measure your bone density to determine if you could benefit from further treatment.
- Remember, osteoporosis does not have to be a normal part of aging.
- Start treatment early and you can improve your bone health!
- It's never too late to prevent bone fractures so start treatment early.

Websites for further information on:

Osteopenia and Osteoporosis

Osteoporosis-Diseases & Condition-Web Health Network:
http://www.webhealthnetwork.com/disease/13-553/osteoporosis

NCBI, Bone Health and Osteoporosis:
https://www.ncbi.nlm.nih.gov/pubmedhealth/PMHT0024680/

National Osteoporosis Foundation: **https://www.nof.org/**

Women's Health Initiative:
https://www.nhlbi.nih.gov/whi/update_ht2002.pdf

Osteopenia-Overview-WebMD:
http://www.webmd.com/osteoporosis/tc/osteopenia-overview#1

Vitamin D

Vitamin D Background-Mayo Clinic:
http://www.mayoclinic.org/es-es/drugs-supplements/vitamin-d/background/hrb-20060400?p=1

Vitamin D: The "sunshine" vitamin:
https://www.ncbi.nlm.nih.gov/pmc/articles/PMC3356951/

Chapter 7

BREAST HEALTH

Chapter Dedication

I am dedicating this chapter to Cheryl Briggs who lost her battle with breast cancer on March 24, 2015. Cheryl was one of my reviewers for this book and one of the many grammar lessons she taught me was that quotation marks and parenthesis are commonly placed after the period in a sentence.

She was a real fighter and did well for several years after the initial surgery and treatment for breast cancer. Unfortunately the cancer reoccurred and spread throughout her body.

Cheryl would want you to use the information in this chapter to become proactive, do your monthly self-breast exams and have your routine screening mammograms to help detect breast cancer at an early stage and obtain the necessary treatment for a better outcome.

I am forever grateful for all that Cheryl taught me and feel blessed to have had her in my life!

Cheryl's sincere kindness and genuine concern for those whom she was close to came naturally and effortlessly. She was always positive toward everyone and every situation. I know of no other whom was as sincere and as caring as Cheryl. She is missed and will always be remembered.

Anatomy Of The Breast

Your breasts are made up of fat and breast tissue. Breast tissue is made up of lobes, lobules and ducts. The larger portions are the lobes and the smaller

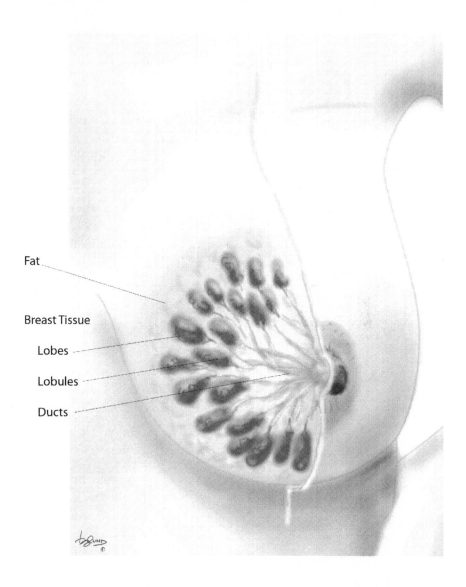

portions are subdivided into lobules, which produce milk for breast feeding. Ducts are the vessels which carry milk from the lobules to the nipple.

Breast Conditions

Fibrocystic Breasts

Development of lumps along with abnormal tissue growth in your breasts is a common condition termed *fibrocystic breasts.*

Symptoms

The symptoms of this condition are usually present the week prior to the onset of your menstrual period and can change throughout your menstrual cycle. This condition is referred to as *benign breast disease.*

Tenderness and swelling of breast tissue are the most common symptoms reported.

Many women with a condition called *estrogen dominance* have fibrocystic breast disease. Estrogen dominance is when a woman has relatively more estrogen and less progesterone. (This condition is discussed in further detail in Chapter 2.)

Treatment

Estrogen dominance is commonly treated with supplemental progesterone.

Vitamin E in low doses may help reduce breast tenderness.

Reducing caffeine consumption has been reported to be helpful for reducing breast pain. (Caffeine may promote growth of fibrous tissue and cyst fluid production.)

Vitamin B6, Magnesium, Chaste Tree and Evening Primrose oil have been reported to help reduce symptoms associated with fibrocystic breasts.

Breast Cancer

Lifetime probability for women is 1 in 6 overall and 1 in 8 for invasive disease.

The incidence of breast cancer has increased since 1980 due to the increased use of screening mammograms, which has resulted in an increased detection of early breast cancer. Over the past decade the incidence of breast cancer has leveled off due to the decreased use of hormonal replacement therapy.

Breast cancer can form either in the lobules or the ducts of your breasts. The cells divide and grow at an abnormally fast rate. They form into odd shapes and clump together forming (cancerous) malignant tumors.

Risk Factors Associated With Developing Breast Cancer

- Caucasian women tend to have a higher incidence of breast cancer, especially after age 40. This may be related to diet and lifestyle, as well as better access to care.

- African-American women have a relatively decreased incidence, although mortality rates are increasing.

- Asian and Hispanic women have a further decreased rate, although second and third generation migrants show a relative increase in incidence due to lifestyle.

- If someone in your immediate family has breast cancer, your risk nearly doubles, especially if the relative was less than forty years of age. This risk decreases for relatives older than sixty years of age. If both your sister and mother have had breast cancer your risk is 2.5 times greater than that of an individual without a family history. Only five percent of breast cancers are linked to identification of a genetic mutation called *BRCA1* and *BRCA2*.

- The amount of exposure to estrogen in a lifetime correlates with the risk of developing breast cancer. It is considered to be a moderate risk if you start menstruating before 12 years of age and enter menopause after 50 years of age. Risk decreases the later you start menstruating and the earlier you enter menopause. The increased level of the weaker form of estrogen called *estriol* found during pregnancy and breast feeding may be protective.

- A woman who has never been pregnant or achieves a pregnancy after age thirty does have a modestly increased risk of developing breast cancer. Oral contraceptive use has no proven risk, although the use of hormone replacement therapy after menopause does increase breast cancer risk, especially if used long term.

- Benign breast disease can be associated with an increased risk for developing breast cancer if a biopsy of the cells reveals *atypical hyperplasia.* Otherwise benign fibrocystic disease and adenomas do not increase risk.

NOTE: Features associated with dense breast tissue, although not a disease, do have an increased incidence of breast cancer reported.

Many radiology departments will send with the mammogram report, a generic paragraph describing how dense breast tissue lowers the sensitivity of a mammogram. Patients often do not realize this is a form letter sent to everyone and misinterpret this as pertaining to an abnormality of their own breasts.

• Diet and lifestyle have had variable reports as it pertains to their role in the development of breast cancer. Increased weight is detrimental to a women's health and does carry an increased risk of developing breast cancer beyond menopause, but not before. In fact, underweight women may have an increased risk.

• Excess fat in the diet, particularly animal fat and excess red meat consumption may increase your risk.

• The use of soy or phytoestrogen products does not convincingly increase your risk.

• Alcohol consumption *does increase your risk.*

• Tobacco studies are conflicting.

• Caffeine use may or may not affect your risk.

Types Of Breast Cancer

Carcinoma In-Situ: This is like a pre-cancer. In-situ means "In place". The cancer has not spread from the original location. The typical location of carcinoma in-situ is in a breast duct or lobule.

Infiltrating Ductal Carcinoma: This is the *most common* type of cancer and occurs in about 80 percent of individuals diagnosed with breast cancer. This type of cancer begins to develop in the ducts and spreads to the surrounding tissues.

Invasive Lobular Cancer: This type of cancer begins in the lobules and spreads to the surrounding tissues.

Inflammatory Breast Cancer (IBC): You have probably heard about this form of breast cancer in the news. This is a *rare* type of breast cancer that shows up differently than the other forms. You may first think you have a bug bite or notice swelling of one breast with redness and it may feel warm and this is why it is called inflammatory breast cancer. The skin of the breast may look pink, red or have a bruised appearance or it may have a dimpled, pitted or ridged surface similar to an orange. This appearance is called *peau d'orange,* resembling an orange rind.

Paget's Disease Of The Breast: This is a very uncommon form of infiltrating intraductal carcinoma which occurs in the nipple and ducts of the nipple. The first symptom can be itching or burning of the nipple. It is important to have a biopsy of any persistent non-healing lesion.

NOTE: Inflammatory breast cancer:
- *Can appear to be an infection and may commonly be treated as one with a course of antibiotics.*
- *Is extremely aggressive and can be diagnosed early with a biopsy in the office.*

Invasive ductal, lobular and inflammatory breast cancer can move through the breast tissue into the blood vessels and travel throughout the entire body. The term used to describe this process is called metastasize, meaning to spread.

Breast cancer, when diagnosed and treated early, can have a better outcome. Early detection is extremely important, if not crucial! Treatment options and survival rates lessen the later cancer is detected.

Early Detection And Prevention
Self-Breast Exam (SBE): You should examine your breasts once a month and at the same time of the month. You then become familiar with your own breast tissue and will be able to notice a change early on.

If you are still menstruating, perform the exam about one week after your cycle begins.

If you are no longer menstruating, pick a day and perform the exam at the same day each month.

I instruct my patients to feel for a lump ranging from a small "piece of gravel" up to the size of a "peanut M&M" or larger when performing a breast exam. (In over thirty years of practice, I have not yet encountered a woman who hasn't had a peanut M&M in her hand.) Report any unfamiliar lump to your clinician and schedule an exam as soon as possible. Most cancerous lumps do not move well when you push on them but even that can fool you. These lumps may or may not be painful.

Be sure to check for nipple changes such as:

- Turning inward (inverted nipple)
- Nipple discharge

Follow These Steps To Perform A Self-Breast Examination

Inspect Before Touching

- First look in the mirror for any changes in size, shape or appearance of your breasts.
- Check for any dimpling, rashes or denting of the skin or nipple.
- Check for any nipple discharge or any change from normal.

Inspect Your Breasts In Four Different Positions

- Hold your arms at your sides
- Hold your arms over your head
- Press your hands on your hips to tighten your chest muscles
- Bend forward with your hands on your hips and look for any changes in your breasts.

NOTE: Why are we inspecting before touching? A breast lump can change the inner architecture of the breast and sometimes result in a visible change on the outside like a flat spot or a dimple, lump, or a nipple pointing in a direction that it wasn't pointing before! These can be valuable clues even when the breast exam might feel normal.

Lying Down Method

You are checking for *any change* in your breast tissue.

- To begin, lie down on your back with a pillow under your right shoulder.
- Use the pads of your left middle fingers to examine your right breast.

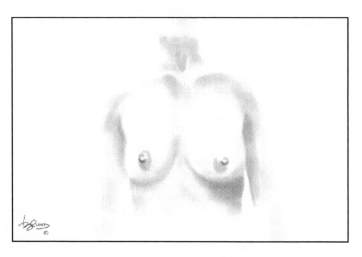

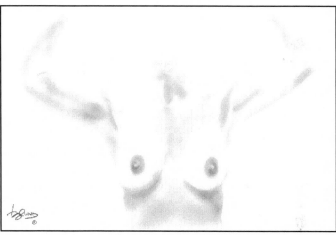

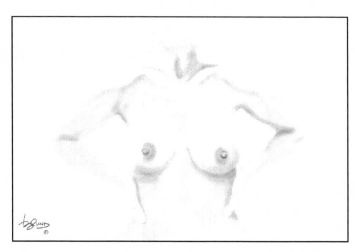

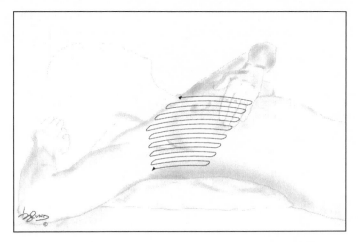

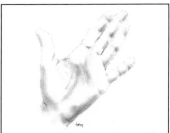

- Press using light, medium and firm pressure in a circular motion.

- Follow up and down in a linear fashion keeping in line with your body.

- Check for any changes from your armpit to below your breast, follow in a linear fashion similar to mowing a lawn, working your way from the outside of your breast to the middle of your chest.

- Repeat the same exam on your left breast using your right hand.

- This method is referred to as the *vertical strip pattern.*

NOTE: *You may also do this same exam with soapy hands while bathing or showering.*

Screening Tests

Conventional Mammograms: These are black and white x-rays of a flattened breast to detect any changes in your breast tissue. Mammograms are useful in detecting breast cancer 80% of the time.

Digital Mammography: These are pictures stored on a computer as opposed to film. The computer analyzes changes from year to year. This is good for imaging dense breasts, commonly found in pre-menopausal women and is now the preferred method.

Ultrasound: This method is used to image soft tissue changes, such as fluid filled cysts. Ultrasound is not helpful to screen for the calcifications associated with cancer.

Magnetic Resonance Imaging (MRI): This method is used for better visualization with breast implants and also to take a closer look at calcifications.

Thermography (Heat Detection): This is an old method used with new technology for detecting breast changes. This is based on the idea that cancerous lumps are hotter than normal breast tissue and may show up on thermography.

NOTE: Mammography is considered the gold standard for detecting the micro-calcifications seen in early breast cancer. Ultrasound, MRI, thermography and other imaging methods are not recommended substitutes for a mammogram but are better used as adjuncts when needed.

Genetic Testing For BRCA1 And BRCA2

A breast cancer *(BRCA)* gene test is a blood test that checks for specific changes (mutations) in genes that control normal cell growth. Identifying changes in these genes, called *BRCA1* and *BRCA2* can help determine your chance of developing breast cancer and ovarian cancer. These harmful *BRCA1* and *BRCA2* gene mutations are relatively rare in the general population and most experts agree that screening should be done only when an individual's personal or family history suggests the possible presence of these harmful gene mutations.

The following criteria may be helpful in determining if screening may be necessary:

• Breast cancer diagnosed before 50 years of age
• Cancer in both breasts in the same individual
• Both breast and ovarian cancers in either the same woman or the same family
• Multiple breast cancer diagnoses
• Two or more primary types of *BRCA1* AND *BRCA2* related cancers in a single family member
• Diagnosis of male breast cancer
• Ashkenazi Jewish ethnicity

> **NOTE:** *Your clinician can assess your individual and family risk and determine if this screening blood test will be necessary.*

Diagnosis

Needle Biopsy: This is a procedure where a needle is used to draw up a sample of the fluid and/or tissue from a mass in the breast to look for cancerous cells.

Open Biopsy: An open biopsy, also called a lumpectomy, is a surgical procedure in which all or part of the lump is removed to look for cancerous cells.

Treatment For Breast Cancer

If you receive a diagnosis of breast cancer, the treatment team will usually consist of an oncologist, radiologist, pathologist, cancer surgeon and possibly a reconstructive surgeon. Sometimes an occupational therapist, lymphedema physical therapist, psychologist and dietician will also be included as part of the team.

The team will look at several factors when deciding on the best treatment plan which could include:

- The type of breast cancer
- The stage ranging from 0 to 4 and grade of the breast cancer (how large is the tumor and has it spread to other parts of the body)
- Whether or not the cancer cells are sensitive to hormones
- Patient's overall health and age (has she been through menopause yet)

The main treatment options may include:

- Surgery
- Radiation therapy (also called radiotherapy)
- Systemic Therapy

Surgery

Most commonly, women will undergo surgery to remove the cancerous tissue. The surgeon will also remove some of the lymph nodes (axillary node dissection) from under the arm to see if any cancerous cells have spread there. A common procedure for this, in more recent years, is called a sentinel lymph node biopsy. In years past they would take 10 or more nodes from the underarm. Now they are more likely to take just one as it "represents" the other nodes. The sentinel lymph node is the hypothetical first lymph node or group of nodes draining the cancer. This procedure provides valuable information about possible spread without the disruption of the tissues and helps guide further treatment. Removing fewer lymph nodes can also help decrease long term effects, such as lymphedema.

NOTE: If the sentinel node is found to have cancer cells, the surgeon may recommend removing several more lymph nodes in the armpit.

Lymphedema (swelling of the tissues) is a condition which can occur in some patients as a result of having had an axillary node dissection or from radiation treatment to the lymph nodes.

Early gentle exercises and wearing a well-fitting compression garment may help reduce some of the swelling. There are also massage therapists that specialize in treating lymphedema. They use a technique called manual lymph drainage which helps move the lymph fluid away from the affected extremity.

The type of breast surgery performed depends on the stage and severity of the breast cancer:

- *Lumpectomy:* Removal of a lump/tumor and a small portion of normal tissue surrounding it.
- *Mastectomy:* A **partial** is when part of the breast is taken to remove the cancerous tissue. A **complete** or **radical** is when the entire breast is removed.

NOTE: In many cases breast reconstruction surgery may be considered to reshape or recreate a breast following surgery.

After surgery one or any combination of the following treatments may be necessary to destroy any remaining cancerous cells - Radiation, Chemotherapy, Hormone therapy and/or Immune therapy.

Radiation
Following a lumpectomy or partial mastectomy, the remaining breast tissue may often need to undergo radiation treatment. Many women do not need radiation treatment following a complete mastectomy. However, it is important to understand that the type of surgery per-

formed, whether lumpectomy or mastectomy, does not influence the decision on whether further hormone or chemotherapy is needed.

Radiation therapy is an adjunct treatment for most women who have undergone a lumpectomy and for some women who have had mastectomy surgery. The purpose of radiation therapy is to eliminate the microscopic cancer cells that remain near the area where the tumor was removed to prevent a recurrence. The type of breast cancer diagnosed will help determine what type of radiation therapy is needed and your doctor will then determine the length of treatment needed.

Systemic Therapy
Systemic therapy uses medications to treat cancer cells throughout the body. Any combination of systemic therapies may be used to treat breast cancer. These therapies include chemotherapy, endocrine (hormone) therapy and immune therapy.

There are many different factors in addition to the type and stage of the cancer that your doctor will need to look at before determining the need for systemic therapy.

Important Markers To Identify
If you have been diagnosed with breast cancer, there is an increased risk for developing a second primary breast cancer tumor compared to the risk of the general population, and certain markers can guide further necessary treatment.

Hormonal Receptor Status
About two-thirds of women diagnosed with breast cancer have tumors that contain hormone receptors. This means a tumor has receptors for estrogen (called ER positive) or progesterone (PR positive) or may even contain both. Patients with estrogen and/or progesterone receptor positive tumors typically will receive endocrine therapy (formerly called hormone therapy) after radiation and chemotherapy is completed, to decrease the risk of recurrence.

HER2 Protein Status
A protein called human epidermal growth factor receptor type 2 (known as HER2) can cause breast cancer cells to grow and spread quickly. Elevated levels of the HER2 protein are caused by having too many copies of the HER2/neu gene. This HER2 protein tells cells

to grow and divide. Positive (HER2+) breast cancer is found in about one in four breast cancers diagnosed and is associated with a more aggressive disease process.

Chemotherapy
There are many different types of drug treatments used to kill the cancer cells and these are referred to as cytotoxic drugs. The oncologist may recommend chemotherapy if there is a high risk of the cancer spreading to other parts of the body. When cancer spreads to other parts of the body it is referred to as metastatic disease. If the tumor is large, chemotherapy may be recommended before surgery to shrink the size making it easier to remove.

Hormone Therapy (Endocrine Blocking Therapy)
Breast tumors typically require estrogen and/or progesterone hormones for growth. The use of oral hormone treatments (endocrine therapy) focuses on blocking the body's naturally occurring estrogen to slow down or stop the cancer's growth.

There are two types of hormone therapy used for treating breast cancer.

• Medications that block estrogen and progesterone from promoting breast cancer cell growth.

• Medications to turn off the production of hormones from the ovaries.

NOTE: *Do not confuse the term "hormone therapy" used for treating breast cancer with the term "hormone replacement therapy" used for replacing hormones in postmenopausal women!*

Hormone Therapies Used To Treat Breast Cancer
Common agents used are called **Selective Estrogen Receptor Modulators (SERMs).** These medications work by blocking estrogen receptors in cancer cells, which prevents estrogen from stimulating cancer cell growth.

• Tamoxifen is a common medication that has been used to treat breast cancer for the past thirty years. This medication is used to reduce the chance of a recurrence and for treatment of new breast cancers in women with ER-positive or ER-unknown breast tumors.

• Evista is another similar medication and can also be used to prevent and treat osteoporosis.

• Fareston is another medication in this class used to treat advanced cancer in postmenopausal women.

Another class of drugs called *Aromatase Inhibitors* work by interrupting the conversion of the hormone androsterone into estrogen, lowering the amount of circulating estrogen. This type of medication is typically given to postmenopausal women because it interferes with this conversion process so breast cancer cells no longer have the estrogen to promote their growth.

Arimidex (anastrozole), Aromasin (exemestane) and Femara (letrozole) are medications in this class used to treat estrogen-receptor-positive breast cancer in postmenopausal women, either following tamoxifen treatment or as initial therapy.

Ovarian Ablation or Suppression Therapy
Some women may benefit from this form of therapy if they have not gone through menopause yet, and their breast cancer is estrogen-receptor positive (ER-positive). This procedure stops the ovaries from making estrogen that promotes cancer cell growth.

This can be accomplished by:

• Using radiation to the ovaries

• Removing the ovaries surgically (oophorectomy)

• Administering a luteinizing hormone-releasing medication called a LHRH agonist given alone or in combination with Tamoxifen.

Biological Or Immune Therapy
Cancer may develop when the immune system is not working properly. Immune therapy, also called biological therapy, uses your body's own immune system to fight the cancer.

If you are diagnosed with HER2 positive breast cancer, an immune therapy such as **Herceptin (trastuzumab)** may be used. This monoclonal antibody targets and destroys cancer cells that are HER2-positive.

Tykerb (lapatinib) is another drug that targets the HER2 protein. It is also used to treat advanced metastatic cancer and used for individuals who did not respond well to Herceptin.

Avastin (bevacizumab) is used to stop the cancer cells from acquiring new blood vessels, essentially starving the tumor from nutrients and oxygen.

NOTE: Cancer vaccines are another type of immune therapy because they can trigger an immune response to fight cancer cells.

Breast Health Recommendations

Stop Smoking

A study published in the Archives of Internal Medicine, reported that "Any history of smoking increases a woman's chance of developing breast cancer by 6 percent." The analysis, which is believed to be the largest ever to address the question, is based on data from the Nurses' Health Study, and included more than 111,000 women followed from 1976 to 2006.

Dietary

Eat at least five to nine servings of whole foods, fresh fruit and vegetables daily.

Avoid simple sugars and carbohydrates to help prevent insulin resistance, which may be linked to increased risk for developing breast cancer. *(See Chapter 10 for more information on insulin resistance.)*

Eat healthy, low-fat organic animal and dairy fats and avoid saturated fat, whenever possible.

Nutritional Supplements

Breast health relies on a rich supply of nutrients, antioxidants, and essential fatty acids, like omega-3 fatty acids and vitamin D, to help boost the immune system and decrease inflammation. Recent studies are showing that the role of inflammation is becoming increasingly important in the development of cancer and heart disease.

Omega-3 fatty acid fish oil: A study suggests that postmenopausal women who take fish oil supplements, high in omega-3 fatty acids, may reduce their breast cancer risk. *(July issue of Cancer Epidemiology 2007, Biomarkers & Prevention, A Journal of the American Association for Cancer Research)*

Vitamin D: Take 1000 IU of Vitamin D3 daily. It would be best to have your vitamin D blood level checked and your clinician can determine the correct dosage for you.

Whole ground flaxseed is a great source of omega 3s, and has the added benefit of helping prevent constipation. Take 1-2 tablespoonfuls

per day. Begin with one-half a teaspoonful daily and gradually increase to 1-2 tablespoonfuls if tolerated.

Alcohol

Drink alcohol in moderation. Drinking more than one to two glasses
of wine, beer or spirits per day has been possibly associated with an
increased risk of breast cancer. The mechanisms of increased risk of
developing breast cancer from alcohol may be:

- Interference with your liver's ability to metabolize extra estrogens.
- Increased mammary gland susceptibility to carcinogenesis
- Increased mammary DNA damage
- Increased metastatic potential of breast cancer cells.

*NOTE: Researchers studied 105,986 women through the famous
Nurses' Health Study and collected data on their alcohol consumption from 1980 to 2008. They found that women who consumed
three to six drinks of alcohol per week had a 15 percent increased
risk of developing breast cancer, while women who consumed two
drinks per day had a more than 50 percent greater risk than wom-
en who did not drink. There was no difference among women who
drank wine, beer or hard liquor.*

Exercise

Studies have shown that exercising five days a week both before
and after menopause can help reduce a woman's risk of developing
breast cancer.

Body Weight

Women who maintain a healthy body weight have a lower chance
of developing breast cancer compared to those who are obese and
overweight.

Early Detection

- Do monthly breast self-exams beginning at 20 years of age.
- Be sure to schedule a yearly well-woman exam with your clini-
  cian, beginning at age 20.
- Get a mammogram as recommended by the American Cancer
  Society and/or your clinician.

NOTE: *Remember, an early diagnosis of breast cancer can lead to an excellent outcome with a five year survival rate of 97%!* **See cancer screening recommendations in Chapter 19 and personal testimonies in Chapter 21.**

Websites for further information on:

Breast cancer

Breast Cancer-Patient Version Overview-National Cancer Institute: **https://www.cancer.gov/types/breast**

Breast Cancer Awareness Resources-American Cancer Society: **https://www.cancer.org/content/cancer/en/latest-news/ special-coverage/how-acs-fights-breast-cancer.html**

Breast cancer information: **http://www.cancercenter.com/breast-cancer/learning/**

City of Hope: **https://www.cityofhope.org/homepage**

WebMD Breast Cancer Health Center: **http://www.webmd.com/breast-cancer/default.htm**

Foundation for Women's Cancer: **http://www.wcn.org/**

Chapter 8

THYROID CONDITIONS

The Link Between Thyroid Disease And Menopause

According to the American Association of Clinical Endocrinologists (ACE), millions of women with persistent menopausal symptoms, even when taking estrogen replacement, may be suffering from undiagnosed thyroid disease.

There appears to be a connection between a woman's estrogen and thyroid hormone levels, especially when estrogen levels fluctuate, such as during pregnancy and menopause.

Symptoms such as fatigue, depression, weight gain, hair loss, mood swings, poor concentration and sleep disturbances, along with hot and cold intolerance that are frequently associated with menopause may also be signs of hypothyroidism.

The incidence of hypothyroidism does increase with age and certainly can co-exist with other conditions.

One out of every four postmenopausal women may have thyroid disease, which can go undetected.

You should have your thyroid checked by age thirty-five and then every five years. If you have any symptoms or a known family history of thyroid disease you should be checked sooner.

The Thyroid Gland

The thyroid gland resembles a butterfly in shape and is located in the lower part of your neck. This gland can be thought of as "the control tower". This master gland makes hormones that regulate your metabolism and deliver energy to cells throughout your body.

When your thyroid is out of balance it can affect many bodily functions from thickness of the hair on your head to the texture of your toenails.

Your brain and thyroid communicate with your body to keep these hormones in balance. The two main hormones made by the thyroid gland are triiodothyronine, abbreviated as T3, and thyroxine, abbreviated as T4. T4 is the most abundant and inactive form of thyroid hormone in your system, and T3 is the active form that enters your cells.

The thyroid gland regulates:
- How many calories you burn (body's metabolism)
- Your body temperature
- Your body weight
- Your heart rate
- Your skin texture
- Your menstrual cycles (periods)
- Your reactions to hot and cold
- Use of other hormones and vitamins
- Growth and maturation of body tissue

How Thyroid Hormones Work In Our Body
(**Warning:** *This section can become a bit technical*)
When your body is in a state of healthy balance, the part of the brain

called the hypothalamus sends out a chemical messenger called *thyro-tropin releasing hormone (TRH)* to the anterior pituitary gland located beneath it, and **thyroid stimulating hormone (TSH)** is produced.

NOTE: The hormone estrogen enhances the function of TRH.

TSH directs the production and the release of thyroid hormones T3 and T4. TSH also controls the conversion process of T4 into T3 in the liver. (More detail on this conversion process to follow.)

The TSH heads for the thyroid gland and upon it's arrival an enzyme called *thyroid peroxide (TPO)* is made. TPO combines with hydrogen peroxide to help create the two thyroid hormones, T3 and T4.

T4 is made in the thyroid gland when a protein attaches to four molecules of iodine creating the thyroid hormone T4, called *thyroxine*. The majority of hormone made in the thyroid gland is the inactive form, T4, (approximately 93%) and the remainder is the active form, T3 hormone (triiodothyronine). T4 is also considered to be a storage form of thyroid hormone that our body converts to the active form T3.

T4 thyroid hormone must be converted to T3 before our body can use it. The thyroid gland makes approximately 7% to 15% of the T3 hormone. Our body has to make more T3 with the help of our liver and intestines. One molecule of iodine is removed from the T4 molecule to make T3. A properly functioning liver is essential for this process to occur.

Our intestines can also help convert about 20% of the circulating T4 into T3. We do need to have healthy gut bacteria for this process to happen.

T3 and T4 are present in your bloodstream in two forms, bound and free.

The bound T3 and T4 are attached to proteins to keep them from having an action on your cells. T3 and T4 must be in the free form to have an effect on your cells.

Once your cells have used the free T3 and T4 hormones, then the bound T3 and T4 can break away to become free, replacing what the cells have just used. T4 is slow acting and T3 is fast acting and your body needs both forms to function properly.

Our bodies will continually adjust minute to minute to meet the changing demands we place on it every day.

NOTE: I hope you can now see how important it is to achieve and maintain proper health for our body to function well and maintain balance throughout the day!

Types Of Thyroid Imbalance

Hypothyroidism

The most common thyroid imbalance is an underactive thyroid and is frequently diagnosed in menopausal women. Elderly patients and those who have received radiation treatments to the head and neck are also at risk for developing this condition.

When hypothyroidism occurs, the thyroid gland does not make enough of the hormone called thyroxine.

Thyroxine helps control your body's metabolism. Remember, a well-functioning metabolism allows your body to make and use energy efficiently. A low thyroxine level can adversely affect many of your biological processes.

It has been estimated that one in seven adults or 12-30 million Americans suffer from an underactive thyroid.

"Hashimoto's Thyroiditis" is the most common cause of hypothyroidism in the United States and worldwide. The name comes from the doctor who first identified this disease, Dr. Hakaru Hashimoto. This is an auto-immune disease. When this occurs your body does not recognize the tissue of the thyroid gland and sees it as foreign. Your immune system reacts by sending cells to attack your thyroid gland, causing inflammation and swelling. Some patients may develop significant swelling known as a goiter.

Causes

Most thyroid disease is autoimmune in nature, so it's not surprising that women, who are more likely to develop autoimmune disease, are diagnosed with this condition. It is six times more commonly found in women than in men.

The symptoms typically found to be associated with puberty, pregnancy and menopause can mimic symptoms of an underactive thyroid. Our thyroid and reproductive hormones are very closely related.

Hypothyroidism can also be associated with a lack of iodine in your diet and with the use of certain medications.

Surgery, radiation therapy, and infection can also cause the thyroid gland to become underactive.

Common Signs And Symptoms

Brain and Head

- Depressed mood
- Decreased ability to focus and concentrate, or "brain fog"
- Slowed thinking and trouble remembering things
- Coarse and brittle hair that breaks easily
- Hair loss from your head and eyebrows
- Swelling of your face and puffiness around the eyes
- Hoarseness and a raspy voice
- Fullness of neck and throat

Heart

- Slow heartbeat

Joints and Muscles

- Aches and pains in joints, hands, and feet
- Muscle cramps
- Slowed reflexes

Nails

- Brittle nails that split easily

Ovaries and Uterus

- Infertility
- Irregular and heavy menstrual periods

Skin

- Overly dry and scaly. Peeling, flaking and cracking can eventually develop.
- Increased sensitivity to cold and temperature change.
- Lack of/or decreased sweating, even with intense exercise.

Thyroid

- Hard, rubbery and enlarged thyroid gland (fullness in neck or throat)
- Sometimes nodules may be present

Other Changes

- Changes in cholesterol and triglyceride levels
- Constipation
- Difficulty losing weight, even when adhering to a strict diet and exercise program
- Decreased energy, feeling fatigued or exhausted

NOTE: *Hypothyroidism may become more difficult to diagnose during the menopausal years because the typical presenting symptoms may not be present. These symptoms may be confused with those found in menopause.*

Postpartum Thyroid Disease

It is common for women to develop hypothyroidism during or immediately following pregnancy. The high level of hormones along with the strain pregnancy places on the thyroid gland is probably the cause. This condition is referred to as *Postpartum Thyroiditis.*

Many times the thyroid function will be restored once the hormones related to pregnancy and lactation return to normal.

Some women may continue to have hypothyroidism if they have a family history or an auto-immune condition.

The symptoms of postpartum thyroiditis may go unnoticed since they can mimic:

- Postpartum depression
- Adjusting to life with a newborn

Common symptoms are:

- Fatigue
- Insomnia
- Nervousness
- Irritability

You can certainly see how easily these symptoms could be justified as "life with a newborn".

NOTE: It is very important that hypothyroidism be treated and monitored closely during pregnancy to prevent brain damage to the fetus!

Hyperthyroidism

This condition occurs when your body makes too much thyroid hormone.

Graves' Disease, which is also called *toxic diffuse goiter*, is the most common cause of an overactive thyroid in the United States. It is eight times more commonly found in women than in men and typically diagnosed between twenty to forty years of age.

This condition is also considered to be an auto-immune disease (when the body sees the thyroid gland as foreign and creates antibodies against its own tissues or organs). In this case, antibodies attack the thyroid and too much thyroid hormone is produced.

Causes Of Hyperthyroidism

Toxic nodular goiter is a non-cancerous tumor. The thyroid gland contains a small rounded growth or growths called *nodules* with this condition. These nodules make too much thyroid hormone. This condition may occur from having a simple goiter and occurs usually in women over 60 years of age. Painful thyroiditis is caused by a virus and the gland becomes inflamed. When the viral infection resolves, so does the thyroiditis.

Painless thyroiditis can occur when the thyroid gland becomes inflamed temporarily, such as after giving birth, and usually resolves on its own.

Thyrotoxicosis factitia can occur from supplementing with too much thyroid hormone.

Thyroid Storm (Thyrotoxicosis) is rarely seen today and can occur from a stressful illness, thyroid surgery, iodine administration and most commonly undiagnosed or under treated hyperthyroidism.

Signs And Symptoms

The additional thyroid hormone affects the body by speeding up many processes, causing many or all of the following symptoms:

• Puffy eyes (swelling of the tissues surrounding the eyes) Your eyes can also become red, irritated and you may experience double vision. It may appear to others as if you have a fixed blank stare.

NOTE: About 25% to 50% of those with Graves' disease develop thyroid eye disease, which is called Graves' orbitopathy.

- Thickening of the skin over the lower extremities
- An irregular heartbeat and/or palpitations (a sensation that your heart is beating rapidly)
- Fatigue
- Insomnia (inability to sleep) and restlessness
- Anxiety and nervousness
- Intolerance to heat (always feeling hot)
- Light or absent menstrual cycles
- Tremor of the hands and/or muscle weakness
- Warm moist skin
- Hair loss
- Weight loss with an increased appetite
- Diarrhea or frequent bowel movements

Other Thyroid Conditions

Thyroid Nodule
A nodule occurs from growth of cells within the thyroid gland and can be cystic or glandular. These growths are usually benign (non-cancerous).

Symptoms
- A lump may be felt on the thyroid gland
- Difficulty swallowing and/or hoarseness
- Pain or fullness in neck or throat
- Breathing problems

Thyroid Cancer
A painless mass occurs on the thyroid gland, and is a malignant tumor. This condition can occur due to a previous history of radiation to the head and/or neck, or to a family history of having a goiter.

Types Of Thyroid Cancer
- Papillary cancer is the most common type of thyroid cancer found. It usually affects women of childbearing age, and is the least dangerous type.
- Follicular cancer is the most likely to recur and spread.
- Anaplastic cancer is very rare and is also called *Giant Cell* or *Spindle*

Cell Cancer. This is the most dangerous form and spreads quickly.

• Medullary cancer is a cancer of the non-thyroid cells found present in the thyroid gland, and tends to occur in families.

Making The Diagnosis

Blood Tests Can Determine If You Have A Thyroid Condition

We now have blood tests that can tell us how well the thyroid produces inactive T4 and how well our body converts T4 into active T3 hormone. We can also test for how our body uses T3, and if there are antibodies present that can attack the thyroid gland.

A **TSH** test is the most common thyroid test ordered and measures the amount of thyroid-stimulating hormone you have circulating in your blood. In review, *thyroid-stimulating hormone* is released from your pituitary gland and alerts your thyroid gland to release thyroid hormones.

A low level of TSH means you have too much circulating thyroid hormone.

A high level of TSH means you have too little circulating thyroid hormone.

NOTE: The interpretation of this test can be confusing, because one tends to think, if the TSH level is low then the thyroid must be low. It is just the opposite. Measuring only the TSH does not tell us if the pituitary gland is working properly or if you have an autoimmune disorder, although in most healthy individuals a TSH test is sufficient to screen for thyroid dysfunction.

Free T4 (FT4): This test measures the amount of free or unbound thyroxine (T4) circulating in your blood. The free T4 level represents the amount of hormone available for uptake to be used by cells in your body. Since free levels of T4 represent immediately available hormone, it is thought to better reflect the patient's hormonal status.

• A low level indicates an underactive thyroid.

• A high level indicates an overactive thyroid.

• This test is commonly done with a TSH to confirm that you have an underactive thyroid.

Total T4 (Total Thyroxine): This test measures the total thyroxine level, free and bound and tells you how much inactive thyroid you have circulating in your blood.

- A low T4 level can indicate an underactive thyroid.
- A low T4 and a high TSH indicates an underactive thyroid.
- A low T4 and a normal TSH indicates a problem with the pituitary gland, rather than the thyroid gland. (The pituitary gland is not sending out TSH.)
- A high T4 indicates an overactive thyroid gland.

NOTE: If you are pregnant, currently taking a birth control pill or hormone replacement therapy, you may have an elevated T4 and NOT have hyperthyroidism. Remember, estrogens used in the birth control pill and hormone replacement can cause a decrease in thyroid binding, so there is an increased amount of free thyroid hormone available to your cells.

Free T3 (FT3): This test measures the amount of free (unbound) T3 circulating in your blood.

- A low level indicates an underactive thyroid.
- A high level indicates an overactive thyroid.

NOTE: T3 levels are more sensitive and change more quickly than T4 levels. A Free T3 is considered to be more accurate than a Total T3 level.

Total T3 (Total Triiodothyronine): This test measures the total triiodothyronine level, free and bound, and tells you how much active thyroid is circulating in your blood.

- A high T3 level indicates an overactive thyroid.
- A low T3 indicates an underactive thyroid.
- The T3 is more sensitive than T4 and it may rise quickly even when the T4 is still normal.
- Medications such as steroids and certain blood pressure pills can falsely lower the T3 level.

Antibody Blood Tests Can Help Diagnose Autoimmune Thyroid Disease

Antibodies are proteins your body uses to protect itself from foreign entities. Sometimes the body will create antibodies against its own organs, referred to as autoimmune disease. This test measures the presence of antibodies against thyroid tissue.

Antibodies can cause your thyroid to work harder, block thyroid hormone or cause harmful inflammation.

Thyroglobulin antibody (TgAb): This is one type of antibody the body creates after the thyroid gland becomes inflamed or has been injured. This test is used to check for antibodies in your body that attack the thyroid.

These levels are usually low or undetectable when your thyroid is functioning normally. These levels are found to be elevated with thyroiditis, Graves' disease and/or thyroid cancer.

The thyroglobulin antibody (TgAb) damages thyroglobulin and interferes with production of thyroid hormone.

When these antibodies are detected and have been elevated for a length of time, destruction of the thyroid gland can eventually occur.

This test can be done initially to measure antibodies that are present when you have an auto-immune process, such as Hashimoto's Thyroiditis or Graves' disease.

If you have been diagnosed with Graves' disease and have a high thyroglobulin antibody level, you are more likely to eventually become hypothyroid.

Thyroglobulin antibodies are positive in about 60% of individuals with Hashimoto's, and 30% of individuals with Graves' disease.

This test is also used to monitor the effectiveness of thyroid cancer treatment, and to identify any thyroid cancer recurrence.

Thyroid Peroxidase (TPO Ab): This antibody disrupts peroxidase, the enzyme that maintains proper chemical balance for the production of thyroid hormone.

(Thyroid peroxidase is a type of enzyme that helps produce T3 and T4 hormones.)

In autoimmune thyroid disease, your body can attack the thyroid gland itself, or the thyroid peroxidase enzyme, and both conditions can cause thyroid imbalance and disease.

A high TPO antibody level is usually found in association with thyroiditis (inflammation of the thyroid gland).

In patients with hypothyroidism a high TPO level indicates a diagnosis of Hashimoto's disease.

In hyperthyroid patients an elevated TPO level indicates a diagnosis of Grave's disease.

TPO antibodies may also become elevated with postpartum thyroiditis.

A moderate level of TPO antibodies may also be found in association with thyroid cancer, anemia, rheumatoid arthritis, and/or Type 1 diabetes.

NOTE: It is important to treat these thyroid conditions to prevent reproductive problems such as infertility, miscarriage, premature delivery and pre-eclampsia (toxicity of pregnancy).

Thyroxine-binding globulin (TBG): This test measures the amount of tyrosine-containing protein in the blood that binds to iodine and carries the thyroid hormones T3 and T4. This test is NOT routinely done.

If this level is too high or too low, it may cause your thyroid hormone levels to look falsely abnormal. A low level of this protein could also indicate hypothyroidism.

Congratulations, you made it through this section. Are you still with me?

Painless Tests That Can Take A Closer Look At Your Thyroid Gland

Thyroid Ultrasound
This test is commonly done and uses high-frequency sound waves to create a dimensional image of your thyroid gland.

A thyroid ultrasound is usually ordered if a lump or nodule is felt on examination. This test can easily determine if a nodule is fluid filled or a solid mass of tissue. This test also gives useful information to help determine if further testing is needed.

Radioactive Iodine Uptake Scan (RAIU)
This test requires that you take a pill that contains radioactive iodine.

Several hours later the iodine is circulating in your blood, and your thyroid absorbs it (takes it up).

Your thyroid gland is the only tissue in your body that absorbs iodine. Since the iodine is radioactive, special cameras can show how it concentrates in your thyroid gland, which gives clinicians useful information about how your thyroid is functioning.

If the thyroid gland is not absorbing the iodine a "cold spot" will appear. This may be a sign of a non-functioning nodule or even cancer.

A "hot spot" in contrast, appears when the thyroid tissue is taking up more iodine than it should and is considered to be overactive. This could possibly be a sign of a toxic nodule.

Radioisotope Scan

This test contains another radioactive substance named *technetium*, which is used along with iodine and provides even more detailed information about your thyroid gland.

These substances together light up your thyroid gland on the scan. Different patterns visualized on the scan correlate with how well your thyroid is functioning.

These scans can be used when a low TSH is found along with thyroiditis and/or a toxic nodular goiter.

All radiation has possible side effects. There is a very small amount of radiation in the tracer pill swallowed during these tests. Your clinician will consider your individual risk versus the benefits of taking the test. In most cases the benefit outweighs the risk.

Further Testing May Be Necessary If A Lump Is Found

Fine Needle Aspiration (FNA) Is Used To Examine Individual Cells

When a lump or nodule is found on examination, your clinician may decide to look at the cells under a microscope to determine if there is any cancer. This procedure is called a fine needle aspiration, and involves using a very small needle to obtain cells from the lump to examine. Sometimes an ultrasound may be used to guide the needle during this procedure.

A fine needle aspiration procedure is less painful than having your blood drawn. Remember, most thyroid lumps are NOT cancer!

Treatments To Restore Thyroid Balance

Medications Used To Treat Hypothyroidism

Synthetic "Levothyroxine" (L-Thyroxine)

This medication replaces only the inactive T4 and your body breaks it down into the active form T3. Common trade names you may recognize:

- Levothroid
- Levoxyl
- Synthroid

Achieving the correct dosage of thyroid replacement can be a bit challenging, especially during the menopausal years. It may take some time.

In pregnancy, only T4 replacement should be used because the fetus cannot use T3 and is dependent on the T4 to T3 conversion for normal growth and development.

Thyroid requirements may go up significantly during pregnancy and thyroid levels should be followed very closely.

The TSH target for patients ages 65 and older on thyroid replacement should range from 4mIU/L to 6mIU/L due to the risk of adverse effects on the heart, mood and bone. The TSH target for individuals less than 65 years of age on thyroid replacement should typically range between 1mIU/L to 2mIU/L.

NOTE: Take your L-thyroxine first thing in the morning on an empty stomach with water only and wait a half hour before putting anything in your stomach, including food, vitamins and supplements.

Synthetic Triiodothyronine (Liothyronine Sodium)

This medication replaces only the active form T3. Common trade name you may recognize is Cytomel. Many Endocrinologists do not replace T3 alone. Complications of over supplementation are more common with T3, including irregular heart rhythms, anxiety and bone loss.

Natural "Desiccated" Thyroid Hormone

This medication replaces both active T3 and T4. Common trade names you may recognize:

- Armour Thyroid
- Nature-Throid

Endocrinologists typically do not recommend these natural therapies because they bypass the body's highly regulated T4 to T3 conversion process, where the appropriate amount of T4 is converted depending on the body's needs. T3 has a much shorter half-life, so a medication containing T3 provides a less stable dose than taking just a T4 replacement medication.

A recent study suggests there may be a subgroup of people with a certain genotype that are more likely to feel better on a T3-T4 combination therapy medication. It may be that those individuals do not convert T4 to T3 efficiently.

Discuss your individual treatment needs with your clinician.

Natural Triiodothyronine
This medication replaces only T3. Alternative medicine clinicians often recommend replacement with T3 (triiodothyronine), to treat a condition called *Wilson's Syndrome*. This condition has many symptoms of thyroid disease, in spite of normal thyroid function tests.

Traditional clinicians have expressed concern that treatment with triiodothyronine can be potentially harmful and do not recommend replacement with just T3 thyroid hormone.

How Often Should Your Blood Levels Be Tested
Initial blood testing is done between six to eight weeks and again at three and six month intervals to ensure that you are taking the correct amount of thyroid replacement. If your thyroid level is balanced at six months, you will then be checked annually to be sure the level remains stable. Some recent information states that you may only need to check the TSH every other year once you have achieved a balanced level.

Research has shown that women taking estrogen replacement or the birth control pill may have lower levels of thyroid hormone and need to have their blood checked more often. (Estrogen therapy can interfere with thyroid medication, reducing the amount of available thyroid hormone as discussed earlier in this chapter.)

Research has also shown that taking too much thyroid can lead to osteoporosis (thinning of the bones) due to excessive calcium loss.

Remember, it is important to be sure that you are taking enough calcium and vitamin D and doing weight bearing exercises. Please refer to Chapters 3 and 6 for more information on exercise and osteoporosis.

Medications To Treat Hyperthyroidism

These medications belong to the thioamide drug family and prevent your thyroid gland from producing and releasing thyroid hormone.

These anti-thyroid medications work more quickly than radioactive iodine.

Propylthiouracil (Propyl-Thyracil Or PTU)

This medication blocks production of thyroid hormones and the conversion of inactive T4 to active T3 hormone.

This medication is no longer commonly used to treat hyperthyroidism, due to recent reports of liver failure in patients taking PTU.

PTU may be the preferred recommended treatment for a short duration in early pregnancy. Your endocrinologist will recommend the lowest effective dose and monitor you closely throughout the pregnancy.

Methimazole (Brand Name Is Tapazole)

This medication is the preferred treatment to use because it can be given once a day and has fewer side effects. Methimazole also works by blocking production of thyroid hormones.

Both medications (PTU and Methimazole) cross the placental barrier, although PTU is thought to cross less so than methimazole.

NOTE: Anti-thyroid medications do not work right away. Symptoms may get better or go away in about eight weeks or even sooner. You may need to keep taking this medication for up to twenty four months to help restore thyroid balance. If you take this medication you may develop hypothyroidism. These medications may possibly lower your white blood cell count, which you need to fight infection. You should see your clinician at the first sign of any infection.

Beta Blockers

Medications like propranolol and atenolol may also be prescribed to control symptoms such as tremor (shaking), irregular heartbeat and anxiety.

Radioactive Iodine

Radioactive iodine is taken in capsule or liquid form and destroys part or most of the thyroid gland. The thyroid gland typically no longer produces thyroid hormone and you then need to take thyroid replacement.

Individuals who do not respond to medication therapy or who are unable to handle the side effects may decide to have radioactive iodine.

• Radioactive iodine is the most common and effective treatment for hyperthyroidism. This is the preferred treatment if you are found to have a "hot nodule" (an area of the gland that is too active).

• This treatment is typically not used when you have been diagnosed with Graves' disease. Graves' eye disease can progress rapidly after treatment with radioactive iodine.

• Individuals diagnosed with thyroid cancer may receive radioactive iodine therapy after having surgery (thyroidectomy) to destroy any remaining thyroid cancer cells. This therapy is also used to prevent thyroid cancer recurrences.

Surgery
Surgery is indicated when you have cancer. The surgeon may need to remove part or all of your thyroid gland, depending on where the tumor is located. This surgery can be very tricky due to the small parathyroid glands that are located above the thyroid gland. The parathyroid glands release the hormone calcitonin, which is responsible for calcium metabolism.

NOTE: Total removal of your thyroid gland may affect the parathyroid glands, which could result in calcium abnormalities, so you will be closely monitored by your clinician.

Recommendations To Help Keep Your Thyroid Healthy
• Eat foods with moderate amounts of iodine such as shell fish, tuna, kelp, asparagus and dairy products.

• Eat more protein and foods rich in tyrosine, like soybeans, chicken, fish, almonds, avocados, bananas, legumes, dairy products. (Tyrosine is an essential amino acid that your body forms from another essential amino acid called phenylalanine.) Your body receives essential amino acids from consuming protein. Your thyroid gland needs iodine and tyrosine to work properly.

- Eat foods rich in vitamins A (beta carotene), B, C, and E.
- Eat foods rich in calcium, selenium, and zinc.
- Eat 6 small meals a day, which can help stimulate your metabolism.
- Exercise at least 5 times a week for at least 30 minutes.
- Reduce the stress in your life by trying yoga, massage, and meditation.
- Take your thyroid hormone first thing in the morning on an empty stomach and wait at least a half hour before putting anything else in your stomach, including food, vitamins, and all supplements. So many substances can interfere with the absorption of thyroid.
- Make sure you have regular check-ups, so any changes can be recognized and treated early!

NOTE: Schedule your appointment today to help maintain thyroid hormone balance.

Websites for further information on:

Graves' Disease

Endocrine Web-Graves' Disease Overview:
https://www.endocrineweb.com/

Graves' Disease Brochure PDF-American Thyroid Association:
http://www.thyroid.org/wp-content/uploads/patients/brochures/Graves_brochure.pdf

Patient Bulletings About Graves' Disease and Thyroid Foundation:
http://www.gdatf.org/

Hypothyroidism

Hashimoto's Thyroiditis: **https://www.endocrineweb.com/**

Hypothyroidism-American Thyroid Association:
http://www.thyroid.org/wp-content/uploads/patients/brochures/ata-hypothyroidism-brochure.pdf

Overview-Hypothyroidism-Mayo Clinic:
http://www.mayoclinic.org/diseases-conditions/hypothyroidism/home/ovc-20155291

Hyperthyroidism

Hyperthyroidism-Mayo Clinic:
**http://www.mayoclinic.org/diseases-conditions/
hyperthyroidism/basics/definition/con-20020986**

Hyperthyroidism Brochure-American Thyroid Association:
**http://www.thyroid.org/wp-content/uploads/patients/brochures/
ata-hyperthyroidism-brochure.pdf**

Hyperthyroidism-Topic Overview-WebMD:
**http://www.webmd.com/women/tc/hyperthyroidism-topic-
overview#1**

Thyroid Cancer

ThyCA: Thyroid Cancer Survivors Association:
http://www.thyca.org/

Chapter 9

URINARY TRACT CONDITIONS

Anatomy of Kidneys and Bladder

The urinary tract is the system that makes urine and carries it out of your body. The basic plumbing consists of:

- Two kidneys (The organs that clean the blood by making liquid waste known as urine.)
- Two ureters (The tubes that carry urine from the kidneys to the bladder.)
- The bladder (A hollow organ shaped like a balloon that holds urine and has muscle lined walls allowing it to expand and contract.)
- The urethra (The opening where urine passes out of the body.)

I guess you could say I have a special interest in piping, since my husband is a plumber—Ha! Ha!

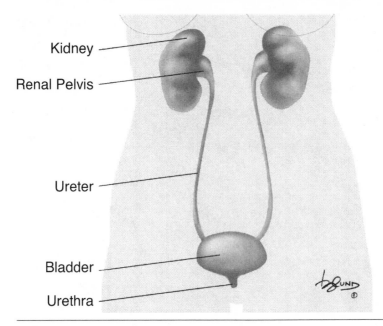

Kidney

Renal Pelvis

Ureter

Bladder

Urethra

Figure 9.1

Urinary tract conditions are more common in women after menopause. The urethra is dependent on estrogen to maintain its elasticity.

When estrogen has been declining or low for a period of time, the urethra tube becomes less flexible.

The connective tissue and collagen (which is the pink fleshy tissue that surrounds the urethra and supports your plumbing) becomes thinner, and you may leak without any warning.

Thinner tissue allows for microscopic tears to occur, especially with intercourse, and bacteria can easily enter the urethra, leading to a possible urinary tract infection.

> *NOTE: Women are more prone to developing bladder infections due to an improper wiping technique that can possibly introduce bacteria from the feces (bowel movements) into the urethra. The most common bacteria found, known as E. coli, can travel to your bladder and kidneys if left untreated.*

Remember These Simple Tips:
• Always wipe from front to back.
• Urinate after sex! (It is also a good idea to urinate before sex!)

If you think you might have a urinary tract infection, be sure to go see your clinician!

Urinary Tract Infections

Signs And Symptoms

• *Burning sensation or pain when urinating.*

• *Urgency (a feeling that your bladder is so full that it could actually burst)*

• *Frequency (The feeling of having to urinate with only small amounts of urine released at a time)*

• *Suprapubic pain (discomfort felt over the bladder)*

• *Sometimes blood may be present in the urine.*

• *A low grade fever may also be present.*

If the infection travels to your kidney, it is called pyelonephritis and you could experience any of the following symptoms:

• *Fever*

• *Chills*

• *Back pain (flank pain)*

• *Nausea and vomiting*

• *Joint pain and muscle aches*

NOTE: If you experience any of the above symptoms, you need to go see your clinician as soon as possible, or head to the emergency room!

Diagnosis

You will first need to give a urine specimen so it can be examined for possible bacteria and white blood cells.

A urine culture will then be sent to the lab to check for the presence of bacteria. Additional sensitivity testing can be done if necessary, to identify which antibiotic will work best to treat the infection.

If your clinician suspects that your kidneys are involved, you may need additional testing, such as an ultrasound, or other diagnostic tests. (If a UTI is left untreated, you could possibly end up in the hospital on intravenous antibiotics.)

Treatment

When you receive a prescription for antibiotics to treat the infection, be sure to take all the pills. Your clinician will determine the length of treatment needed.

Sometimes a urinary tract analgesic may be given. This is a medication that produces a numbing sensation of the urethra (dulls the discomfort). Phenazopyridine is available over-the-counter and popular names you may recognize are AZO and Uristat. You can expect your urine to turn a bright orange color while taking this medication.

A newer medication called Uribel is considered to be a multi-symptom pain relief medication because it contains an analgesic, an antispasmotic, and an antiseptic. This medication can help relieve urinary pain, spasms, and burning.

Drink sufficient water (half your body weight in ounces) and cranberry juice or an extract, which makes your urine more acidic. Remember, bacteria do not like to grow in an acid environment.

NOTE: Be sure to go and see your clinician at the first sign of an infection.

Interstitial Cystitis

Interstitial cystitis (IC) is a painful chronic condition possibly caused by repeated immune system attacks on the bladder lining. Infection and allergic reactions may also play a role in the etiology of this condition. IC is sometimes referred to as "painful bladder syndrome" (PBS).

Recent studies revealed that between 2.7 and 6.53 million women in the United States have symptoms of interstitial cystitis (IC).

IC is often misdiagnosed as a urinary tract infection because the symptoms can be very similar, although urine cultures are usually free of bacteria.

The average age of receiving a diagnosis of "IC" is about 42 years of age. The symptoms can begin as early as 30, and as late as 70 years of age. There may be an association with lower levels of estrogen.

Symptoms

• Pain when urinating and/or generalized pelvic pain that is relieved with voiding (urinating) and recurs with bladder filling.

- Pressure and/or tenderness on or around the bladder (suprapubic tenderness)
- Pain with intercourse

The above listed symptoms may often become worse one week prior to menstruation.

They may also come and go throughout the month and at times may become debilitating for some individuals.

It is important to keep a bladder diary recording the amount you drink and the volume of urine you pass.

Certain foods may aggravate symptoms such as those with a high acid content.

Diagnosis

Making the diagnosis of interstitial cystitis can be challenging and is considered one of exclusion. This means that other gynecologic and/or urologic conditions must be considered first and excluded.

Cystoscopy

A procedure using a scope to visualize the bladder called cystoscopy should be done. Cystoscopy involves an examination of your bladder using a thin tube with a tiny camera (cystoscope) and is inserted through the urethra. This procedure can visualize the bladder walls looking for any microscopic tears or scarring. If you have had a previous infection or infections, scar tissue can form and eventually microscopic tears can occur.

Hydrodistention With Cystoscopy

Hydrodistention may be used with cystoscopy in complicated cases, where the bladder is visualized after the walls of the bladder have been stretched. Hydrodistention is used with caution as this procedure can cause tiny hemorrhages (bleeding) within the bladder wall.

If the above described changes are found with cystoscopy, you could possibly have interstitial cystitis.

Biopsy

During cystoscopy under anesthesia, your doctor may need to remove a sample of tissue (biopsy) from the bladder and/or the urethra to be examined under a microscope. This procedure is done to check for cancer when the tissue shows changes that look suspicious.

Treatment

Unfortunately, there is no cure for this condition. Supportive therapies, patient education, lifestyle modifications and medications have been shown to provide some benefit.

Uribel, as mentioned above in the urinary tract infection section, may provide relief from bladder discomfort associated with this condition.

Lifestyle Modifications

• Decrease your alcohol, coffee, and soda consumption.

• Quit tobacco!

• Decrease consumption of sharp cheeses.

• Avoid artificial sweeteners, preservatives, and acidic foods.

• Avoid dyes in foods and medications.

Physical Therapy

Pelvic floor muscle spasms may be relieved with physical therapy techniques that can relax and lengthen these muscles reducing the discomfort.

Prescription Medications

DMSO (dimethyl sulfoxide) is a prescription medication and a dietary supplement used to treat inflammation. DMSO can be instilled into the bladder through a thin flexible tube (catheter) inserted through the urethra. This solution may be mixed with other medications like lidocaine, which is an anesthetic, to help treat the chronic inflammation and pain associated with interstitial cystitis.

Elmiron (pentosan polysulfate sodium) can be taken by mouth or instilled into the bladder to help repair some of the damage within the walls of the bladder.

Pain Control Therapies

Neuromodulation
TENS Unit (Transcutaneous Electrical Nerve Stimulation) This is a device that uses electrical wires which are placed on your lower back and pelvic region, and electrical pulses are given for minutes to hours in attempt to reduce the discomfort.

Percutaneous Sacral Nerve Root Stimulation (PTNS)
This is another nerve-stimulation treatment. A thin wire is placed

near the sacral nerve in your lower spine which delivers electrical impulses to your bladder in attempt to reduce urinary urgency associated with IC.

Acupuncture is where a practitioner places many tiny needles in your skin at specific points on your body, to relieve pain and other symptoms by rebalancing the flow of life energy.

Biofeedback is a relaxation technique which can help control functions of the autonomic nervous system and has shown some benefit in controlling pain when combined with other treatment modalities.

Other Treatments

Botox

Botox is not an FDA-approved treatment, although it is used by urologists to treat the discomfort associated with IC. Botox is injected directly into the bladder through a needle, and is thought to work by blocking the sensory nerves in the bladder that transmit pain, spasticity and inflammation.

Bladder distension (Hydrodistention) as described above is used with low pressure for a short duration. This procedure may help reduce urinary frequency and discomfort.

Surgery

Laser surgery has been used to treat ulcers (Hunner's ulcers) or patches associated with IC.

Bladder surgical interventions are rarely used and are considered to be the last option in attempt to repair the bladder walls, or in some cases remove the entire bladder.

Urinary Incontinence

Lower levels of estrogen contribute to weakened muscle tone of the urethra, so you can lose bladder control. One in three women over the age of sixty experience some form of urinary incontinence.

The urethra (the tube where urine flows from the bladder out of your body) functions by having greater pressure around the urethra than in the bladder, keeping it closed.

Estrogen helps increase muscle tone and maintains an increased pressure, preventing leakage.

Lower estrogen levels lead to decreased flexibility and elasticity of the muscle fibers, and therefore the urethra is unable to make a tight seal, closing off the bladder. Pregnancies and previous surgeries can make this condition even worse.

> ### Time For A Brain Break!
> Speaking of a tight seal, why did the Walrus go to the Tupperware party?
> *Yes, you guessed, "To find a tight seal!" Ha! Ha!*

If you *laughed*, congratulations, you just raised your serotonin level (the feel good hormone), but my apologies if it made you leak.

If you did experience leakage, you need to see your clinician!

Remember, many women experience some form of urinary incontinence.

Questions To Ask Yourself
- Do you ever leak urine when you cough, sneeze or lift a heavy object?
- How many times a day do you feel the urge to urinate?
- How quickly do you need to get to the bathroom when you feel the urge to urinate?
- Do you ever leak when you feel the urge to urinate?
- How many times do you wake up at night to urinate?
- Do you need to wear a pad to protect your clothing from urine? If you answered yes, how many wet pads do you change daily?
- Do you experience pain when you urinate?
- Do you ever feel that you cannot fully empty your bladder?

Four Major Types Of Incontinence

Total Incontinence
This type of incontinence occurs at any time and in any position. It is typically found in association with anatomical abnormalities such as:
- Congenital defects
- Nerve damage
- After surgery in the pelvic region
- Vesico-vaginal fistulas (an abnormal connection between the bladder and the vagina)

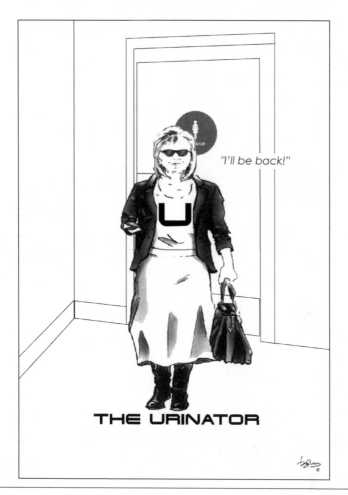

Figure 9.2

Stress Incontinence

This type of incontinence is the most common form and allows small amounts of urine to be lost during a sudden increase in abdominal pressure. Urine may leak when you laugh, exercise, sneeze or cough. This is because the muscle that seals off the bladder fails without warning. Stress is placed on your bladder when pressure is created in your abdomen, such as when laughing or coughing.

This is commonly associated with child bearing, previous trauma, or surgery in the pelvic region.

Stress incontinence occurs in approximately sixty-six percent of postmenopausal women.

Urge Incontinence (Overactive Bladder)

This type of incontinence allows a large amount of urine to be lost when you experience an abrupt urge to urinate "urinary urgency". You feel you have to urinate right now, and are unable to make it to the bathroom without leaking. This type of incontinence is unrelated to a certain position or activity, and is due to spasms or contractions in your bladder.

This type of incontinence can be associated with a more serious medical condition, such as a neurologic disorder, so you need to see your clinician if you experience this symptom.

Overflow Incontinence

This type of incontinence allows a small but nearly continuous amount of urine to be lost. This occurs when you have weak bladder muscle tone or a possible blockage, causing the bladder to become overfilled before the urge to urinate occurs.

Scar tissue formation from a previous infection, trauma or surgery can affect the inner musculature and nerves of the bladder, interfering with a normal signal to urinate.

Women may also experience this type of incontinence following a hysterectomy.

NOTE: Overflow incontinence is more common in males.

Symptoms

• A sudden uncontrollable need to urinate
• An involuntary loss of urine
• Urinating frequently (greater than eight times in twenty-four hours)
• Inability to make it to the bathroom in time

Treatment

Kegel Exercises

These exercises are commonly recommended and work well when you have **stress incontinence** (weakened muscles in the pelvic floor). The pelvic floor muscles and connective tissue form a structure similar to a hammock. These exercises strengthen your pelvic and sphincter muscles surrounding your urethra, and can help reduce some of the symptoms.

How to do Kegel exercises

First identify the correct muscles that help you stop the flow of urine. The use of a water douche may be helpful to confirm the correct muscle use. The muscles that hold the water in are the target muscles to exercise.

Tighten these muscles quickly and then release and rest for about 10 seconds.

Next tighten these same muscles slowly and then release. Make it a goal to hold it for 10 seconds and then release. Try doing 10 repetitions at least three times a day.

Kegel exercises may also help enhance sexual pleasure.

Urinary Devices

Silicone caps

These are rubber caps that are placed over the urethra and apply pressure to the urethral opening. This device must be removed to urinate and has been reported to decrease leakage by approximately fifty percent in women.

Pessaries

Vaginal pessaries are small devices that fit into the vagina and support the neck of the bladder and compress the urethra, preventing leakage. This device is shaped like a ring or a dish, and holds the bladder in place by lifting other organs away from it. This is typically used when you have a prolapsed bladder and/or uterus. You must remove this device and clean it two to three times a week to prevent infection. If you are unable to remove the device then you should schedule an office visit every six to eight weeks for a pessary check and cleaning.

NOTE: *Vaginal inserts need to be fitted by a clinician.*

Acupuncture

This treatment helps improve muscle tone and increases blood flow to the bladder. This may also help you do Kegel exercises correctly.

Bladder Training

This helps you regain control of your bladder by increasing the capacity to hold more urine and overcome the urge to urinate. This also helps lengthen the amount of time between trips to the bathroom. If you make the commitment, you may see results within 4-6 weeks!

Biofeedback
This method of treatment uses audio and visual relaxation techniques to help strengthen the pelvic muscles, which helps improve bladder control.

Pelvic Floor Muscle Exercises With Vaginal Cones Or Weights
Vaginal cones are packaged in a case containing a set of small cones which are the same size and volume although contain different weights. These small weights can help strengthen the muscles, to help you control your bladder flow and are recommended to treat *stress incontinence*. You insert a tampon-like cone into your vagina and hold it as long as you can.

The goal is to gradually increase the weight and amount of time you can hold the cone in place and then release it. A reasonable goal would be about fifteen minutes daily or twice daily. These exercises can be performed in the comfort and privacy of your home.

Apex M is a new over-the-counter FDA approved device to help with urinary incontinence in the privacy of your own home. This device provides gentle muscle stimulation to the pelvic floor muscles for both strengthening and relaxing targeted muscles surrounding your bladder, decreasing symptoms of urinary incontinence. You use the device for ten minutes six days a week until desired results are achieved and then use it once or twice a week for maintenance.

Pelvic Physical Therapy
This treatment includes pelvic massage, relaxation training, biofeedback, bladder training, and home exercises. This therapy has been shown to be effective with some difficult cases.

Electrical Stimulation
Low frequency pulsed electrical shocks are delivered to the pelvic floor muscles, which can reduce bladder contractions and the symptoms of urgency and frequency. These electrical impulses stimulate your pelvic muscles to become stronger and tighter.

Electrical stimulation is often referred to as pelvic floor electrical stimulation (PFES). This procedure places electrodes in the vagina and/or rectum either at a clinic or in the privacy of your own home. An electrical current stimulates the involuntary muscles to contract. A typical session usually lasts 15-20 minutes and is given daily or every other day for several weeks or months.

PFES is used along with pelvic floor muscle exercises and biofeedback therapy to help:

- Identify and isolate the pelvic muscles
- Increase pelvic muscle contraction strength
- Decrease bladder muscle contractions
- Promote normal pelvic muscle relaxation

This method of treatment is used to treat both *urge and stress incontinence.*

Neuromodulation Therapies

Percutaneous Tibial Nerve Stimulation

This outpatient procedure is also referred to as posterior tibial nerve stimulation (PTNS) and is a form of neuromodulation therapy used to treat overactive bladder (OAB). A fine needle electrode is placed near the ankle to stimulate the tibial nerve that goes up your leg to the pelvis. This needle electrode is then connected to an external pulse generator which delivers an adjustable electrical pulse that travels to the sacral plexus (via the tibial nerve), which regulates bladder and pelvic floor function.

A typical session lasts for 30 minutes and is continued for 12 weeks. Patients have reported that urinary leakage was reduced to half the amount they previously experienced after receiving this treatment.

This method of treatment is used to treat *urge incontinence (overactive bladder).*

Sacral Nerve Stimulation

This is another form of modulation therapy where a device similar to a cardiac pacemaker is implanted under the skin near the hip, called a sacral nerve stimulator. This device is programmable and delivers weak electrical impulses stimulating the sacral nerve which influences bladder and surrounding pelvic floor muscle function.

The sacral nerve stimulator device was recently found to also be effective in the treatment of interstitial cystitis.

The FDA has approved the InterStim II device by Medtronic for treatment of *urge incontinence.*

Magnetic Chair Therapy

This procedure involves sitting in a magnetic chair fully clothed and magnetic waves stimulate muscle contractions in the bladder.

A typical session lasts approximately 20 minutes and is given twice weekly for a total of 10 to 20 sessions.

This treatment works by strengthening the pelvic muscles through magnetic stimulation of the nerves, improving urinary control. Complete bladder control has been reported in one-quarter of the patients treated with this procedure.

Emotional Treatment
The brain and bladder are connected!

Gaining an awareness and understanding of hidden fears, anger and reluctance to "let-go" can be very effective in treating incontinence. The Feldenkrals method is a mind-body technique, which can help heal physical conditions by releasing emotional blockages, and can be effective in treating incontinence.

If the above treatment recommendations are ineffective, you may need to consider trying a medication.

Medications
There are a variety of medicines available in pill and gel form which can help prevent leakage by blocking the nerve signals that are responsible for:

• Making the bladder contract at the inappropriate time

• Relaxing the bladder

These medications work by relaxing the smooth muscles of the bladder and decreasing unwanted spasms and involuntary contractions.

Anticholinergic drugs
These medications are in the anticholinergic family of drugs and are used for *urge incontinence (overactive bladder)*. (Anticholinergic medications do have annoying side effects such as a dry mouth.) They have their best effect when combined with behavior therapy such as pelvic floor muscle exercises, healthy lifestyle changes, fluid consumption timing and scheduled toilet trips.

Beta 3-adrenergic agonist drug
A new class of medication is now available which targets a different pathway called the Beta 3-adrenergic receptor pathway.

This medication works by relaxing the detrusor smooth muscle as the bladder is filling, promoting an increased bladder capacity.

The brand name of this medication is *Myrbetriq* and the generic name is *mirabegron.*

Tricyclic antidepressant drugs
These medications can help treat **urge incontinence** by reducing night time urinary leakage.

Hormonal Therapies
Hormone therapy may help boost the immune system and restore hormonal balance.

Estrogen Therapy
Topical estrogen, when applied to the vagina, can help strengthen the sphincter muscles. Topical estrogen therapy is available in ring form, cream and tablets.

Natural estrogen, such as "estriol" when applied to the vaginal wall and near the urethra, can also help improve elasticity and flexibility of the pelvic floor, with minimal systemic absorption. Estrogen cream inserted into the vagina can also help decrease vaginal dryness and hot flashes.

Progesterone Therapy
Progesterone cream can help reduce urinary and vaginal infections by enhancing the sensitivity of estrogen receptors, promoting an improved response to estrogen therapy.

Progesterone is part of our immune defense system that can help prevent bladder infections.

Testosterone Therapy
Testosterone cream in low doses may help improve stretched and weakened tissues. Testosterone is considered the tissue building hormone for ligaments and muscles.

NOTE: You should not use hormone therapy if you have had cancer of the breast or uterus. Consult with your clinician for recommended treatment!

Bulking Agents
These are agents made of synthetic materials, bovine collagen or your own fat which are injected around the urethra or into the base of the bladder. This treatment enables your sphincter muscles to close and hold in urine. This treatment is considered to be minimally invasive and is performed as an outpatient procedure.

If other treatments have been ineffective, you may need to discuss the option of surgery with your clinician.

Surgical Treatment

Most surgeries help *stress incontinence*. If thinning of the bladder tissue is responsible for incontinence, surgery may be the appropriate treatment.

Sling Procedure

A strip of muscle, ligament or tendon from your body is wrapped beneath the urethra to reduce the opening and to help improve closure.

Synthetic material or a mesh can also be used to create a hammock around your bladder neck and urethra.

Burch Suspension Procedure

This procedure can now be performed using a laparoscope as opposed to the traditional open incision surgery. The vagina is sutured to the pelvic ligaments, which provides support to the lower portion of the bladder. This corrects the weakness by not allowing the bladder to move down during a stress activity such as sneezing or coughing. This procedure is used to treat *stress incontinence*.

Bladder Neck Suspension

This surgical procedure involves creating an area of thickened muscle where the bladder connects to the urethra, providing support to the bladder neck and decreasing leakage.

Bladder Cancer

Cancer of the bladder is the most common malignancy of the urinary tract. Most cases are diagnosed between 50 and 70 years of age. The urothelium is the layer of tissue that lines the urethra, bladder, ureters, renal pelvis and the prostate in men.

There are three types of cancer that begin in the cells of the bladder.

Transitional Cell Carcinoma

Most bladder cancers begin in the transitional cells. These cells termed the urothelium line the inside of the bladder. These cells stretch when the bladder is full and shrink when the bladder is empty.

Squamous Cell Carcinoma

These are the thin and flat cells that may form in the bladder urothelium after many years of persistent irritation and infections.

Adenocarcinoma

This type of cancer forms in the glandular cells of the bladder. These cells produce mucus.

Risk Factors For Developing Bladder Cancer

• Using tobacco, especially smoking cigarettes

• Advanced age, 60 years or older

• Males are at higher risk than females

• Exposure to certain chemicals such as coal soot, aniline dyes, textiles and chemicals used when making rubber products

• Employment at a dry cleaner and/or factories where clothes, paper, rope and twine are made

• Drinking water with a high arsenic content

• History of numerous bladder infections

• Long-term use of urinary catheters

• Past treatment with certain chemotherapy agents and/or radiation to the pelvic region

• History of having a kidney transplant

• Being diagnosed with Lynch syndrome (also known as hereditary non-polyposis colorectal cancer or HNPCC). This syndrome is also linked to an increase risk for cancer of the ureters as well.

• Taking a Chinese herb called *A. fang chi*

NOTE: There is not a standard or routine test used currently to screen for bladder cancer.

Signs And Symptoms

Hematuria (red blood cells in the urine). You may notice that your urine looks darker in color, or you may see frank red blood in the toilet bowl after urinating.

Hematuria can be caused by cancer and/or other conditions of the bladder. You need to be seen by your clinician as soon as possible should you experience blood in your urine.

Tests To Identify Bladder Cancer

Urine Sample

The sample of urine is placed under a microscope to look for red blood cells.

Special test strips are also available to dip the urine and it will change color if blood cells are present.

Keep in mind that there may be other non-malignant reasons to have microscopic blood in the urine, including menopause. You need to be examined to determine the cause.

Cytology Of Urine
This is when a sample of urine is placed under a microscope to look for abnormal cells.

Ultrasound
This procedure uses sound waves to take a picture of your bladder, kidneys and urethra.

Cystoscopy
This procedure as discussed earlier in the chapter is used to look inside the bladder and urethra to check for any abnormal tissue, growths and cells.

A thin lighted tube called a cystoscope is inserted through the urethra into the bladder.

Tissue samplings (biopsies) may be taken with this procedure.

A Quick Note On Kidney Cancer
Renal (kidney) cancer is rare and usually affects about 2 percent of the population in the United States, occurring most commonly in the 6th decade of life. It is more commonly seen in males, with a 2 to 1 ratio of males to females.

Advanced age and cigarette smoking are risk factors for developing renal carcinoma.

Patients rarely have symptoms and commonly present with advanced disease at the time of diagnosis. My father passed away from kidney cancer at the age of only 56. Prevention is key so schedule your routine health assessment exams.

Tips For Keeping Your Bladder Healthy

Stay Hydrated
When you don't drink enough water your urine becomes concentrated, which can irritate your bladder. Sufficient fluid intake also flushes

bacteria. Recent studies showed that drinking cranberry juice (preferably with no added sugar) actually helped prevent urinary tract infections. Cranberry juice and/or an extract supplement can lower the ph of urine keeping it more acidic (bacteria prefer a basic or also referred to as an alkaline environment).

Supplements
D-Mannose is a supplement that has been reported to possibly prevent the occurrence of a urinary tract infection. It works by coating the bacteria, thereby preventing it from adhering to the bladder wall and causing an infection.

D-Mannose is now available combined with a cranberry extract which can provide even greater results.

Don't Hold It!
Holding your urine can contribute to stretching and weakening the bladder muscles. You should attempt to urinate 4-8 times a day.

Quit Smoking
Tobacco can alter the tissue cells of the bladder and lead to an increased risk of developing cancer. Prolonged coughing associated with smoking can weaken the pelvic muscles.

Lose Weight
Carrying extra weight can increase the pressure placed on your bladder and surrounding muscles. Losing just 5% of your total weight can reduce leakage by 50%. The greatest benefit is seen when you have stress incontinence.

Make Sure You Urinate Completely
• Try to relax and let it all come out naturally. Do not strain.

• Stand up after urinating and try again to be sure your bladder is empty.

• You can also stand and squat to urinate, which helps strengthen your pelvic floor muscles.

I had better "go" now and practice what I preach—ha! ha!

NOTE: In India, older women who do not wear underwear and squat to urinate have a very low incidence of urinary incontinence.

Avoid Becoming Constipated

Having regular bowel movements prevents strain on the pelvic muscles when passing a bowel movement (BM). If you are constantly straining during BMs, you may weaken the muscles that support your bladder and urethra. Straining can also irritate the nerves that control the bladder, colon and rectum, resulting in an urge to urinate. Drink plenty of water and eat fiber rich foods. Try whole ground flax seed meal, 1-2 tablespoons daily over cereal or salad - it really works! Flax seed can also help reduce your cholesterol and your risk of colon cancer.

Avoid Certain Foods

The following foods can irritate the bladder:

• Caffeine (chocolate, coffee, tea and carbonated beverages such as Coke and Pepsi)

• Alcoholic drinks (wine, beer and hard liquor)

• Acidic foods (tomatoes, citrus, spices and vinegar)

• Artificial sweeteners and corn syrup

Avoid Drinking Any Liquid A Few Hours Before Bed

This can help reduce the number of times you urinate through the night.

Practice Good Hygiene

• Urinate before and after sex.

• Keep clean and practice good hygiene to prevent skin irritations.

• Wipe front to back and do not use perfumed products.

Get Moving And Exercise

If you have **stress incontinence** you may be afraid to exercise due to fear of leakage. Core workouts like Pilates and yoga can help strengthen the pelvic muscles that help with bladder control. Low impact exercises like swimming, biking and walking can also help.

Keep A Bladder Diary

Log on paper how often you urinate, experience leakage, and keep track of your fluid intake.

Bring this diary to your follow-up appointment so you can discuss it with your clinician.

NOTE: Be sure to have your annual check-up, which includes a urinalysis!

Websites for further information on:

Bladder cancer

American Bladder Cancer Society: Bladder Cancer:
https://www.bladdercancersupport.org/

Bladder cancer Symptoms-Mayo Clinic:
https://www.mayoclinic.org/diseases-conditions/bladder-cancer/home/ovc-20308744

Bladder Cancer-Patient Version-National Cancer Institute:
https://www.cancer.gov/types/bladder

What is Bladder Cancer? -American Cancer Society:
https://www.cancer.org/cancer/bladder-cancer.html

Urinary incontinence

Urinary Incontinence-Mayo Clinic:
https://www.mayoclinic.org/diseases-conditions/urinary-incontinence/diagnosis-treatment/expertise-ranking/orc-20326118

Bladder Control Problems in Women (Urinary Incontinence)-National Institute of Health:
https://www.niddk.nih.gov/health-information/urologic-diseases/bladder-control-problems-women

Urinary Tract Infections

Urinary Tract Infection (UTI)-Mayo Clinic:
http://www.mayoclinic.org/diseases-conditions/urinary-tract-infection/basics/definition/con-20037892

Urinary tract infection in women-self-care: MedlinePlus:
https://medlineplus.gov/ency/patientinstructions/000391.htm

Chapter 10

DIABETES AND MENOPAUSE

Definition

Diabetes is a group of diseases associated with high levels of sugar circulating throughout the body. When we eat food, it is converted to sugar known as *glucose* and this is our body's main source of energy. When sugar is unable to enter the cells to create energy, it will continue circulating through the bloodstream affecting all that it comes in contact with. This disease process can result in damage to many different body systems and functions.

Insulin

Insulin is a hormone that is needed to convert sugar, starches and other food into energy needed for daily life. Insulin is a carrier, somewhat like a truck that delivers its load of sugar to its destination, your body's cells. It then acts like a key fitting into a lock (known as a cell receptor) on a variety of cells in your body. When the connection between insulin and the cell receptor is working, the door to the cell opens allowing sugar from your bloodstream to flow in and be converted into energy. If the door to the cell does not open, sugar builds up in your bloodstream causing damage and then begins spilling into the urine.

Pancreas

The *pancreas* is a gland located behind your stomach that contains beta cells which are responsible for making and releasing insulin. Beta cells function by delivering just the right amount of insulin at the correct time to keep the blood sugar level normal.

Insulin Response After Eating A Meal

After ingesting a meal your blood sugar normally goes up, and a healthy insulin response returns it back down to a normal range (approximately 70-110mg/dl), within two hours. One of the first defects to develop in diabetes is the failure to bring this number down to normal within that 2 hour window.

Insulin Resistance

When you have insulin resistance, your body's cells have a decreased ability to respond to the action of the hormone insulin. The ability of your cells to respond to insulin is called *insulin sensitivity*. This sensitivity declines early in the development of diabetes and your pancreas produces more insulin to try and compensate. This may work for a while but then the cells become more and more resistant and the pancreas works harder and harder until it eventually burns out. The more overweight you are, the *more resistant* the cells become to insulin and the *less sensitivity* you have for insulin and its effects.

How Insulin Resistance Develops

Today many of the calories consumed in our daily diet come from carbohydrates, most being simple carbohydrates, sugars that quickly enter the blood stream. The pancreas has to work overtime to keep the level of glucose from skyrocketing out of control in the bloodstream. The cells of the pancreas eventually tire out and can no longer crank out the high levels of insulin required. At the same time the cells are not accepting insulin the way that they should. They are *resistant* to insulin knocking at the door. This is what we call *insulin resistance* which usually leads to diabetes. This process can occur for years prior to being detected as diabetes.

NOTE: Some individuals have a genetic predisposition to develop insulin resistance.

Signs Of Insulin Resistance

If you have been diagnosed with high blood pressure, elevated triglycerides and/or cholesterol, you should be checked for insulin resistance, regardless of your weight, as it is often associated with these conditions. The following can be associated with insulin resistance.

• *An impaired fasting blood sugar or an impaired glucose tolerance test.*

• *High blood pressure:* Studies show a link between high blood pressure and insulin resistance. The higher the blood pressure the worse the insulin resistance.

• *Abnormal cholesterol levels:* The typical abnormal cholesterol levels found in an individual with insulin resistance are a low HDL (good cholesterol) and a high level of triglycerides (fat in the blood). We are now also looking at the non-HDL level which is often elevated.

• *Heart disease:* Insulin resistance can promote atherosclerosis (hardening of the arteries) and increase the risk for developing blood clots.

• *Obesity:* Obesity plays a major role in the development of insulin resistance, especially with abdominal fat or belly fat. Obesity promotes insulin resistance and decreases insulin's responsiveness (insulin sensitivity).

NOTE: Insulin resistance will lead to diabetes if left untreated!

Insulin Resistance And Hormonal Imbalance

The hormone fluctuations that occur during perimenopause and menopause can interfere with maintaining good blood glucose control.

During perimenopause, when a woman has more testosterone in proportion to the declining levels of estrogen and progesterone production, she may be at risk for *insulin resistance* and blood sugar problems.

• Too much testosterone combined with an estrogen deficiency increases your risk of becoming *insulin resistant.*

- Low estrogen and progesterone levels typically found in peri-menopause and menopause can cause sleep deprivation, which can also promote *insulin resistance.*

Menopause And Fat Distribution

As women approach perimenopause and menopause, they find it difficult to lose weight and can become *intolerant of carbohydrates.* This often occurs due to less exercise and increased abdominal fat called sarcopenia (decreased lean muscle mass that naturally occurs as we age). The extra weight tends to migrate around the waist, referred to as truncal obesity. Some women deposit more fat around their waistline due to an inherited body shape, referred to as an *apple* body type. Apple-shaped women tend to show less sensitivity to insulin and its affects.

Women who have insulin resistance have a problem with fat metabolism. The cells in your body are not absorbing the excess glucose (sugar) and the liver turns it into fat. You not only gain weight, but your cells are starving for glucose. The sugar is circulating in the blood instead of entering the cells to be turned into energy. You feel tired and tend to eat carbohydrate-rich foods in search of energy. What a catch 22! These extra fat cells can make estrogen (estrone) causing *estrogen dominance,* which can produce many perimeno-pausal symptoms. (I discuss estrogen dominance in further detail in Chapter 2.)

Women who are *insulin resistant* are at greater risk for developing diabetes, hypertension (high blood pressure), heart disease, high cholesterol, breast cancer and polycystic ovarian disease.

Over time, individuals with *insulin resistance* develop high blood sugars and/or eventually diabetes.

Preventing Insulin Resistance

If you make lifestyle changes to include a healthy diet, proper sleep and exercise you may be able to prevent insulin resistance.

- Try exercising and just walk 30 minutes a day five times a week. You can divide the 30 minutes into smaller increments if needed, such as three 10 minute sessions or two 15 minute sessions. Try whatever will work best for your schedule.
- Try to maintain a healthy weight.

- Try to eat smaller meals every three hours or six times a day.
- Try to get at least eight hours of restful sleep per night.

Hyperinsulinemia

This term refers to high levels of insulin in the bloodstream. This process occurs early in the disease due to the demand for sugar by the body's cells. Remember that the cells are not letting insulin and sugar enter normally, so the pancreas continually receives messages from the cells saying that they are sugar deficient. The poor pancreas tries to increase production not realizing that there is a problem at the cellular level.

Prediabetes

Prediabetes (now referred to as "increased risk for diabetes" by the American College of Endocrinology, ACE) is defined as an *impaired fasting glucose* and/or *impaired glucose tolerance,* which typically may *not* have any symptoms.

About 79 million Americans over the age of 19 now have prediabetes. The rate of prediabetes and diabetes is even higher in many racial and ethnic minorities. This represents about 30% of Americans and these statistics are quite alarming.

You are considered to have *prediabetes* when your fasting blood glucose (sugar) levels consistently fall in the range of 100mg/dl to 125 mg/dl. Prediabetes raises your risk for developing Type 2 diabetes, heart disease and stroke. *Further detail to follow in the diagnosis of diabetes section.*

> *NOTE: We need to increase the awareness of this condition, so that we can prevent diabetes from ever occurring and treat those who already have the disease early to help prevent complications. New recommendations for treatment of prediabetes include diet, exercise and possibly a medication called metformin.*

Diabetes

Type 1 Diabetes

This type of diabetes (previously called juvenile diabetes) is typically found in children and young adults, although it can start at any age. This condition begins when the beta cells that produce insulin are damaged and do not produce insulin, so you have to take insulin on a regular basis. This is not necessarily diet related.

Type 2 Diabetes

This type of diabetes occurs when your body is unable to make a sufficient amount of insulin or if your body's cell receptors for insulin aren't working well (resistant to insulin's signal). This type of diabetes (previously called "adult-onset diabetes") is the most common form of diabetes.

- Type 2 diabetes is on the rise and more than 20 million individuals in the US currently have it. Many more individuals are expected to develop this disease in the next 20 to 30 years.
- Type 2 diabetes can run in families and is increasingly being diagnosed in children and young adults. This disease is commonly found in individuals who are overweight.
- Type 2 diabetes is not just a problem with blood sugar but can affect blood pressure, cholesterol and triglycerides (fats in the blood), blood clotting and cause inflammation in the body.

Gestational Diabetes

This is another form of diabetes which occurs during pregnancy.

Pregnancy is thought of as a "stress test" for females predisposed to developing diabetes later in life. A blood sugar test is typically done between the 24th and 28th week of pregnancy to screen for gestational diabetes. This form of diabetes occurs in approximately 5% of all pregnancies. Recent studies show that children born to mothers with gestational diabetes tend to become obese.

Organs Affected By Diabetes

Pancreas: Insulin production decreases as the pancreas gets tired of putting out so much insulin.

Liver: Receives a message to produce extra sugar called glycogen and then dumps it into your bloodstream.

Gastrointestinal System: Hormones that regulate your appetite and sense of feeling full after a meal are impaired by the disease, resulting in increased hunger.

Genitourinary: The high sugar content in the blood causes increased thirst and urination. Kidney function can become impaired which can lead to failure if untreated. *Diabetes is the leading cause of kidney failure!*

Cells: All the body's cells including muscle tissue become less responsive to insulin and sugar does not enter the cells, resulting in fatigue.

Arteries: High sugar levels in the bloodstream promote build-up of plaque in the artery walls increasing the risk for developing a stroke, heart attack and/or peripheral vascular disease. Plaque build-up in the extremities may cause pain, loss of sensation and in some cases even amputation of a limb.

Eyes: High blood sugar causes blurred vision and can lead to blindness if untreated! Diabetes is the leading cause of new cases of blindness among adults ages 20 to 74!

Nervous system: The continued high sugar content in the blood causes mild to severe forms of nervous system damage resulting in decreased sensation, numbness and tingling in the extremities called peripheral neuropathy.

Brain: Diabetes is considered a risk factor for developing vascular dementia which is caused by reduced or blocked blood flow to the brain. New research has found a possible link between type 2 diabetes and Alzheimer's dementia. This is thought to be associated with the complex ways that type 2 diabetes affects the ability of the brain and other body tissues to use sugar (glucose) and respond to insulin.

Skin: The continued high sugar content in the blood eventually causes damage to skin and can result in numerous infections.

Complications Associated With Diabetes
When your blood sugar is not in balance and remains elevated, damage can occur to both the large and small blood vessels in your body. These complications are classified into two categories:

• *When small vessels are affected:* Diabetes can damage small blood vessels in the eyes, nerves and kidneys. This can lead to blindness, loss of sensation in hands and feet and kidney failure. These are serious complications and can lead to the loss of a limb or even a possible amputation.

• *When large blood vessels are affected:* Diabetes can damage large blood vessels causing "hardening of the arteries" (atherosclerosis) that feed your heart, brain and body. These complications are very serious and can cause a heart attack and/or stroke, which is the major cause of disability and death in the diabetic population.

The Link Between Menopause And Diabetes
Women approaching menopause are at risk for developing insulin resistance due to metabolic changes associated with fluctuating hormone levels, such as a decline in estrogen.

- Women typically gain five to 10 pounds during menopause which can increase your risk of developing type 2 diabetes.

- Gaining extra abdominal fat carries a greater risk of developing type 2 diabetes than if the fat was distributed in other areas of the body.

- Symptoms of type 2 diabetes and menopause can be similar, such as feelings of fatigue and not sleeping well.

- Sleep deprivation can slow down your metabolism promoting more weight gain. Not getting enough sleep can also result in *insulin resistance* which can lead to the development of Type 2 diabetes. The hormones that regulate hunger and satiety (feeling full after a meal) are also affected by the length and quality of your sleep. When you feel tired, you tend to eat more in search of energy. The hormone *leptin* is responsible for telling you to stop eating when you are full. When you do not get enough sleep, leptin does not work properly and you continue to eat.

- Sometimes menopausal women who have diabetes (especially if they have recently been diagnosed) may confuse the signs of menopause with some of the signs of low or high blood sugar. Dizziness, fatigue, sweating, vision changes, feeling irritable and finding it difficult to concentrate can all be signs of both menopause and diabetes. Testing the blood sugar will help to determine if your glucose is under control.

- In type 2 diabetes, fluctuating hormone levels during perimenopause and menopause can cause fluctuations in blood sugar levels and testing more frequently may be necessary.

- In type 1 diabetes, declining hormone levels associated with perimenopause and menopause may lower blood sugar levels and frequent insulin adjustments may be necessary.

Screening For Diabetes
Many women with type 2 diabetes have **no** symptoms or any warning signs and may not find out they have it until they develop a complication like heart disease.

All women ages 45 and older should be screened for diabetes every three years or earlier if you have any of the diabetes risk factors outlined below.

Risk Factors For Developing Diabetes

- A positive family history or type 2 diabetes in a parent or sibling.
- If you are one of the following racial or ethnic groups:
  - African American
  - Alaska Native
  - Asian American
  - Hispanic and Latin American
  - South Pacific Islander
- If you are over age 45
- If you are overweight and do not exercise regularly
- If you have signs of *insulin resistance* or conditions associated with *insulin resistance* such as high blood pressure, elevated triglycerides (fats) and/or non-HDL and low HDL cholesterol.
- Women who have had gestational diabetes or a baby weighing nine pounds or more at birth.

Signs And Symptoms

Type 1 Diabetes

- Frequent urination
- Unusual thirst
- Extreme hunger
- Unusual weight loss despite increased appetite
- Extreme fatigue and irritability
- Often presents with an onset of infection
- Possible loss of consciousness (fainting) or even coma

Type 2 Diabetes

- Any of the above symptoms listed for Type 1 diabetes
- Frequent infections
- Blurred vision
- Cuts or bruises that heal slowly

- Tingling and/or numbness sensation in the hands and feet
- Recurring skin, gum and/or bladder infections

NOTE: Many individuals may not have any symptoms!

Type 2 Diabetes Can Be Prevented

Making changes in your lifestyle such as healthy eating; increasing physical activity and losing weight have been shown to help prevent type 2 diabetes.

Clinical trials have shown that losing just 5-7% of your body weight (about 10-14 pounds, if you weigh 200 pounds) along with at least two and a half hours of moderate exercise per week, can reduce the risk of developing type 2 diabetes by 60%.

Hormones Which Help Control Blood Sugar

CAUTION: This section contains detailed information for those individuals who have been diagnosed with, or are at risk, for developing diabetes.

GLP-1

When we eat food, a hormone called *GLP-1* is made in the stomach. This hormone slows down the emptying of food from the stomach by telling your brain you are no longer hungry and it helps the pancreas make the right amount of insulin. This hormone also helps regulate the amount of sugar that is made by the liver, keeping blood sugar in balance.

Glucagon

Glucagon is the hormone that tells the liver to release stored sugar when the blood sugar drops too low.

NOTE: These hormones work together to keep your blood sugar in balance.

Know The Numbers For Making The Diagnosis

Prediabetes

The diagnosis of *prediabetes* according to a 2010 publication from the American Diabetes Association is made when one of the following is present:

- A fasting blood sugar result of 100 mg/dL to 125 mg/dL

- A hemoglobin A1C result between 5.7% to 6.4%

- A two hour blood sugar result between 140 mg/dL to 199 mg/dL during an oral glucose tolerance blood test

NOTE: Remember, you may not have any symptoms when your blood sugar is at these levels.

Diabetes

The diagnosis of *diabetes* according to this 2010 publication from the American Diabetes Association is made when one of the following is present:

- Two fasting blood sugar results greater than or equal to 126 mg/dL on different days

- A hemoglobin A1C result greater than or equal to 6.5%

- A non-fasting (random) blood sugar result greater than or equal to 200 mg/dL with symptoms

- A two hour blood sugar result greater than 200mg/dL during an oral glucose tolerance test

A Hemoglobin A1C Blood Test

When you have been diagnosed with diabetes your endocrinologist or primary care clinician will order a hemoglobin A1C blood test to monitor your treatment.

An A1C test represents the attachment of glucose (sugar) to hemoglobin (the oxygen-carrying protein in our red blood cells). Think of it this way, the hemoglobin molecule and the sugar in the blood are attracted to each other but are a little shy and take time, up to 3 months, to actually hook up together. By measuring how many of them are "married" together at any time, you can determine how long they've been exposed to each other and how much sugar has been present as indicated by how many hemoglobin/sugar "pairs" are counted at the time of the test. The average life of a red blood cell is about three to four months. The hemoglobin A1C blood test can measure your average sugar level for the past 3 to 4 months.

This test is very useful in that it "tells the truth" about the average amount of sugar in the blood and is less influenced by what you did or didn't eat prior to the blood test.

The American Association of Clinical Endocrinologists recommends your treatment target level be at 6.5% or less for healthy individuals. *Please see treatment of diabetes section for further details.*

An A1C level of 5.6% or less is considered to be normal. A border-line A1C level is 5.7% to 6.4% (prediabetes). An A1C level of 6.5% or greater is consistent with having diabetes.

Lowering your A1C level to 7% or less has shown to help reduce the risk of developing complications associated with diabetes as outlined below. *Please see Treatment of Diabetes section for further detail on new treatment guidelines from the American Association of Clinical Endocrinologists, AACE.*

NOTE: An A1C test should not be used in pregnancy and/or if you have been diagnosed with a vitamin B12 deficiency, iron deficiency and/or thalassemia. If you have any other bleeding disorders, kidney disease, liver disease or any recent blood loss, this test will not be accurate.

Diabetes And Heart Disease

Insulin resistance paves the way for developing type 2 diabetes and is a strong risk factor for developing heart disease. I discuss heart disease in great detail in Chapter 5.

Diabetics develop *atherosclerosis* (the build-up of fatty substances like cholesterol), which is plaque formation adhering to the inner lining of their arteries. A blood clot can develop where plaque has formed in the arteries and cause a partial or total blockage, resulting in a stroke or heart attack and sometimes even sudden death.

Postmenopausal women may have a higher level of homocysteine, which is an unstable protein (toxic amino acid molecule) that makes your arteries sticky, allowing cholesterol to adhere to the artery walls, promoting plaque buildup.

Consuming foods rich in B vitamins (B-6 and B-12) and/or taking a daily supplement of these vitamins, may help decrease homocysteine levels. Fruits, vegetables, fish and nuts (almonds and walnuts) are all rich in B vitamins.

NOTE: Consumption of red meat has been associated with elevated homocysteine levels.

Risk Factors For Developing Heart Disease In Women

- A positive family history of heart disease
- History of insulin resistance, metabolic syndrome and/or diabetes
- A positive history of smoking (past or present)
- High blood pressure (hypertension)
- Elevated lipids (including non-HDL and LDL-P)
- Obesity and inactivity
- Protein detectable in your urine (also called albumin)
- Age 30 years and older

The presence of *a single risk factor at 50 years of age* is associated with a substantially increased lifetime absolute risk for developing cardio-vascular heart disease and a shorter duration of survival.

Chapter 5 outlines further detail on cardiac risk factors and heart disease.

Ask Yourself These Four Questions:

- Have you been diagnosed with diabetes or high blood pressure?
- Are you overweight, obese and never exercise?
- Do you consume an unhealthy diet?
- Do you currently or have you smoked in the past?

If you answered yes to any or all the above questions, you may have atherosclerosis (thickening or hardening of the artery walls), which is a major cause of heart disease.

NOTE: Three out of every four women with diabetes are unaware of the connection between diabetes and heart disease.

Women with diabetes are four times more likely to develop heart disease and have a heart attack. Heart disease is the leading cause of death in diabetics and the number one killer of women! Please see Chapter 5 for more detailed information on heart disease.

Treatment Of Diabetes

There is *no* cure for diabetes, although it can be controlled with proper treatment.

Controlling your blood sugar early and aggressively may help preserve your insulin producing cells in the pancreas (beta cells), slowing the progression of diabetes. Typically by the time you are diagnosed with diabetes, almost half of the beta cell function is gone and over time may progress to the point where insulin is needed. The goal of treatment is to keep your blood sugar level within a normal range and prevent complications. It is a good idea to buy a home monitor device so you know what your numbers are. The goal of treatment numbers should be:

- The ADA now recommends an A1C treatment goal of 7.0% for most Type 2 diabetics. The AACE recommends a target A1C of less than or equal to 6.5% to minimize diabetes-related complications in otherwise healthy individuals not at risk for hypoglycemia (low blood sugar).

- The ADA suggests a target A1C of closer to 8.0% for individuals with any of the following: History of severe hypoglycemia (low blood sugar), a limited life expectancy, advanced microvascular and macrovascular complications and multiple other illnesses.

- A glucose reading before meals (preprandial glucose) to be between 90 and 130 mg/dl

- A glucose reading after a meal (postprandial glucose) to be less than 180 mg/dl

You should check your blood sugar:

- When you wake up in the morning
- Before meals or a large snack
- Before and after physical activity
- 90 minutes to two hours after eating

You should keep a log of your blood sugar results and take it with you when you see your clinician.

You can learn to check your urine for ketones, which is a sign that your body is using stored fat for energy instead of glucose. This process occurs when not enough insulin is available and more commonly found in association with type 1 diabetes.

Blood Pressure Control

Try to maintain a normal blood pressure of 130/80.

Lipid (Cholesterol) Management

LDL-C Cholesterol Levels

Keep your **LDL-C** at less than 100 mg/dL for those with diabetes and a moderate cardiovascular (CVD) risk and/or are less than 40 years of age.

Keep your **LDL-C** at less than 70 mg/dL if you have diabetes, cardiovascular disease or major CVD risk, family history of CVD, hypertension (high blood pressure), a low HDL-C and/or are a smoker.

Non-HDL-C Cholesterol Levels

Keep at less than 130 mg/dL for those with diabetes and a moderate cardiovascular risk and/or age less than 40.

Keep at less than 100 mg/dL if you have diabetes, cardiovascular disease or major cardiovascular risk, family history of CVD, hypertension, a low HDL-C and/or are a smoker.

Triglyceride Level

Keep your *triglyceride* level less than 150 mg/dL and 100 mg/dL would be even better.

TC/HDL-C (triglyceride to HDL) Ratio

Keep your *TC/HDL-C (triglyceride to HDL ratio)* at less than 3.5 if have diabetes, cardiovascular disease or major CVD risk, family history of CVD, hypertension, a low HDL-C and/or are a smoker.

ApoB Levels

Keep your *ApoB* level at less than 90 mg/dL for those with diabetes, moderate CVD risk and/or less than age 40.

Keep your *ApoB* level at less than 80 if you have diabetes, cardiovascular disease or major CVD risk, family history of CVD, hypertension, a low HDL-C and/or are a smoker.

LDL-P Levels

Keep your **LDL-P** level at less than 1,200 mmol/L (millimoles per litre) for those with diabetes and a moderate CVD risk and/or age less than 40.

Keep your **LDL-P** level at less than 1,000 mmol/L, if you have diabetes, cardiovascular disease or major CVD risk, family history of CVD, hypertension, low-HDL-C and/or are a smoker.

Keeping these numbers within this range can help prevent heart disease! *You will find further detail on heart disease and lipids (cholesterol) in Chapter 5.*

Diet, exercise and weight control are also very important in the treatment of diabetes.

Weight loss along with a balanced diet and regular exercise may:
• Prevent diabetes from ever developing
• Prevent progression to full blown diabetes
• Delay the onset of diabetes
• Reverse prediabetes

Diet Recommendations
Try eating a healthy diet consisting of:
• 7 to 13 servings of fruits and vegetables daily
• Complex carbohydrates (beans, whole grains and low fat dairy products)
• Choose brown over white carbohydrates, which can help you achieve glycemic (glucose) control
• Less sweets and starchy foods (they raise your blood sugar level)
• High fiber (25-50 grams a day), which can help control your blood sugar by slowing down sugar absorption
• Sufficient daily water intake (drink half your body weight in ounces of water daily) unless you have a medical condition that requires fluid restriction. Consult your clinician to be certain! Water helps rid the body of toxins and can promote weight loss. Remember, hunger can be a sign of dehydration.
• Eat six small meals a day, follow the American Diabetic Association (ADA) diet and become aware of the glycemic index. (Glycemic index discussion to follow.) Your clinician will determine the number of daily calories you will need to lose weight and achieve your ideal body weight.

- Avoid salty snacks, processed foods and fatty foods (saturated and trans-fats). Limit saturated fat intake to less than 7% of the total daily calories.
- Eat fresh, not processed from a box.
- Work with a registered dietician and/or a certified diabetes educator to help guide with meal planning and teach you how to stay healthy.
  - An insulin controlled diet (slow release sugar foods), such as fruits and vegetables help lower the insulin response.
  - Excess insulin promotes fat storage. *Insulin is a fat storage hormone. A high level of insulin takes your sugar and processed food calories and locks them into fat cells.*

Please read the following section on glycemic index and diet tips to help you lose weight.

The Glycemic Index

The glycemic index is an important factor to consider and can help you lose weight. Not all carbohydrate foods behave the same way in our body. The glycemic index describes this difference by ranking carbohydrates according to their effect on our blood sugar (glucose) levels.

The glycemic index measures the amount of glucose in an individual's blood after consuming foods containing carbohydrates. This value is measured using real people and real food and commonly referred to as the GI index.

Each volunteer is fed a serving of food containing 50 grams of carbohydrate and then monitored continuously to determine what effect the food has on their blood sugar. The blood sugar is measured every 15 minutes over a three hour period and the food is given an index number. The reference food used is white bread containing 50 grams of carbohydrate which equals 100. Each food's glycemic index is compared to white bread.

- Foods that break down quickly produce a fast and high blood sugar response.
- Foods that break down slowly release glucose (blood sugar) gradually into the bloodstream.
- Foods with a GI index of greater than 70 have a high glycemic index.
- Foods with a GI index of less than 55 have a low glycemic index.

NOTE: The body requires less insulin to process low glycemic index foods. Consuming less glucose means less insulin is needed, which translates to less fat around your waist.

The glycemic index represents the impact that various carbohydrates (sugars) have on blood sugar levels and the insulin response. Remember, the higher the GI index the greater the glucose and insulin response.

Examples Of Foods With A High GI Index

White bread	100
Bagel	72
Watermelon	72
Saltine crackers	74
French fries	75
Gatorade	78
Potatoes, mashed	86

Examples Of Foods With A Low GI Index

Yogurt, non-fat	14
Yogurt, non-fat (flavored)	33
Oatmeal (old fashioned)	49
Carrots	49
Chocolate	49
Sourdough bread	52

If you graze on small portions of low-glycemic-index foods throughout the day you will receive a constant low level source of glucose (energy) and your body will not need a lot of insulin, avoiding a large spike.

Skipping meals and then eating a large meal once a day makes the body think it is starving, promoting food storage which can become fat.

How Large Spikes Of Glucose Make You Gain Weight

Your pancreas is the organ that makes insulin, which keeps your glucose (blood sugar) in a normal range. This would be easy to do if we ate the way our cavemen ancestors did, only free range meat and fresh vegetation. Unfortunately, many of us consume large amounts of refined sugars and starches and the pancreas has to work hard to keep up.

If you have insulin resistance, your pancreas has to make about six times more insulin to get the job done. When your pancreas repeatedly has to make high levels of insulin, it eventually becomes exhausted and diabetes can develop.

Excessive insulin secretion makes your body store calories as fat.

How Your Body Reacts To Refined Carbohydrates And Starches
Refined carbohydrates and starches travel only a short distance down your digestive tract before being absorbed into your bloodstream. They never make it far enough down the intestine to encounter the "appetite suppressing hormones" which signal the brain we have food, so stop eating.

When you eat starch only a small amount turns into glucose (sugar) in your mouth that you can taste, and the remaining amount heads to your intestines without even encountering your taste buds. Starch then immediately breaks down into glucose once it's in the stomach and this process encourages weight gain.

Believe it or not, sugar you can taste causes less weight gain than sugar you can't taste. You would be better off having a small piece of 72% organic cocoa chocolate to satisfy your sweet tooth than a piece of bread.

NOTE: Refined carbohydrates and starches, referred to as "bad carbs" are unnatural foods and behave unnaturally in our bodies.

The more "bad" carbs we eat the fatter we become and this is particularly true in midlife and beyond. The reason low-carb diets work is because they restrict refined carbohydrates, not carbohydrates in general. In fact, the more fruits and vegetables you eat the less likely you will become overweight. You will feel a lot better too.

Exercise
Regular exercise can:
• Lower insulin levels and enhance insulin function
• Help protect your bones by increasing your bone density
• Help protect your heart by raising the good cholesterol (HDL) and lowering the bad cholesterol (LDL)
• Help lower the risk of heart attack and stroke
• Help you lose fat and maintain a healthy weight
• Help lower your risk for developing diabetes by 58% if you lose 7 percent of your body weight (15 pounds if you weigh 200 pounds)

Individuals with diabetes should exercise at least thirty minutes a day, five days a week. The exercise should be (moderate-intensity) aerobic physical activity and 50% to 70% of your maximum heart rate, unless your clinician tells you otherwise. This should include resistance training three times a week. You may divide it up into two 15 minute sessions or three 10 minute sessions. You can start slow and work up to 30 minutes. Try beginning with 5 minutes and add a minute each day and within a month you will achieve a 30 minute session. Please refer to Chapter 3 in the exercise section to determine how to calculate your target heart rate during exercise.

After age 35, the average woman loses one half a pound of muscle and gains one pound of fat per year. By the age of 55 she will have lost 10 pounds of muscle and gained 20 pounds of fat. Yikes!

• Fat is not metabolically active tissue because it does not burn calories like muscle.

• One pound of fat burns only two calories in 24 hours.

• One pound of muscle burns forty calories in 24 hours, even if you are sleeping. Wow!

NOTE: Weight loss and exercise are potent agents in helping to achieve good glucose control. Some patients have been able to discontinue their medications with just these lifestyle measures alone!

Medications
It is often necessary for many type 2 diabetics to include a non-insulin medication along with healthy dietary changes and exercise to help control their blood sugar.

We are now recommending that some prediabetic individuals begin medication early on along with lifestyle interventions to help prevent serious long term complications.

Medications To Help Lower Blood Sugar
The three types of medications commonly used to treat type 2 diabetes are oral pills, injectable medicines and insulin. These different types of medications work in different ways to help control blood sugar. Combination pills are also available that have two different medications in one tablet and injectable medications are available to help control blood sugar. Two new combination injectable medications which contain long acting insulin were just released.

Oral Diabetes Medication By Class

Secretagogues

These drugs increase the insulin output from the pancreas.

One older class of medication, known as **sulfonylureas,** helps the beta cells in the pancreas to release more insulin when the sugar level rises, like after a meal. Common brand names you may recognize are DiaBeta, Micronase and Glynase (glyburide), Glipizide (glucotrol) and Amaryl (glimepiride). Unfortunately, this class of medication can cause hypoglycemia (low blood sugar) and your pancreas to burn out sooner.

Another class of medication, known as **meglitinides,** help the pancreas produce insulin and are often referred to as short acting secretagogues. Common brand names you may recognize are Prandin (repaglinide) and Starlix (nateglinide).

Biguanides

Metformin is the only medication available in this category and is used to treat prediabetes and diabetes. Brand names you may recognize are Glucophage, Glucophage XR, Glumetza, Riomet and Fortamet. Metformin has a dual mechanism of action:

• Decreases the amount of sugar being released from the liver, therefore decreasing the sugar in the blood.

• Helps the body use insulin more efficiently by increasing the tissue sensitivity to insulin.

CAUTION: It is recommended that you not use this medication in patients with impaired kidney function and that you stop taking metformin 48 hours before having any radiologic study that is performed using contrast media.

Alpha-Glucosidase Inhibitors

These medications work by slowing the digestion of starch in the small intestine, so that glucose from starch enters the bloodstream slowly. Your body is given more time to store extra sugar lowering the level of sugar in your bloodstream.

Brand names you may recognize are Precose (acarbose) and Glyset (miglitol).

Dipeptidyl Peptidase-4 (DPP-4 Inhibitors)

These medications are also referred to as gliptins and they block the action of dipeptidyl peptidase 4 (DPP-4), reducing the level of the hormone glucagon. Glucagon increases blood glucose levels.

The mechanism of DPP-4 inhibitors is to increase incretin levels (GLP-1 and GIP), which prevents the release of glucagon from the liver and increases insulin production from the pancreas, lowering blood glucose levels. This action also slows down gastric emptying and helps promote satiety (helps you feel full after a meal).

This class of medications may help slow down the loss of beta cell function in the pancreas that occurs as diabetes progresses.

Common brand names you may recognize are Januvia (sitagliptin), Onglyza (saxagliptin) and Tradjenta (linagliptin). This class of medication has a low risk of causing hypoglycemia (low blood sugar).

Thiazolidinediones

These medications are referred to as T-Z-Ds or glitazones and work by making the body more sensitive to insulin, allowing glucose to enter the cells for use more effectively. These medications also prevent release of glucose from the liver and help insulin to work better in muscle and fat, decreasing the amount of sugar in the blood.

Common brand names you may recognize are Avandia (rosiglitazone) and Actos (pioglitazone). This class of medication has been associated with serious adverse events such as heart failure, heart attack, stroke and liver failure.

Sodium-Glucose Co-Transporter 2 (Sglt2) Inhibitors (Relatively New FDA Approved Type 2 Diabetes Drug Class)

The names of these medications are Invokana (canaglifozin), Farxiga (dapagliflozin) and Jardiance (empagliflozin).

- These medications work by blocking the action of sodium-glucose co-transporter 2 (SGLT2), which is responsible for directing reabsorption of glucose (sugar) by the kidney. This blocking action of SGLT2 increases excretion (elimination) of the excess sugar in the urine.

- These drugs should not be used in Type 1 diabetics or in individuals with severe kidney disease.

- Your clinician will do blood tests to check your kidney function before you begin therapy and during treatment.
- The most common side effect seen in women who are taking this medication is a vaginal yeast infection.

Other Injectable Medications For Type 2 Diabetes

These non-insulin medications given by subcutaneous (under the skin) injections are administered using a small pen device.

Incretin Mimetics

This class of drugs referred to as the GLP-1 injectables or incretins, work similarly to the hormone GLP-1 by helping the beta cells in the pancreas make more insulin when the sugar level rises. These medicines slow down the digestive process of food, leaving food in the stomach longer, increasing the release of insulin. You also have a sense of feeling full while on these medications which helps with weight loss and can be a real plus.

Byetta (exenatide), Tanzeum (albiglutide) and Victoza (liraglutide) are the names of these injectable medications commonly administered once or twice daily.

New extended-release forms that are given only once a week are now available. Bydureon (exenatide long acting) and Trulicity (dulaglutide), both given only once a week, can be a real benefit for some patients.

Amylin Mimetics

The only medication in this class is called Symlin (pramlintide acetate) and is used to treat type 1 and type 2 diabetes. This medication works like the hormone amylin in the body:

- Increases insulin production
- Slows down digestion which reduces appetite
- Decreases the production of glucose made by the liver

NOTE: Many patients may need to take more than one type of medication to help maintain control of their blood sugar level. Remember, there are now combination medications available in pill and injectable form.

Insulin

Insulin is an important hormone made by the pancreas and is also used as a medication to treat diabetes. Insulin is now made to be genetically just like human insulin and no longer derived from just pork (porcine) and beef (bovine).

- Type 1 diabetics require lifelong insulin treatment to control their blood sugar because the beta cells in their pancreas do not make insulin.

- Individuals with type 2 diabetes eventually may need to take insulin to control their blood sugar. Insulin is recommended when the beta cells burn out over time and no longer work well.

- Pregnant women who have diabetes during pregnancy (gestational diabetes) need to be on insulin to have a healthy baby. All patients with diabetes who are hospitalized for a medical condition will be given insulin to manage their diabetes for the duration of their hospital stay.

Types of Insulin

There are many different types of insulin products and devices available to treat diabetes. Insulin medication is classified by:

- How fast it starts to work

- When it reaches a peak level in the bloodstream (when the concentration of insulin in your blood is the highest)

- How long the effect lasts

Rapid-acting insulin begins working within 15 minutes, peaks in 30 to 90 minutes and lasts for 3 to 5 hours. Names you may recognize are: Humalog (lispro insulin), Novolog (aspart insulin) or Apidra (glulisine).

Regular or short-acting insulin begins working in about 30 to 60 minutes, so it should be administered before a meal, peaks in 2 to 4 hours and lasts for 5 to 8 hours. Names you may recognize are Humulin R (regular insulin) and Novolin R (regular insulin).

Intermediate-acting insulin begins working in 1 to 3 hours, peaks in 8 hours and lasts for up to 12–16 hours. Names you may recognize are Humulin N (human NPH insulin) and Novolin N (human NPH insulin).

Long-acting insulin begins to work in 1 hour, reaches peak levels in 6 to 10 hours and can continue working for an entire day, 20 to 26 hours. Names you may recognize are: Lantus (glargine insulin) and Levemir (detemir insulin). Tresiba (degludec insulin) and Toujeo (glargine insulin) are two newer long-acting insulins now available in higher concentrations than standard insulin for better blood sugar control.

Pre-mixed insulins are often combined with rapid or short acting insulin. These products are a combination of specific proportions of intermediate-acting insulin in one bottle or in an insulin pen. The numbers reflect the percentage of insulin in each product; Humulin 70/30, Novolin 70/30, Novolog 70/30, Humulin 50/50 and Humulog mix 75/25.

Insulin Devices
Insulin pens are available which allow you to select the specific amount of insulin that needs to be delivered and they are almost pain free.

Inhaled insulin powder is now available which is absorbed into the blood through your lungs so it begins working faster and lasts for a shorter time period than regular insulin that is injected under the skin. This new product called *Afrezza* should be inhaled by mouth just before eating a meal or as instructed by your clinician. This medication can be used along with a medium or long acting insulin product and/or with an oral medication like metformin to control blood sugar.

An **insulin pump** about the size of a cell phone can be worn on the outside of the body. A tube connects the reservoir of insulin to a catheter that is inserted under the skin of your abdomen. A tube-less pump is now available. An insulin pump can be programmed to deliver just the right amount of insulin when needed to control the blood sugar level. It can be adjusted to deliver more or less insulin depending on meals, activity and the blood sugar level.

The amount of daily insulin should also be balanced with food intake and exercise. Eating a healthy balanced diabetic diet along with regular exercise and insulin are the three main goals of therapy. Some individuals may even need to take additional medications along with insulin to help adequately control their blood sugar. Your doctor or clinician will determine what type and/or types and the amount of insulin you will need to help control your blood sugar.

NOTE: There are two new combination injectable medications available which contain a higher concentration of long acting insulin and a GLP-1 medication. The names of these new products are: Xultrophy (degludec/liraglutide) and Soliqua (glargine/lixisenatide). This drug combination improves blood sugar control, reduces episodes of hypoglycemia (low blood sugar) and helps keep weight stable.

Metabolic Surgery

If you are morbidly obese and have type 2 diabetes inadequately controlled with oral or injectable medications you may be a candidate for gastric by-pass surgery. Reversal of type 2 diabetes was reported to be found in 78% of individuals who underwent gastric by-pass surgery. Newer studies have reported that the gastrointestinal tract is a key regulator of energy and glucose (sugar) balance. The current surgical recommendations are for those patients with Class lll Obesity with a body mass index (BMI) of greater than or equal to 40 and those with Class ll Obesity with a BMI of 35 to 39.9 with hyperglycemia that is inadequately controlled by lifestyle and optimal medical therapy. See Chapter 3 for further information on BMI.

What Should I Do To Stay Healthy?

Schedule an appointment with your clinician to obtain a detailed history and physical, which can identify any signs, symptoms or risk factors that may be present.

Ask for a fasting glucose blood test (usually a twelve hour fast) and a hemoglobin A1C test if you are at risk for insulin resistance and/or diabetes.

Know Your Numbers

- What are my blood sugar, blood pressure and cholesterol numbers and are they in the normal range?
- Schedule routine dental and annual eye examinations.
- Schedule an annual foot exam with a podiatrist if you have been diagnosed with diabetes.

Protect Your Heart

- Find out if your cholesterol numbers are under control.
- If you smoke, stop!
- Ask your healthcare clinician if you should be taking a daily aspirin.
- Take all prescription medications as directed.

Facts To Remember

- The most common form of diabetes is "Type 2," previously termed *adult onset* or *non-insulin-dependent* diabetes.
- According to the 2015 CDC (Center for Disease Control and Prevention) report, 30.3 million Americans have diabetes (9.4% of the population). Approximately 1.25 million American children and adults have type 1 diabetes.
- 1.5 million Americans are diagnosed with diabetes every year.
- 13.5 million American women aged 20 years or older have diabetes.
- 25.2 percent of Americans age 65 and older have type diabetes.
- One out of every three women who has diabetes does not even know she has it, according to the American Diabetes Association.
- 84.1 million Americans age 18 and older had prediabetes in 2015.
- It is estimated that 30.3 million people in the United States have diabetes, although 7.2 million may be undiagnosed and unaware of their condition.
- Eating healthy along with practicing healthy habits and regular exercise can prevent diabetes from ever developing!
- Diabetes remains the seventh leading cause of death in the United States.
- The U.S. Department of Health and Human services reports that 80% of people with type 2 diabetes are overweight. The more overweight you become, the more insulin it takes to get the sugar in your blood into your cells.
- Twenty-five percent of the population has a gene that prevents them from acquiring insulin resistance and the other seventy-five percent aren't so lucky, which includes some *menopausal women!*
- Two thirds of American women are overweight or obese and more than 25% do not exercise regularly.
- Women with diabetes are two to four times more likely to develop heart disease, have a heart attack and die from it than women without diabetes.

Chapter Summary

I realize this chapter provides a great deal of information to process but if you just remember to eat small meals every three hours throughout the day and avoid processed sugars and carbohydrates you will be a lot healthier.

I truly believe that processed sugars and carbohydrates pave the way for many degenerative diseases, especially insulin resistance, diabetes and heart disease in the menopausal woman.

Remember to exercise five times a week for at least 30 minutes and keep moving! This will help keep your weight down, help insulin work better and reduce your stress. Do not smoke and quit if you do.

I continue to diagnose perimenopausal and menopausal women with insulin resistance, prediabetes and diabetes almost daily. I have also seen too many younger women in my practice experience heart attacks and strokes that could possibly have been prevented.

Schedule your physical and get tested today so you can take charge of your health and not become a statistic as stated above.

Websites for further information on:

Prediabetes and Diabetes

CDC-Centers for Disease Control and Prevention:
https://www.cdc.gov/diabetes/home/index.html

American Diabetes Association:
http://www.diabetes.org/

U.S. National Library of Medicine-MedlinePlus:
http://medlineplus.gov/diabetes.html
http//medlineplus.gov/prediabetes.html

Diabetes and Cardiovascular Disease

Diabetes-American Heart Association:
http://www.heart.org/HEARTORG/Conditions/More/Diabetes/
Diabetes_UCM_001091_SubHomePage.jsp

Chapter 11

SOLVING STOMACH ISSUES

Digestive Disturbances

Our digestive system relies on *hormonal balance* to function properly and proper digestion is key to maintaining *hormonal balance!* Simply stated, hormones such as estrogen guide digestion and proper digestion promotes healthy hormonal activity.

When I began my practice in 1982, I quickly realized that women experience symptoms of *gastrointestinal distress* more often than men.

Common symptoms reported are:

• Constipation

• Diarrhea

• Gas and bloating (especially after eating)

• Heartburn

Over time, a pattern appeared to exist in some women, often associated with their menstrual cycle. Research has now shown that gastrointestinal distress is twice as common in women as in men.

Women also tend to have a greater incidence of conditions that can complicate proper digestion, such as:

• Gastro-esophageal reflux disease (initially felt as heartburn)

• Gastritis (initially felt as heartburn)

• Irritable Bowel Syndrome (which can initially present itself with constipation and/or diarrhea, gas and bloating)

The Digestive System

Functions

• The main role of the digestive system is to break down the food we eat, so the nutrients can be absorbed to fuel our body.

• This system is also responsible for ridding our body of waste products in the form of a bowel movement.

• Specific digestive hormones regulate hunger and appetite.

Anatomy

The *esophagus* is the tube that connects your throat to your stomach. The walls of your esophagus are lined with muscles which help move the food downward into your stomach. There is a valve at the lower end of the esophagus called the lower esophageal sphincter (LES), which prevents stomach acids from flowing upward back into the esophagus.

The *stomach* breaks down the food you eat and monitors its flow into the small intestine.

The *small intestine* is where digestion and absorption of the nutrients from the food we eat occurs and then waste products are passed to the large intestine.

The *large intestine or colon* is where waste products from the food we eat are formed into stool and then pass out of our body. Waste products enter the large intestine as fluid, which is absorbed and then stool is formed. Muscles in the wall of the large intestine contract in a wave like pattern and slowly move the stool downward and eventually out the rectum.

Digestive Hormones

Many of us have an interest in understanding how the two main digestive hormones, ghrelin and leptin, promote a healthy weight by controlling hunger and appetite.

- **Ghrelin** is secreted by the stomach and stimulates our appetite.
- **Leptin** is secreted by our fat cells and alerts our brain when we are full.

In midlife many women find it difficult to lose weight and if you consume high fructose corn syrup (HFCS) products (a sugar substitute used in soft drinks, salad dressings and processed foods) you will gain weight, especially in the belly. HFCS decreases and/or blocks the secretion of leptin, preventing ghrelin from receiving the signal to shut off, so your brain thinks that you are still hungry. Sleep deprivation can also cause this hormone imbalance to occur.

The message is: *Avoid HFCS and get your proper amount of sleep or you may gain weight.*

NOTE: Did you know that eating processed sugars (carbohydrates), salt and fats light up the same area of the brain responsible for addiction?

Common Conditions Of The Upper Digestive Tract

Gastro-Esophageal Reflux (GERD)

Gastro-esophageal reflux occurs when stomach acid is refluxed upward toward the esophagus. Other names for this condition are heartburn, acid indigestion, dyspepsia, esophagitis and gastric reflux. Midlife may become very stressful for many women, which can promote the development of Gastro-Esophageal Reflux Disease (GERD). Ten to twenty percent of individuals with this condition experience symptoms several times a week. If you experience frequent heartburn, you may have gastro-esophageal reflux disease.

Signs And Symptoms

- Heartburn two or more days a week aggravated by meals, bending over and/or lying flat
- Coughing, wheezing, hoarseness or a persistent sore throat
- Food coming back into your throat after you swallow (regurgitation)
- A sour or bitter taste in your mouth
- Nausea

- Belching

- Burning chest pain

NOTE: If you experience any of the symptoms listed above, you should have your heart checked too!

Diagnosis

Endoscopy is considered the "gold standard" test to evaluate individuals with persistent heartburn. This procedure uses a scope with a camera that is inserted into the mouth, through the esophagus and then into the stomach to visualize any abnormal tissue or growths. A tissue sample (biopsy) can be taken and any abnormal growth can also be removed during this procedure.

Treatment

Lifestyle Modifications

Changing your diet and lifestyle could prove to be the best treatment.

Avoid Tobacco

Smoking weakens the lower esophageal valve (LES) and stimulates more stomach acid production, which leads to increased heartburn.

Diet

If you are overweight, losing weight can help reduce your symptoms.

Eating six small healthy meals a day can:

- Stimulate your metabolism and help you lose weight.

- Help reduce the pressure on the LES valve

Do not eat for about three hours prior to going to bed.

Do not lie down right after eating.

Do not wear tight clothing around your waist, especially a girdle because this increases pressure on your stomach.

Avoid foods that trigger heartburn:

- Caffeine containing foods and beverages, including chocolate

- Fatty and spicy foods, including onions, garlic and tomatoes

- Citrus fruits and juices
- Alcoholic beverages
- Milk/dairy products initially may afford relief and then can aggravate heartburn.
- Sodas or carbonated drinks. They may seem to provide relief initially and then can promote heartburn. (Remember "HFCS" is found in most soft drinks and can make you gain weight too!)

Other Modifications
If you experience symptoms at night:

- Sleep in a tilted position to help keep the acid in your stomach.
- Try using a wedge support to elevate the top half of your body. (Be careful when using extra pillows, elevating just your head can increase reflux.)
- You can also try placing four inch blocks under the head of your bed.

If you have changed your diet and lifestyle, and the heartburn persists, you need to make an appointment with your clinician!

Medications to Avoid
Aspirin, non-steroidal anti-inflammatory drugs (NSAIDs) like ibuprofen (Motrin or Advil) and naproxen (Aleve). These medications can promote heartburn!

Tylenol (acetaminophen) is ok to take as an alternative for pain relief, if needed for a short period of time. **(Be careful because too much acetaminophen can affect your liver.)**

Medications to Take
Over the counter medicinal herbs:
Roots of marshmallow can offer protection to the mucous membranes in the stomach.

The following herbs may help reduce inflammation of the stomach lining and relax the tense muscles, promoting less gas and relief from the discomfort:

- Consider making a cup of hot tea with peppermint, chamomile, ginger, aniseed, catnip, fennel or papaya.

- Papaya enzymes, digestive enzymes and licorice are available at natural food stores and can be taken by mouth to help afford relief.

Over the counter antacids:

- Baking soda mixed with water can help neutralize stomach acid, promoting relief.

- Maalox, Mylanta, Gaviscon or Alka-Seltzer and many other available over-the-counter products can help neutralize acid in the stomach.

- *H2 Blockers:* Zantac (ranitidine), Pepcid AC (famotidine) or Tagamet (cimetidine) can help reduce the amount of acid produced in the stomach and help heal the damaged tissue. *(These medications are also available in prescription strength dosages, so consult with your clinician.)*

NOTE: These products should only be used for a short period of time to provide temporary relief.

Prescription medications:

Proton Pump Inhibitors (PPIs) can help stop the acid secretion in the stomach and heal damaged tissue.

- **Prilosec (omeprazole)** is available over-the-counter and by prescription and is recommended to be taken once daily for a short time period. If heartburn persists once you stop the medication you need to set up an appointment with your clinician for further testing and treatment.

- **Protonix (pantoprazole), Aciphex (rabeprazole), Prevacid (lansoparazole), Nexium (esomeprazole)** and **Dexilant (dexlansorazole)** are all prescription medications approved for treating gastroesophageal reflux (GERD).

Carafate (Sucralfate) is another anti-ulcer prescription medication available which acts as an acid buffer protecting the affected area from further injury. This medication comes in tablet and liquid form and coats the lining of the esophagus and stomach, promoting healing of the damaged tissue.

Complications Of GERD

Persistent heartburn can be very serious! If you continue to experience heartburn or acid reflux, your lower esophageal sphincter (LES) is not working properly and stomach acid is flowing back into your esophagus. Your esophagus can become damaged over time if frequently exposed to stomach acid.

The esophagus can become narrowed and an *esophageal stricture* can develop.

A hole in the esophagus can occur and this is called an *ulcer.*

Barrett's esophagus can develop with prolonged exposure to stomach acid and may lead to cancer. The stomach acid changes the normal squamous cells in the esophagus to abnormal glandular type cells, leading to further cellular change and eventually adenocarcinoma (cancer).

Gastritis

Gastritis is an inflammation (swelling), irritation or an erosion of the lining of the stomach. It can occur suddenly or gradually.

Signs And Symptoms

The symptoms may vary among individuals and some may not even experience any symptoms at all. The most common symptoms reported are:

• Nausea

• Recurrent upset stomach

• Abdominal bloating and discomfort

• Vomiting dark brown coffee-like material

• Indigestion

• Hiccups

• Burning sensation in stomach

• Decreased appetite

• Dark colored or black bowel movement

Causes

Gastritis can be caused by an irritation from:

• Coffee (caffeinated and/or decaffeinated)

• Excessive alcohol use, more than two glasses a day

• Persistent stress

- Chronic vomiting

- Taking daily aspirin and/or other anti-inflammatory medications, like Advil and Aleve

- The organism *Helicobacter pylori* (commonly referred to as H. pylori). This bacteria lives in the mucus lining of your stomach and without treatment, could lead to development of an ulcer and possibly even cancer. It can also be associated with a condition called pernicious anemia, which is related to a vitamin B12 deficiency.

NOTE: If you find yourself searching for antacids more than twice a week, you need to be examined by your clinician!

Diagnosis

An upper endoscopy as outlined previously in the GERD section. A thin tube with a small camera is inserted through your mouth and down your esophagus to look at the lining of the stomach.

Blood tests can be ordered to check for anemia from blood loss and to screen for the H. pylori infection and pernicious anemia (vitamin B12 deficiency) as outlined in the GERD section.

A fecal occult blood test (stool guaiac test) may be ordered. This will test for blood in your stool and could be a possible sign of gastritis.

Treatment
Lifestyle Modifications

- Reduce caffeine and alcohol intake
- Eliminate foods from your diet such as:
    - Lactose from dairy
    - Gluten (a protein found in wheat) including: durum, emmer, semolina, spelt, farina, farro, graham spelt, khorasan (Kamut) and einkorn
    - Barley, rye and triticale (a rye/wheat hybrid) that is hard for some people to digest.
    - Citrus and spicy foods
- Reduce stress
- Avoid taking NSAID medications (Aleve and Ibuprofen) and aspirin

Medications

Medications that reduce the amount of acid in the stomach can relieve symptoms associated with gastritis and can promote healing of the stomach lining. Please see above outline in the GERD section for further detail on the following medication therapies:

• Antacids

• Histamine 2 (H2) blockers

• Proton pump inhibitors (PPIs)

Common Conditions Of The Lower Digestive Tract

The Lower Intestine And Colon

The colon is about 5 feet long and connects the small intestine to the rectum and anus. The main function of the colon is to absorb water, nutrients and salts from partially digested foods. Approximately 2 pints of liquid enter the colon from the small intestine daily. The stool volume is equal to about a third of a pint. The difference of the amount of fluid entering the colon from the amount of stool produced is what the colon absorbs every day.

The contraction of the colon muscles and the movement of its contents are influenced by hormones and nerves. Muscle contractions move the contents inside the colon to the rectum. During this passage, water and nutrients are absorbed into the body and the left over material becomes the stool. A few times a day the muscle contractions occur pushing the stool toward the colon, resulting in a bowel movement. If the muscles in the colon, pelvis and sphincters do not work properly, colon contents do not move correctly, causing abdominal bloating, pain, cramping, constipation and/or a sense of incomplete stool movement or even diarrhea.

The bottom line is (no pun intended-ha! ha!) that the lining of the colon (epithelium) is influenced by proper functioning of the immune, endocrine and nervous systems, regulating the flow of fluids in and out of the colon.

Constipation

Constipation is a very common condition experienced by almost everyone at some point in their lifetime.

This condition exists when there is:

• Excessive hardness of the stool

- Infrequent bowel movements
- A sense of incomplete emptying of the rectum
- A decrease in stool size and it may become more difficult to pass.

If you don't have a bowel movement within three days, the stool becomes hard and this leads to constipation. Women and the elderly most commonly experience this condition.

Causes

Hormonal Imbalance can be seen during pregnancy, perimenopause and with hypothyroidism. Constipation can occur during perimenopause and menopause when estrogen is declining along with the level of serotonin.

Stress and/or Anxiety along with sleep deprivation can promote constipation.

Travel can lead to constipation when you are not following your usual routine.

Not drinking enough water can definitely promote constipation. You should try drinking half your body weight in ounces per day.

Not consuming enough fiber in your diet. Try consuming at least 25 grams of fiber each day. (One tablespoon of ground Flax or Chia equals about 2.5 grams of fiber and you can sprinkle the seeds over cereal, yogurt or a salad.)

Eating too much dairy and not enough fiber can lead to constipation.

Not exercising enough. You need to move your body to move your bowels.

Eating disorders and depression can be associated with an improper diet. You need to eat small meals every three hours with increased fiber and decreased sugar.

Irritable Bowel Syndrome with constipation (IBSc) is a condition associated with having chronic constipation. I discuss this syndrome in further detail to follow.

Medication can promote constipation. Narcotic pain medications are one of the most common causes followed by iron supplementation and certain vitamin preparations.

*NOTE: Your bowels will be most active in the morning. It's import-
ant to allow sufficient time to relax and let them move!*

Treatment Recommendations

Lifestyle Modifications

You should **consume** at least 25 grams of **fiber** per day to keep
your intestines healthy and on the move. The goal is to keep going.

Drink water! Did you know that if you become dehydrated your
digestion slows down? Yes, this is true! Again, try to drink half
your body weight in ounces every day.

Eat fresh fruits and vegetables and avoid processed foods. Keep
in mind that bananas can promote constipation.

Consuming pure coconut oil daily can help move your bowels.
Start with a third of a teaspoonful in your hot morning coffee or
tea. You can also stir fry fresh vegetables with coconut oil. Be
careful to limit your daily intake of coconut oil to a half a teaspoonful or less since it is high in saturated fat.

Use a Squatty Potty to help facilitate a bowel movement. The
modern style toilet seat requires us to sit which may narrow the
recto-angle and impair defecation. The use of a squatty potty (a
stool placed under your feet to elevate your legs) changes the anorectal angle associated with squatting and promotes smooth bowel
elimination and helps prevent straining.

Non-Prescription Medications

Stool Softeners

Miralax is an over-the-counter medication that works by gently replenishing the water to your digestive system to help
a bowel movement occur. This water can help increase the
frequency of a bowel movement and soften the stool making
it easier to pass.

Colace is another stool softener that may be used on a short
term basis for relief of constipation and to help prevent straining with stools. It may take up to three days of continued use to
produce desired results. Do not take this stool softener for more
than a week without consulting your clinician.

Stimulants

Senna (Senokot) is an herb that is used as a laxative and is a FDA approved non-prescription laxative. This herb is commonly used to empty the bowels before a medical procedure such as a colonoscopy. It is also used to treat irritable bowel syndrome discussed in further detail later in this chapter. Senna is available in liquid, powder, granules, tea leaves and a tablet form to be taken by mouth usually in the evening to promote a bowel movement. A bowel movement will typically occur within six to twelve hours. Do not take this herb for more than a week without consulting your clinician.

Prescription Medications

Linzess (linaclotide) is a relatively new prescription medication used to treat chronic constipation and irritable bowel syndrome with constipation termed IBS-c. This medication works by increasing fluid in your intestines and helps move food more quickly through your gastrointestinal tract. Linzess may also help decrease symptoms of bloating, abdominal pain/discomfort, straining and feelings of an incomplete bowel movement. The recommended dose for treatment of chronic constipation is 145 mcg once daily and for irritable bowel syndrome with constipation is 290 mcg daily.

Amitiza (lubiprostone) is another prescription medication that is used to treat chronic idiopathic constipation (unknown cause), irritable bowel with constipation and constipation caused by narcotic medications in individuals with ongoing pain, such as with cancer. Amitiza may also help relieve other symptoms such as bloating and abdominal discomfort. This medication works by increasing the fluid in your intestines making the stool easier to pass. It can also help improve the stool texture and decrease feelings of straining and/or having an incomplete bowel movement. This class of drug is known as a chloride channel activator. Amitiza is available in two strengths, 8 mcg and 24 mcg, to be taken twice daily with food or water. Your clinician will determine which dose will be best for you.

Movantik (naloxegol) is a new prescription medication used to treat constipation that is caused by long term use of opioid (narcotic) prescription pain medications. Opioids are commonly used to treat chronic pain. Naloxegol works by attaching (binding) to the mu-opioid receptor in the gastrointestinal tract thereby reducing constipation while not reducing the pain-relieving effects of the narcotic. This medication is available in two strengths, 12.5 mg and 25 mg, to be taken once daily in the morning. Many drugs can interact with naloxegol so be sure to discuss all medications that you take with your clinician.

Relistor (methylnaltrexone bromide) is another opioid antagonist medication recently released for treatment of opioid-induced constipation (OIC) in adults with chronic non-cancer pain. The dosage of this medication is three 150 mg tablets to be taken in the morning. A 12 mg once daily injectable form of this medication is also available. A lower dose is recommended for patients with kidney disease.

Diarrhea

This is a common condition experienced by almost everyone at some point in their life.

Diarrhea exists when there is an increased number of stools (bowel movements) or if the stool contains more water than normal. If your intestines push the stool through the bowel too quickly before the water is absorbed, you will experience diarrhea.

Women commonly will experience diarrhea during perimenopause and menopause due to:

• Increased anxiety and/or emotional stress
• Digestive problems, including lactose intolerance and irritable bowel syndrome

Causes

• Visible lactose found in milk, young cheeses, chocolate, cottage cheese and ice cream
• Fructose found in fresh fruit
• Sorbitol, a sweetener found in sugar-free gum, candy and mints
• Taking over the counter and prescription medications
• Travel
• Some viruses

Treatment Recommendations

Dietary

Bananas are often recommended for diarrhea because they are soft, bland and supply complex carbohydrates which make them easy to digest. Bananas are a rich source of the mineral potassium which is lost from the body when diarrhea occurs. This fruit also contains a starch that is amylase-resistant, so it can help reduce stomach acid while protecting the gastrointestinal mucosa (tissue lining the stomach and intestine).

Rice is another food often recommended for reducing diarrhea. Plain white rice is easily digested and similar to bananas in that it is also high in complex carbohydrates. Rice water can decrease acid production and promote hydration. You can make rice water with one cup of uncooked rice and one quart of boiling water. Let the rice steep for 20 minutes, strain and sip the broth throughout the day as needed.

Other Foods that help relieve diarrhea are apples, applesauce and toast. These foods along with bananas and rice are part of the **b-r-a-t** diet that is commonly recommended for children with diarrhea.

Boiled potatoes, chicken without the skin or fat, crackers, cooked carrots and clear liquids are also helpful for diarrhea.

Non-Prescription Medications
Imodium A-D, Kaopectate II, Maalox Anti-diarrheal Caplets and Pepto Bismol Diarrhea Control are some of the non-prescription medications found over-the-counter that contain the active ingredient loperamide used to relieve the symptoms of diarrhea. Loperamide helps decrease diarrhea by slowing down the propulsion of the intestinal contents and inhibits the action of the intestinal muscles.

Prescription Medications
Lomotil (diphenoxylate and atropine sulfate) is a prescription that contains an antidiarrheal and anticholinergic medication. The diphenoxylate helps reduce diarrhea and the atropine reduces intestinal spasms. This medication is available in both tablet and liquid form.

This medication works by decreasing the motion of the intestinal muscles and prolongs the time it takes to move the contents through the bowels.

Loperamide is also available by prescription to help control chronic diarrhea in individuals with irritable bowel syndrome, Crohn's disease and ulcerative colitis. It can also be prescribed to help with symptoms associated with traveler's diarrhea.

Your clinician will review the side effects and drug interactions of these medications with you and determine the dose and duration of therapy needed.

> *NOTE: Remember the digestive system needs proper nutrients to function and maintain hormonal balance!*

Irritable Bowel Syndrome (IBS)

This is an intestinal disorder characterized most commonly by abdominal pain, bloating, cramping, increased gas, diarrhea or constipation. Symptoms can vary from individual to individual. It is sometimes referred to as a "spastic or nervous" colon.

Individuals with IBS have a colon that appears to look normal (no structural or biochemical abnormalities to explain the symptoms), so it is called a "functional" disorder. The digestive system just doesn't work correctly and this affects how waste is removed from the body.

The good news is that IBS does not lead to a serious illness such as cancer and does not shorten one's lifespan.

IBS affects 1 in 5 adults in the United States and is more common in women than in men, usually beginning before the age of 35.

Definition And Descriptive Terms

Abdominal pain or discomfort: Cramping pain that may result from strong contractions of the intestines and increased sensitivity to pain.

Urgency: A feeling of having to move your bowels right away.

Diarrhea: An increase in the amount of water in the stool and frequency of having a bowel movement. In review, diarrhea is caused by the rapid movement of stool through the intestines.

Irritable bowel with constipation (IBSc) is when you have a hard time passing stool or infrequent stools. These individuals will often experience straining and cramping when trying to have a bowel movement. They may have a very small amount of stool or may not eliminate at all. If they do pass a small amount of stool it may have mucus in it. This mucus is fluid that is made to help moisten and protect the stool during passage in the digestive system.

Irritable bowel with diarrhea (IBSd) is when you have frequent loose or watery stools. These individuals may experience an urge and/or an uncontrollable need to have a bowel movement.

Some individuals may alternate between experiencing diarrhea and constipation. The symptoms can be constant and at other times intermittent. Normal movement may not be present in the colon of an individual with IBS. It may be spasmodic (muscle contractions that come and go) or may even temporarily stop working.

In Review:

If you have IBSd the epithelium (intestinal lining) works properly although the contents inside the colon move too quickly and the fluids are unable to be absorbed. This results in a watery stool.

If you have IBSc, the movement inside the colon is too slow, allowing too much fluid to be absorbed, which results in constipation.

The cause of IBS is unknown, although many factors may play a role:

- The colon or large intestine has a heightened sensitivity to certain foods and stress.
- The immune system which fights infection may also be involved.
- Some researchers report that IBS may be caused by a bacterial infection, "Post infectious IBS" which responds well to antibiotic therapy.
- Other research has reported that the hormone *serotonin* may be linked to normal gastrointestinal functioning. Serotonin is a neurotransmitter (a chemical messenger) which delivers messages from one part of your body to another. Ninety-five percent of the serotonin in your body is located in the GI tract and the remaining five percent in your brain. Cells that line the inside of the intestine work as transporters carrying serotonin out of the GI tract. This receptor activity is decreased in individuals with IBS, allowing abnormal levels of serotonin to remain in the GI tract. This can lead to problems with bowel movements, motility and more sensitive pain receptors in the GI tract.
- Researchers have also found celiac disease in some patients with symptoms similar to IBS. Individuals with celiac disease are unable to tolerate foods with gluten. You can have a blood test done to screen for celiac disease.

Common Triggers

- *Dietary:* Consuming high fat foods, dairy products, carbonated drinks, alcohol and caffeine.
- *Psychological or emotional:* Prolonged periods of stress and anxiety.

• *Hormonal:* Some women experience an increase in symptoms during their menstrual cycle, perimenopause and menopause. This is probably associated with the fluctuation of hormone levels, which may also influence the amount of serotonin you have at that given time.

Diagnosis

A careful history taken by the clinician can identify the possibility of IBS, based on the pattern and duration of symptoms.

A patient should then undergo a complete medical examination with appropriate blood tests and x-ray imaging, if necessary.

Finally, a direct visualization procedure like a colonoscopy should be done to exclude any other causes. IBS is referred to as a diagnosis of exclusion, which means that all other causes have been considered.

Treatment

The treatment for IBS may differ from patient to patient. The following recommendations have been shown to help the symptoms associated with IBS.

Dietary

• Avoid high fat foods, dairy products, caffeine, sugar and alcohol.
• Avoid eating beans, cabbage, apples and other foods which can be hard to digest and this may also help decrease gas and bloating.
• Avoid carbonated beverages.
• Eat smaller meals every three to four hours.

NOTE: If the above measures are ineffective at reducing your symptoms the FODMAP elimination diet may be recommended by your clinician and dietician for a one to two week period of time. If the FODMAP carbs are the culprit, relief of symptoms can occur in just a few days.

The FODMAP Diet: This diet describes a group of poorly absorbed sugars that contribute to the onset of symptoms associated with irritable bowel syndrome (IBS). The FODMAP acronym stands for Fermentable Oligo-saccharides, Di-saccharides, Mono-saccharides and Polyols. These sugars are: **Fructose** found in fruit, honey and juices, **lactose** found in milk and milk products and sugar polyols such as **sorbitol** and **mannitol** found in some fruits, vegetables and artificial sweeteners. **Fructans** are a type of sugar found in wheat, rye, onions and garlic. **Galacto-oligosaccharides (GOS)** are found in legumes such as chickpeas, kidney beans and baked beans and can be a problem for some individuals.

When these sugars are poorly absorbed in the small intestine, increased water can be drawn to the gut, resulting in diarrhea.

When these sugars travel to the large intestine where they are fermented by bacteria, gas can occur. This gas can lead to bloating, flatulence, pain and nausea. This increased gas can also slow down a bowel movement leading to constipation.

Stress Reduction
- Begin an exercise program which includes yoga and stretching
- Acupuncture has been shown to provide relief
- If you enjoy the outdoors, try walking, biking or hiking
- Cultivate friendships that relieve stress
- Join a support group which can help you achieve a better understanding of IBS and reduce your stress
- Try a new hobby or take a new class
- Treat yourself to a massage or manicure and just enjoy it!

Medications
Many of the over-the-counter products are targeted at relieving a single symptom:
- **Imodium AD** for diarrhea
- **Miralax** is a laxative for constipation
- **Fiber supplements** such as **Metamucil** may help with constipation
- **Probiotics** such as **Align** or **VSL#3** helps restore the good intestinal bacteria, alleviating the symptoms of bloating, gas and diarrhea. Many patients have reported a favorable response.

Prescription medications for treating constipation:
- **Amitiza (lubiprostone)** is a chloride channel activator used for treating constipation in individuals with IBSc.

This medication is taken twice daily and promotes fluid secretion into the intestine, decreasing the firmness of the stool.

- **Linzess (linaclotide)** is another prescription medication used to treat constipation associated with irritable bowel syndrome. This medication also works by increasing fluid in your intestines and helps move food more quickly through your gastrointestinal tract.

NOTE: See more about Linzess and Amitza on pages 58 and 59 in the treatment section for constipation.

Prescription medications for treating diarrhea:
Two new medications were approved on May 28, 2015 for the treatment of irritable bowel with diarrhea or IBSd.

- **Viberzi (eluxadoline)** is a narcotic that helps decrease the number of bowel contractions which leads to less diarrhea. This medication has a significant effect on bowel frequency, consistency and ameliorates excess urgency. This drug also improves abdominal discomfort. Viberzi is available in two prescription strengths, 75 mg and 100 mg, to be taken two times daily with food.

- **Xifaxan (rifaximin)** is an antibiotic that fights infection only in the intestines, changing your gut bacteria, which reduces diarrhea. This supports the theory that a bacterial infection may be causing IBSd.

  Xifaxan is different than other antibiotics because it passes through your stomach and into your intestines without being absorbed into your blood stream. It is available in two strengths; 200 mg and 550 mg. The recommended treatment for individuals with IBSd is a 550 mg tablet to be taken three times a day for fourteen days to help provide relief from symptoms which include diarrhea and abdominal discomfort. Your clinician will determine if this medication is right for you after performing a medical examination.

- **Elavil,** which is a tricyclic medication, may help regulate the serotonin level.

- **Zoloft, Prozac** or **Lexapro are selective serotonin re-**

uptake inhibitors (SSRIs) which are used to treat depression and will also help regulate the serotonin level in the digestive system.

• **Buspar** is an antianxiety medication which has been reported to also help regulate the serotonin level.

All of the above mentioned medications have side effects and some of them may potentially have *serious* side effects, so talk with your clinician to determine which treatment will be best for you.

Remember your bowels are most active in the morning, so allow sufficient time to relax and let them go!

Candida Albicans

Overview

Candida Albicans is known to cause the most common type of fungal infection, called a yeast infection.

Candida fungus is present in everyone's mouth, digestive system and skin. Healthy individuals usually have small amounts present because their immune system keeps the fungus from reproducing quickly. Our immune system and the beneficial bacteria in our intestinal tract normally keep these microorganisms in balance. When certain conditions are present an imbalance can occur, promoting rapid growth of this organism which may invade our body tissues and cause an infection. Individuals with immune deficiencies, such as patients with HIV and/or AIDS can develop serious candida infections referred to as systemic candidiasis. This means the fungus grows rapidly and spreads through the blood to certain organs.

Types Of Candida Infection

Vaginal Infections

Sometimes candida will cause a yeast infection in healthy people. The most common presentation of candida overgrowth would be in the form of a vaginal yeast infection.

Symptoms can be vaginal itching, swelling, painful urination along with a thick white cottage cheese type discharge. See Chapter 3 for further detail on vaginal infections.

Mouth and Throat Infections

Yeast infections that occur in the mouth and sometimes the throat are called thrush. Oral thrush may present initially with white or yellow spots on the mouth or tongue which can then form a coating.

Symptoms of thrush can be a discomfort or burning sensation in the mouth and/or throat and sometimes taste can be affected. Thrush may also be present without any symptoms.

Esophageal Infection

Candida that occurs in the throat and esophagus is a serious systemic form of this infection.

Symptoms experienced by patients may be difficulty swallowing, chest pain and nausea. AIDS patients and those receiving chemotherapy for cancer can develop this esophageal manifestation of systemic candidiasis, which can spread through the digestive tract if not diagnosed and treated early on.

Skin Infections

Yeast infections can affect the skin and fingernails in individuals with systemic candida. Yeast grows well in moist environments on the skin such as armpits, groin, beneath the breasts and scrotum. Infected nails can develop a thickened texture, become brittle and turn a yellowish-brown in color.

Diaper rash can commonly occur in babies and young children.

Disseminated Candidiasis

Individuals with a compromised immune system can develop serious candida infections throughout their body called disseminated candidiasis. The brain, heart, eyes, kidneys, liver or joints may become infected and must be treated immediately and many times will require hospitalization!

Candida Overgrowth

Causes

- A common cause of candida overgrowth is from taking prescription medications such as antibiotics, birth control pills, corticosteroid and anticancer medications.

- A weakened immune system due to illness or stress such as HIV, diabetes and many other conditions.

- A diet high in processed sugars and high fructose corn syrup.

Digestive Symptoms

If candida overgrowth occurs in the intestinal tract, symptoms can mimic those of irritable bowel syndrome (IBS):

• Abdominal pain, bloating, gas, burping, especially after eating

• Constipation

• Diarrhea

• Fatigue

• Increased food sensitivities

• Indigestion

Diagnosis

A comprehensive stool test can determine if you have yeast overgrowth in your colon and lower intestines.

Treatment

To successfully treat candida you need to stop the yeast overgrowth and rebuild the essential friendly bacteria so your gut can heal.

Diet

Avoid yeast containing foods:

• Alcohol (beer and wine)

• Carbohydrates (breads, sweet rolls, pastries, pretzels and cookies)

• B-complex and selenium supplements made with yeast. Look for labels which say, "Yeast Free"

• Vinegar containing foods (mustard, salad dressings, pickles, barbeque sauce, mayonnaise)

• Processed foods (soups, potato chips, soy sauce, cider and dry roasted nuts)

Avoid mold containing foods:

• Smoked or pickled meats, fish and poultry

• All cheeses (aged and fresh)

• Mushrooms

• Peanuts and pistachios

• Malted foods

• Soy sauce, tamari, tempeh and miso

• Canned tomatoes

Avoid all concentrated sugars:

- Maple syrup, brown sugar and honey
- All fruit juices and dried fruit
- All processed sugar products, especially those that contain high-fructose corn syrup
- Avoid artificial colors, sweeteners and dyes
- Don't eat processed foods

(Please refer to Chapter 3 for further information on nutrition)

Recommended Foods

- All fresh vegetables such as: Artichokes, asparagus, avocado, broccoli, Brussels sprouts, cabbage, celery, cucumbers, eggplant, garlic (raw), kale, olives, onions, rutabagas, spinach, tomatoes and zucchini. Try to include sea vegetables such as kelp and dulse as well.
- Fresh protein and organic meat such as: fish, shellfish, beef, chicken, lamb, turkey and eggs. Avoid processed meats because they have a lot of sugar, nitrates and sulfates.
- Complex carbohydrates such as:
  - Non-gluten whole grains, buckwheat, millet, oat bran, oatmeal and quinoa
  - Beans (black, red and lima)
  - Whole wheat pasta (a small serving only)
- Limit carbohydrates to 15 grams per meal. I know this seems impossible but you can do it.
- Raw unprocessed nuts and seeds such as: almonds, flaxseed, hazelnuts, pecans, sunflower seeds and walnuts. Remember, no peanuts.
- Unrefined corn, safflower, olive, sesame oil, flax oil, coconut oil. Keep refrigerated after opening.
- A freshly squeezed lemon or lime
- Lemon juice with oil for salad dressing. Remember to avoid any vinegar containing products.
- Soy and unprocessed nut milks
- Mineral and spring water, keep hydrated.
- Fresh fruits three times a day, although avoid grapes, raisins, dates, figs, prunes and dried fruits due to the high sugar content.

Water Intake

It is important to drink sufficient amounts of water to cleanse your body and keep the bowels moving. Try drinking at least half your body weight in ounces daily. (Divide the number of pounds you weigh by two and drink that many ounces of water per day.) Drinking eight glasses of water if you weigh 200 pounds does not equal the same as someone weighing 100 pounds-right?

(Please see Chapters 3 and 6 for further information on vitamins and minerals.)

Exercise

Regular exercise 25-30 minute sessions, 4-5 times a week helps:

• Reduce stress

• Improve circulation

• Enhance your energy level

• Promote a healthy immune system

Supplements

Digestive enzymes: The cell wall of candida is made up of fiber and glycoproteins, which makes enzymes specific for treating yeast infections very effective.

Anti-inflammatory herbs: Cinnamon, turmeric, green tea and ginger are good anti-oxidant supplements to help fight against yeast and candida.

Candex is a dietary enzyme supplement which contains about 200,000 daily units of cellulose and hemicellulase, which can help destroy yeast and candida when taken on an empty stomach. You should consult with a herbologist and/or clinician before starting this supplement.

Probiotics are medical food that boost the beneficial bacteria in the digestive tract to help fight off yeast and other infections. We need sufficient lactobacillus and bifidobacteria to digest food.

Superdophilus (lactobacillus acidophilus) is a bacteria that naturally occurs in the body, intestines and vagina. This type of bacteria is present to help maintain an acid environment, preventing the growth of harmful bacteria in the stomach, intestines and vagina. Your clinician will determine the dosage and duration of treatment you will need.

Bifidobacteria are in a group called lactic acid bacteria. Lactic acid bacteria can be found in fermented foods like yogurt and cheese. This group of bacteria is considered to help boost the immune system and fight infection.

Essential Fatty Acids:

• Flaxseed, preferably whole ground

• Fish oil, omega-3 and 6

• Borage seed oil capsules which contain GLA (gamma-linolenic acid)

These supplements help strengthen the immune system.

Natural Antifungal agents: There are many natural antifungal supplements that work by breaking down the cell walls of the candida yeast. Popular over-the-counter antifungals are caprylic acid, grape seed extract, garlic and oil of oregano. You should consult with a herbologist before beginning an antifungal regimen.

Prescription Medications

Prescription Antifungals:

• *Nystatin (mycostatin)* is an antifungal medication used to treat fungal infections of the stomach, intestines and mucous membranes. This medication is available in a tablet, capsule and liquid form to be taken by mouth and a soft lozenge that can be dissolved on the tongue. Nystatin is also used to treat fungal infections of the vagina and skin. A tablet or cream can be inserted into the vagina and a cream, powder or ointment can be applied to the skin.

• *Diflucan (fluconazole)* is an antifungal prescription medication used to treat fungal/yeast infections of the vagina, mouth, throat, esophagus, lungs, blood and other organs. Fluconazole is also used to treat more serious fungal infections of the lung, eye, prostate (in men), skin and nails. A potentially serious fungal infection known as meningitis which involves the membranes that cover the brain and spine may also be treated with fluconazole. This medication is available in a tablet or liquid form that can be taken by mouth.

Should you ever be diagnosed with a serious candida infection there are many other prescription medications available that can be used and your clinician will determine which medication is appropriate for your condition.

NOTE: Remember, it is very important to consume a healthy diet because our digestive system relies on healthy nutrition to maintain hormonal balance to function properly!

Websites for further information on:

Digestive System

National Institutes of Health: **https://www.niddk.nih.gov/health-information/health-topics/Anatomy/your-digestive-system/Pages/anatomy.aspx**

Constipation

Mayo Clinic: **http://www.mayoclinic.org/symptom-checker/constipation-adult/related-factors/itt-20009075**

Squatty Potty: **https://www.squattypotty.com/**

Candida Infections

Candidiasis-CDC-Centers for Disease Control and Prevention: **https://www.cdc.gov/fungal/diseases/candidiasis/**

Candida Overgrowth: **http://www.healthy-holistic-living.com/10-signs-candida-overgrowth.html**

Diarrhea

Mayo Clinic: **http://www.mayoclinic.org/symptom-checker/diarrhea-adult/related-factors/itt-20009075**

MedlinePlus: **https://vsearch.nlm.nih.gov/vivisimo/cgi-bin/query-meta?query=diarrhea&v%3Aproject=nlm-main-website**

Heartburn-Gastrointestinal Reflux Disease (GERD)

WebMD: **www.webmd.com/heartburn-gerd/your-digestive-system**

Irritable Bowel Syndrome (IBS)

Irritable Bowel Syndrome Association: **http://www.ibsgroup.org/ibsassociation.org/**

Medicine Net: **https://www.medicinenet.com/irritable_bowel_syndrome_ibs_triggers_prevention/article.htm**

Irritable Bowel Syndrome-Symptoms and Causes-Mayo Clinic: **https://www.mayoclinic.org/diseases-conditions/irritable-bowel-syndrome/symptoms-causes/syc-20360016**

Women's Health-IBS Fact Sheet: **https://www.womenshealth.gov/a-z-topics/irritable-bowel-syndrome**

Chapter 12

EATING DISORDERS IN MIDLIFE

Eating disorders can affect you at any age and may range from binge eating to compulsive exercise and/or calorie restriction. New studies have shown that eating disorders and the need to exercise compulsively are on the rise among **middle-aged** women. Approximately ninety percent of individuals diagnosed with an eating disorder are female and a significant number of these women are over 50. Could you be one of them?

In June of 2012, a study was published in the **International Journal of Eating Disorders** which looked at the prevalence of eating disorders in midlife and beyond. This study lead by Cynthia Bulik, Ph.D., revealed that 13 percent of women 50 and older experience symptoms of an eating disorder; 60 percent report that their concerns about weight and shape negatively affect their lives, and 70 percent are currently trying to lose weight. These same figures can also be found in teens and young women when female hormones are fluctuating, as they do during the perimenopausal period. The psychological and physical changes that a woman experiences during puberty and menopause can be very similar and the development of new eating disorders may occur at these times. Yes, women in their twenties, thirties and forties are still showing signs of anorexia and bulimia as well. Some individuals recover in their teens and twenties where others may struggle well into midlife and beyond.

An eating disorder is considered to be a mental illness and can be closely associated with anxiety and depression. Most of us think of bulimia and anorexia nervosa when an eating disorder comes to mind. Some individuals may have other symptoms that do not meet the criteria of anorexia or bulimia and this is referred to as OSFED (other specific feeding and eating disorder). An eating disorder, if left untreated, can also become a serious medical illness.

Eating disorders do tend to run in families. One study revealed that the risk for anorexia is about eleven times greater for a relative of an individual with this disorder than for the average woman.

These disorders were once thought to be most prevalent in just adolescent single, Caucasian individuals from well-educated and upper middle class backgrounds, but this is no longer true.

Eating disorders can definitely affect your quality of life! There is an increased risk of suicide and death associated with some eating disorders. Almost *four out of every five deaths* that involved anorexia nervosa occurred *in individuals more than forty five years of age.*

Midlife Stressors And Weight Gain

Midlife stressors that can trigger these disorders appear to be:

• Divorce

• Aging parents

• Children leaving home

• Menopause, aging bodies and other midlife problems

The average woman gains about fifteen pounds during the menopausal period. This weight gain can actually be beneficial in some women by helping to boost the immune system, aiding in fighting off infections, and decreasing the risk for bone fractures. Weight gain beyond ten to fifteen pounds can be detrimental to your health.

Anorexia Nervosa

Anorexia nervosa is a type of eating disorder that affects both the mind and body. These individuals think about food, dieting and their weight all the time with a distorted body image. It often begins so subtly that neither the individual nor her family realizes what is happening. It may simply begin with just a diet and then becomes out of control!

Women are often living productive lives and just want to avoid "midlife weight gain" so they may:

- Begin to skip meals or take only tiny portions, often avoiding all but a few kinds of foods
- Weigh and measure their food, chew it at length and spit it out, or secretly pocket it and throw it away
- Use laxatives and/or water pills or even make themselves vomit after a meal
- Exercise compulsively
- Say that they look or feel "fat," although they may be becoming emaciated. As weight continues to drop and their health deteriorates, the individual may persist in denying that anything is wrong. They often will wear baggy clothes or avoid other people to conceal the problem.

Today's society can certainly promote concerns about body image and weight. Unfortunately, too much emphasis can be placed on pursuing the fountain of youth with fixes of multiple Botox injections and cosmetic procedures. A good example would be the characters depicted on popular TV shows such as "Desperate Housewives." Women on TV are almost never overweight and if they are overweight they usually are in a comic relief role. There is definitely an overt message from programmers that if you are overweight there is something wrong with you. Many women feel the pressure to remain thin and look as young as they can forever.

Some women have struggled with an eating disorder for many years, while other women find it began at the start of **menopause,** which coincided with the onset of midlife stressors.

Unfortunately, eating disorders, if not recognized and treated can potentially be life-threatening.

Screening Questions To Ask

1. Do you feel guilty about eating?
2. Do you eat in secret?

3. Do you eat until you feel uncomfortably full?

4. Are you satisfied with your diet?

5. Do others tell you that you are thin when you feel fat?

Signs And Symptoms

Individuals diagnosed with anorexia nervosa have a distorted body image and exhibit an intense fear of becoming fat, even though they are underweight. This results in a self-imposed starvation, despite having a normal appetite and craving for food.

An individual with anorexia is likely to have:

- Disturbed ideas about weight or body shape, or deny that weight loss is a serious problem
- Not menstruated for at least three consecutive cycles, if she is in her reproductive years
- A desire to exercise compulsively
- Food-related obsessions (hoarding food or collecting recipes)
- Feelings that losing weight is a desired achievement of self-control, whereas gaining weight is thought of as an unacceptable lack of discipline
- A depressed mood, feel anxious (irritable) and/or experience insomnia. There appears to be a 75% risk of developing a major depressive episode and a 25% risk for developing an obsessive compulsive disorder.

Other symptoms may develop over time to include:

- Swollen joints, brittle nails, dry skin and hair
- Osteopenia (thinning of bones) and osteoporosis
- Dry and yellowish appearance of skin
- Growth of fine hair all over the body called lanugo
- Anemia and muscle wasting with weakness
- Constipation
- A decrease in body temperature making one feel cold all the time
- Extreme fatigue, sluggishness and lethargy
- Infertility
- Low blood pressure, slowed breathing and pulse
- Damage to the heart structure and function

- Multi-organ failure
- Brain damage

These individuals refuse to maintain a normal weight and show an intense fear (they become terrified) of gaining any weight or becoming fat. Their weight is typically 15% below the healthy minimum and/or they have a BMI less than 17.5%. Remember, a healthy BMI range is between 18.5 and 24.9.

See the Body Mass index (BMI), under the Weight Maintenance section in Chapter 3 on page 56, for further information.

Types Of Anorexia Nervosa

Restrictive

- Dieting, restricting calorie intake, or just tasting food
- Excessive or compulsive exercise

Purging

- Chronic use of laxatives and/or vomiting
- Binge eating/burping (deliberate vomiting or misuse of laxatives, enemas, or diuretics in addition to dieting, fasting and excessive exercise)

NOTE: Individuals with anorexia have a high rate of bulimia, the bingeing and purging syndrome.

Bulimia Nervosa

Bulimia nervosa is another of type of eating disorder characterized by a cyclic pattern of binge eating followed by inappropriate compensatory behaviors. Weight is usually in the normal range. An individual with bulimia nervosa often fears gaining weight and desperately desires to lose weight. They are intensely unhappy with their body size and shape. This behavior is typically done secretly and can be accompanied by feelings of guilt and shame. The binge-eating and purging cycle can occur several times a day or many times a week.

Types Of Bulimia

Purging Type

An individual with this type of bulimia will regularly engage in self-induced vomiting or the misuse of laxatives, diuretics or enemas. They will typically consume a large amount of food in a short period of time (binge). A typical binge consists of ingesting high calorie sweet foods with an average caloric intake of approximately 3,400 calories. A binge can range anywhere from 1,200 to 11,500 calories. They will then do something to get rid of the food (purge), such as vomit, over-exercise, or use a medication such as a laxative.

The most common compensatory method is induction of vomiting seen in approximately eighty to ninety percent of individuals with this disorder.

Non-Purging Type
An individual with this type of bulimia uses other inappropriate compensatory behaviors, such as fasting or excessive exercise.

Approximately thirty percent of individuals with bulimia misuse laxatives and diuretics. Between binges, individuals may restrict their diet to low-calorie foods while avoiding high fat foods or those that may trigger a binge.

Bulimia may also be associated with depressive symptoms, obsessive compulsive traits, substance abuse and/or other impulse control problems.

NOTE: Substance abuse and dependence (frequently alcohol and/ or other stimulants) were reported in approximately thirty percent of eating disorder cases.

Signs And Symptoms
- Persistent sore and inflamed throat
- Swollen salivary glands in the neck and throat
- Decreased tooth enamel with increased sensitivity and decaying teeth as a result of ongoing exposure to stomach acid
- Acid reflux disorder and other gastrointestinal problems. (See Chapter 11 for further detail on gastrointestinal disorders.)
- Intestinal distress and irritation from chronic laxative abuse
- Severe dehydration from purging of fluids
- Electrolyte imbalance (too high or too low levels of sodium, potassium, calcium and other minerals) which, if persists, may lead to a heart attack

Binge-Eating Disorder

An individual with binge-eating disorder loses control over their eating. Unlike bulimia nervosa, periods of binge eating are not followed by purging, excessive exercise or fasting. As a result of this behavior, individuals with binge eating disorder are overweight or obese. They also experience guilt, shame and distress about their binge eating which often times promotes further binge eating.

Diagnosis

Eating disorders are treatable medical illnesses. They can be found to coexist with other illnesses such as depression, anxiety and/or substance abuse. Some symptoms associated with an eating disorder can be life-threatening and death may result if treatment is not received!

Treatments

Eating disorders impact the whole person including mind, body and spirit. Effective treatment can be unique to each individual.

Most eating disorder treatment programs implement a comprehensive plan, including medical care, psychotherapy (talk therapy), nutritional education and medications when needed.

Eating disorders can affect every system of the body, especially the heart and kidneys. If left untreated, permanent damage and even death can occur. Some individuals may need to be hospitalized to treat these problems caused by malnutrition and to ensure they receive sufficient calorie intake.

Treating Anorexia Nervosa

Three important components of treatment are:

- Restoring a healthy weight. Weight gain of one-half to one pound a week is a good target goal. Keep in mind this is a very challenging disease to treat.
- Addressing the psychological issues related to the eating disorder
- Developing goals which eliminate behaviors and thoughts that promote insufficient eating.

Inpatient treatment becomes necessary when:

- Ideal weight falls below 75%
- Cardiac (heart) abnormalities and electrolyte imbalances occur and persist
- Outpatient therapy has failed

Medication therapy with use of antidepressants, antipsychotics and/or mood stabilizers may be effective in treating anorexia nervosa. These medications may also help improve mood and anxiety symptoms found to co-exist with anorexia nervosa. Different forms of psychotherapy including individual, group and family therapy can help address psychological concerns associated with this illness.

Treating Bulimia Nervosa

The goal of treatment is to reduce and eliminate binge-eating and purging behaviors.

Three forms of therapy may be effective:

• Nutritional counseling

• Psychotherapy to include cognitive behavior therapy (CBT). The therapist helps the individual to identify distorted thinking patterns and corrects inaccurate beliefs so they can change behaviors associated with this disorder.

• The antidepressant fluoxetine (Prozac) is the only FDA approved prescription medication for treating bulimia nervosa and may also help treat the depression and anxiety. Fluoxetine appears to help decrease the binge-eating and purging behaviors, reduce the chance of relapse and improve eating attitudes.

Treating Binge-Eating Disorder

• The goal of treatment is to reduce and eliminate binge-eating behaviors.

• Psychotherapy to include cognitive behavior therapy (CBT) which can be tailored to the individual. Individual and group therapies are both effective.

• Fluoxetine and other serotonin re-uptake inhibitors (SSRI) medications may help reduce binge eating episodes and improve mood in depressed individuals.

NOTE: Caution should be used when prescribing SSRIs like Fluoxetine in adolescents and young adults. The FDA warns that all patients receiving treatment with SSRIs should be closely monitored for adverse side effects such as depression that gets worse and/or thoughts of suicide.

Details On Different Therapies Used For Treating Eating Disorders

Art Therapy

Art therapy allows individuals to express themselves in a non-verbal manner, without the pressure of one-on-one therapy. This type of therapy can be an outlet to explore body image and provide a new perspective on viewing their distorted self-image.

Art therapy allows the individual to express their creativity and can serve as a journal to record the journey to recovery.

Culinary Therapy

Culinary therapy includes cooking classes, planting a garden, and grocery store and restaurant outings to help change their previous relationship with food.

This type of therapy can help individuals view food as a tool for achieving optimal health and look at meal time as an opportunity rather than a threat.

Dialectical Behavior Therapy (DBT)

This is one of the most effective therapies used to treat eating disorders. DBT teaches new coping skills to handle difficult emotions. Rather than resorting to previous eating behaviors, individuals develop a set of life skills they can use to maintain lasting recovery.

The four DBT skill sets are:

- *Mindfulness:* Staying in the present moment with a deep awareness of one's thoughts, feelings and actions. Rather than judging a thought or feeling, mindfulness practice helps individuals accept whatever they are experiencing in a given moment. This greater awareness allows individuals to regulate their thoughts and feelings, shifting their attention in another direction when their thought pattern is becoming unproductive or unhealthy.

- *Distress Tolerance:* Learning to accept distress and other difficult emotions that are an inevitable part of life, rather than resorting to eating disorder behaviors. Part of distress tolerance is delaying gratification and avoiding impulsive behaviors, thereby finding healthier ways to cope such as self-soothing, distracting and assessing pros and cons.

- *Emotional Regulation:* Identifying emotions and working to let go of painful feelings to make room for positive ones.

- *Interpersonal Effectiveness:* Improving interpersonal relationships by increasing assertiveness and communication skills. Individuals learn skills such as asking for what they need, setting healthy boundaries and coping with conflict effectively without hurting others or jeopardizing their self-respect.

Family Therapy

Eating disorders affect the entire family causing frustration and concern which can draw attention away from other members. Recovery is a process that unfolds each day in the presence of family and friends.

Studies have shown that family involvement is essential for successful eating disorder recovery. Family therapy affords the individual an opportunity to discuss any underlying issues and conflicts with their family in the presence of an objective therapist. Conflicted, controlling and over organized family environments can impede recovery.

Borderline personality disorder may be seen along with anorexia and can be associated with poor emotional expression and problem solving abilities in families.

Family therapy can accomplish the following goals:

- Educate family members about eating disorders and the recovery process

- Instill new conflict resolution skills and communication strategies

- Prepare family members for the individual to return home (if prior in-patient therapy was needed)

- Help family members learn how to support their loved one's recovery

- Increase communication among family members to offer support

- Ensure that family members have a supportive network of their own in place and a healthy sense of self

- Provide guidance so members can take care of their own needs while also providing support

Group Therapy

Group therapy is a critical part of eating-disorder treatment. Hearing about other individuals experiences and that they are facing similar struggles can be a beneficial aspect of treatment.

Individuals are able to share their pain in a safe nurturing environment and realize that they are not alone. Group therapy can help the individual build self-esteem and serve as a model for developing trusting and supportive relationships. The group setting is a safe place to try new communication skills and learn to accept both themselves and others.

Individuals can also help one another identify and resolve problems with the guidance and expertise of a professional therapist. A caring spirit can encourage one to question distorted thoughts and destructive behaviors and promote the process of change.

Group therapy is a great place to learn about nutrition, the process of recovery, relapse prevention, assertiveness techniques and coping skills.

Individual Therapy

Eating disorder treatment is a journey of self discovery. Individual therapy provides an opportunity to explore sensitive personal issues with feedback from a therapist. One-on-one therapy creates an opportunity for healing by directly addressing the specific issues such as childhood experiences, difficult relationships and emotions associated with the eating disorder. This therapy combines psychoanalysis and cognitive-behavior therapy.

Cognitive-Behavior Therapy (CBT)

This treatment focuses on changing distorted cognitions associated with body images and food intake. CBT is used as a practical approach for solving problems and changing thought patterns. This therapy can help an individual learn new skills to reduce eating disorder symptoms, recognize triggers and avoid relapses.

Movement Therapy

Many eating disorder programs offer some type of movement therapy. While exercise can trigger or exacerbate eating disorder behaviors, movement therapy can help individuals become aware of their bodies and feel more comfortable in their own skin.

Movement therapy can provide:

- A healthier body image
- A greater appreciation for one's physical health
- A positive outlook when movement therapy is combined with music
- Relaxation through breathing exercises
- A greater acceptance of self and others

Nutrition Therapy

Nutrition education and counseling is offered by most eating disorder treatment programs.

A registered dietitian works with the individual to encourage normal food intake and a healthy relationship with food. The dietitian will assess eating patterns, weight, exercise habits, medical concerns and body image.

Nutrition counseling sessions can teach the individual about:

- Different types of food, including carbohydrates, proteins and fats and why the body needs these foods
- Portion sizes and the need to eat a variety of foods in moderation
- The consequences of eating disorder behaviors
- Recognizing the body's hunger cues
- How to create balanced meal plans
- Eating in social situations
- Overcoming fears associated with certain foods
- Healthy exercise routines
- Nutritional supplements that can be of benefit

The dietician and the individual can work together to create achievable goals while providing support, encouragement and understanding. Once the nutritional needs have been met, the individual may often experience improved energy and sleep, which clearly helps them feel better.

Psychiatric Care

Psychiatrists and psychologists work together with individuals to assess, diagnose and treat eating disorders.

Many times individuals will have other co-existing anxiety and depression which require dual treatment from a team of healthcare professionals.

Psychiatrists may need to prescribe medications to aid in weight maintenance or to treat symptoms of co-occurring mental health issues.

Individual psychotherapy can address weight through the use of contingent management programs. Weight gain is rewarded with privileges, which reinforces the positive aspects of treatment and aides in progress for the individual.

Support Groups
All individuals diagnosed with an eating disorder need support. Family and friends can certainly provide support, although structured eating disorder support groups can also be beneficial.

Support groups combined with other forms of therapy can help individuals develop relationship skills and promote motivation needed for maintained recovery.

Some of the well known eating disorder support groups you may recognize:
• Overeaters Anonymous
• Anorexics and Bulimics Anonymous
• Eating Disorders Anonymous

Summary
The goal of treatment for anorexia is weight gain and subsequent maintenance.

Inpatient treatment is recommended to address the behavioral patterns which often lead to the severe physical consequences outlined earlier in this chapter.

Outpatient treatment and follow-up care may be appropriate in less severe cases.

Fluoxetine (Prozac) and other SSRIs (Selective Serotonin Re-uptake Inhibitors) have shown some effectiveness for weight maintenance.

Antidepressant medications have been found to be effective in reducing the frequency of binge-purge behaviors seen with bulimia.

Many individuals who have been diagnosed with bulimia may also experience depression.

Binge Eating Disorder has been shown to respond favorably to SSRIs like fluoxetine (Prozac).

Eating disorders can take a toll on the body. The longer the behaviors take place, the greater the risk of developing serious and sometimes life threatening health consequences.

The following medical complications can occur as a result of anorexia, bulimia and related eating disorders:

• Heart disease and/or heart attack
• Ongoing depression and anxiety
• Irregular menstrual periods
• Bone loss, osteoporosis
• Seizures
• Kidney damage
• Diabetes
• High or low blood pressure
• Dental problems
• GERD, hiatal hernia and gastrointestinal bleeding
• Death

If you see changes in a individual's weight, eating behavior and conversations dominated by food or weight, be suspicious and on the alert to direct them to the right path for obtaining help.

Keep in mind that it may take several years for middle aged women to respond to treatment for eating disorders and achieve a full recovery. Middle-aged and older individuals tend to have a higher level of maturity and more life experiences which can be a real plus in reaching the goal to recovery. Increased awareness of eating disorders in older women can lead to better treatment outcomes so do not wait until it is too late!

A Few Words About Overeating And Obesity

Obesity has become commonplace in our culture, yet it destroys the lives of thousands of individuals each year. More than one in three adults are now obese, which translates to 37.9%. The percentage of adults aged 20 and over who are overweight is about 32.5%. So Americans who are overweight and obese is approaching 70 percent and the highest incidence is among middle-aged adults.

The prevalence of obesity in 2014 was 36.5 percent in US adults. Overall the prevalence among middle-aged adults aged 40-59 was 40.2 percent and among older adults aged 60 and older was 37.0 percent. The overall prevalence of obesity in women for this age group was 38.3 percent compared to 34.3 percent in men. In individuals over 60 the percentages are very similar among both sexes.

Definition
You are classified as being obese when you are more than twenty percent over your ideal weight, based on age, gender and activity level and/or have greater than thirty percent body fat for women and twenty-five percent for men.

Causes
• Genetics
• Overeating
• Consuming too many high-fat, high sugar and high caloric foods
• Sedentary lifestyle
• Social and cultural expectations
• Emotional and/or psychological issues
• Hormonal fluctuations and imbalance

Health Risks Associated With Obesity
• Heart disease
• Stroke
• High blood pressure and cholesterol
• Diabetes
• Certain types of cancer
• Depression
• Pregnancy complications
• Eating disorders

Treatment
If you are struggling with excess weight, you are not alone. Weight loss can improve your life dramatically.

- Learn new skills, adopt new lifestyle habits and become physically active. You have to move your body to burn fat and lose weight.
- Begin psychotherapy to address underlying emotional issues.
- Enroll in a weight loss program like Weight Watchers to help you get started and learn how to make better food choices so you can enjoy long term success.
- There are several medications available to help facilitate weight loss.
  - Orlistat (Xenical and Alli) works in the gastrointestinal tract by preventing absorption of about 30 percent of ingested fat.
  - Newer prescription medications are available that target specific serotonin receptors in the brain associated with appetite and others that decrease cravings and promote feelings of satiety (feeling full) and satisfaction. The names of these medications are Belviq (lorcaserin), Contrave (naltrexone HCL and bupropion HCL) and Qysmia (topiramate extended-release and phentermine). These medications are approved for treatment of obese individuals with a body mass index (BMI) of 30 or higher or individuals with a BMI of 27 or more who have at least one weight-related health condition such as type 2 diabetes, high blood pressure and/or high cholesterol. These drugs can have dangerous side effects and can interact with other medicines so your clinician will determine if one of these medications would be appropriate treatment for you.
  - Saxenda (liraglutide) is the fourth new drug to receive approval from the FDA to be used for weight loss. This medication mimics a hormone in the intestines called GLP-1 (glucagon-like peptide) which tells your brain that you feel full. Saxenda is administered by an injection and titrated over several weeks to reach a 3 mg dose given once daily. This medication is approved for individuals with a BMI (body mass index) of 30 (considered to be obese) or a BMI of 27 with one weight-related condition such as high blood pressure, high cholesterol and/or type 2 diabetes. A lower dose of this same medication (1.8 mg daily) is currently being used to treat type 2 Diabetes and the brand name is Victoza.
- Bariatric Surgery: If you are morbidly obese and all attempted treatment measures for weight loss have failed, you may be a candidate for gastric by-pass surgery. This type of surgical procedure is performed on the stomach or intestines to promote weight loss.

NOTE: Your clinician can determine which weight loss treatment will be best for you and can prescribe a medication or recommend surgery if needed.

Do not delay and get started today! It could possibly save your life!

NOTE: Please see Chapters 3 and 10 for more information on healthy eating choices, lifestyle recommendations and diabetes.

Websites for further information on:

Anorexia Nervosa

Facts, Signs and Symptoms of Anorexia-Bulimia: **https://www.bulimia.com/topics/anorexia/**

Eating Disorders

American Psychiatric Association: **http://www.psychiatry.org/patients-families/eating-disorders**

Bing Eating Disorder (BED): **https://www1.bingeeatingdisorder.com/**

National Institute of Mental Health: **https://www.nimh.nih.gov/health/topics/eating-disorders/**

Binge-eating, Anorexia nervosa and Bulimia nervosa: **http://www.mayoclinic.org/diseases-conditions/eating-disorders/symptoms-causes/dxc-20182875**

National Eating Disorders Association: **https://www.nationaleatingdisorders.org/**

Obesity

Obesity Resources- Public Health: **http://www.publichealth.org/resources/obesity/**

Centers for Disease Control and Prevention: **https://www.cdc.gov/obesity/data/adult.html**

Chapter 13

Mood And Sleep Disturbances

Relieving Anxiety

Definition

Anxiety is defined as free floating fear or a state of apprehension and can be a normal reaction to stress and an important part of life. It can help us get out of harm's way, prepare for important events and warns us when we need to take action. Everyone has experienced feeling worried, anxious or nervous at some time in their life but when it continues and affects your daily life, it is time to seek treatment.

Menopause And Anxiety

Anxiety affects your mind and body and is a common symptom of perimenopause and menopause. It seems to be associated with declining estrogen levels. The lower levels of endorphins and serotonin that follow along with low estrogen levels may trigger anxiety.

Think of it as your threshold to deal with stressors in your life has just been lowered. Some days you may find yourself having no patience at all. It is OK and you are not alone! There are a lot of us baby boomers out there. Just inform the people around you that your mood could change suddenly and they have now been warned! Once the fluctuating hormones calm down, this too shall pass.

Women are twice as likely as men to experience anxiety that interferes with daily living.

Anxiety can also be associated with:

• Depression

• Insomnia (inability to sleep)

• Excessive fatigue

• Overwhelming stress

• Angry outbursts

• Substance abuse

Some women may experience "panic attacks" during perimenopause.

Emotional symptoms:

• Intense fear or worry

• Anger

• Irritability

• Panic accompanied with a sensation of losing control.

Physical symptoms:

• Shortness of breath

• Feeling restless, trembling or twitching

• Sweaty, cold and clammy hands

• A choking sensation

• Heart pounding (palpitations)

• Lightheaded or dizziness and/or disorientation

NOTE: You need to see your clinician if you experience any of the above symptoms, as it could also be your heart. Heart disease is the number one killer of women! If these feelings continue and interfere with daily functioning, an anxiety disorder may develop.

Try These Simple ABCs To Help Manage Anxiety

• Accept yourself

• Be yourself and take care of yourself

• Control yourself when possible

If you have been experiencing anxiety it would be a good idea to see your clinician and have a complete physical exam with blood work, which could identify an underlying condition that may cause anxiety.

Treatment

Prescription Medications: If you are diagnosed with a general anxiety disorder, many times a selective serotonin reuptake inhibitor (SSRI) medication may be prescribed such as Zoloft (sertraline), Paxil (paroxetine) or Lexapro (escitalopram). Another class of medications referred to as serotonin norepinephrine reuptake inhibitors (SNRIs) may be prescribed instead. Common medications used are Effexor (venlafaxine) and Cymbalta (duloxetine). Benzodiazepines such as Xanax (alprazolam) and Ativan (lorazepam) are commonly prescribed for a short term. This class of drugs can be very addictive, so use with caution! A different type of medicine used to treat anxiety is called Buspar (buspirone) and is non-habit forming. Your clinician will determine which medication will be best for you.

Talk Therapy: We refer to this as psychotherapy.

Hypnotherapy: This therapy involves hypnotizing the individual during the treatment session and has been reported to be effective for reducing anxiety.

Acupuncture: This treatment uses tiny needles placed over different parts of the body which can soothe and relax tense muscles, restoring a sense of well-being.

NOTE: Anxiety disorders are real, treatable and can be very serious. Untreated anxiety disorders may lead to depression and even substance abuse. You need to seek treatment as soon as possible, so you can begin to enjoy life. Be sure to read the lifestyle modification section in Chapter 3 and look at "The Twelve Prevention Steps" for managing a stressful life.

Tips For Relieving Stress When You Work

• Go to bed early and wake up with the sun, so you can get things done. This gives you a little quiet/private time before everyone gets up.

- This is a great time to exercise and get energized to start your day.
- Leave the house early to anticipate any delays.
- Listen to relaxing music while you are in traffic and try the slow breathing exercises. You can car pool which saves gas and you can chat. I am very fortunate to work with my sister, so we can catch up on everything when we car pool. Remember the *cuddle hormone* to tend and befriend?
- Arrive early at the office so you will have a little time to get organized and relax before you start work. (Anyone who knows me well will laugh at this one!) I need to take my own advice and leave now. Have a great day and safe driving!

Depression

One out of every four women will develop clinical depression during her lifetime, according to the National Mental Health Association.

Women are more than twice as likely as men to develop depression.

Smile, it is almost entirely treatable! Believe it or not, only about one third of the individuals with depression seek treatment.

Description
Depression is real and a common medical illness that affects your mind and body. Hormonal changes associated with menstrual cycle changes, miscarriage, childbirth, menopause and perimenopause can all contribute to mood changes. Depression is especially common during the perimenopausal and menopausal years. Depression is not a moral failure or *"only in your mind."*

Major depression interferes with the ability to work, sleep, eat and enjoy activities. Once you have had an episode of major depression, you are at risk for having another!

Menopause And Depression
Many women experience insomnia, anxiety and irritability during perimenopause and if these symptoms continue the risk of developing a major depression increases.

Women seem to be more vulnerable to developing depression because of hormonal imbalances during their lifetime, coupled with increased demands at the work place and at home.

Menopause does not cause depression per se, although the hormonal imbalances that occur during the perimenopausal period coupled with midlife events can certainly contribute to the onset of depression.

Factors That Can Trigger Depression

• Grief (death of a loved one, divorce, loss of job and/or a parent's illness)

• Unresolved emotional issues (conflict with a boss or co-worker)

• Transitions (moving, job change or retirement)

• Hormonal imbalances (pregnancy, perimenopause and menopause). Women who have had a hysterectomy may be more likely to experience menopause related depression than women who go through natural menopause. Women who abruptly stop estrogen therapy rather than tapering off slowly may also experience depression.

NOTE: Estrogen assists in the making of serotonin (a chemical which helps regulate mood) so lower estrogen levels can mean lower serotonin levels.

• Having a chronic illness, such as heart disease, arthritis, diabetes and/or cancer.

• Having a permanent disability from an injury or illness such as a stroke

• Having a personal or family history of a depressive disorder

• Having a personal history of an anxiety disorder

• If you think you might be depressed, ask yourself these few questions. Over the past couple of weeks have you felt:

  • Down, depressed or hopeless?

  • Little interest in doing things?

  • Do you want to sleep all the time?

Common Symptoms

• Little interest or pleasure in doing things

• Feelings of depressed mood and hopelessness

• Unable to sleep or you may sleep too much

• Feeling tired and a lack of energy

- Poor appetite or overeating
- Negative feelings about one's self or a perception that you have let people down
- Difficulty concentrating and/or focusing
- Slowness in movement or speaking, which is evident to others
- Restless or fidgety movements
- Thoughts of self-harm or feelings that you would be better off dead
- Low self-esteem despite contrary information

If you have experienced five or more of the above mentioned symptoms on most days for two consecutive weeks, you need to see your clinician as soon as possible for an evaluation and treatment.

Treatment
Depression is treatable and the sooner the better!

Prescription Medications
There are many different medications used to treat depression.

The selective serotonin reuptake inhibitors (SSRIs) and the serotonin and norepinephrine reuptake inhibitors (SNRIs) medications are commonly prescribed to treat depression and anxiety.

Selective Serotonin Reuptake Inhibitors (SSRIs)
Common names you may recognize are: Prozac (fluoxetine), Celexa (citalopram), Zoloft (sertraline), Paxil (paroxetine) and Lexapro (escitalopram).

This class of medications carries a black box warning that it can be associated with suicidal thinking and behavior in children, adolescents and young adults.

Serotonin and Norepinephrine reuptake inhibitors (SNRIs)
Common names you may recognize are: Effexor (venlafaxine), Pristiq and Khedezla (desvenlafaxine), Cymbalta (duloxetine), Fetzima (levomilnacipran) and two newer SNRIs, Trintellix (vortioxetine) and Viibryd (vilazodone).

NOTE: Sexual side effects can occur with both the SSRI and SNRI antidepressants. Trintellix is reported to have less sexual side effects and improves cognition. Cymbalta has an added benefit of relieving chronic pain.

Tricyclic antidepressants (TCAs)

This is an older group of medications and not commonly used to-day due to unwanted side effects such as dizziness, blood pressure changes and dry mouth. Names you may recognize are: Elavil (amitriptyline), Adapin and Sinequan (doxepin), Tofranil (imipramine), Pamelor (nortriptyline) and Vivactil (protriptyline).

Wellbutrin and Aplenzin (bupropion)

This is a different type of antidepressant medication that affects the brain chemicals norepinephrine and dopamine. This medication is not associated with the side effect of a decreased libido although it has an increased risk for the possibility of developing a seizure.

Remeron (mirtazapine)

This medication is used more commonly in the elderly because it promotes weight gain and sleep.

Desyrel (trazadone)

This is an older antidepressant medication that was also used to promote sleep. It has many other unwanted side effects such as dizziness, blurred vision, constipation and dry mouth.

It is very important to take your medication daily and to continue for six to nine months, even though you are feeling better. Taking your medication daily can help prevent another episode of depression from occurring.

Your clinician can assess you and then recommend a medication that is right for you and will determine the length of time the medication is needed.

NOTE: These medications are not addictive. Never stop taking your medication abruptly and always talk to your clinician about how to slowly taper off a medication. During perimenopause and menopause you may also need to take hormone replacement therapy to correct the hormonal imbalance, which can certainly affect your mood. Once the hormonal imbalance has been corrected, your clinician can adjust the dosage as needed. According to the North American Menopause Society, women are more likely than men to consume more alcohol when they are depressed, so be careful! Alcohol is a depressant, addictive and can make depression even worse.

Psychotherapy

Talk therapy may be recommended, referred to as "psychotherapy." This includes individual and group counseling.

Individual therapy provides an opportunity to explore sensitive personal issues with feedback from a therapist. One-on-one therapy also creates an opportunity for healing by addressing specific issues such as childhood experiences, difficult relationships and emotions associated with experiencing a depressed mood.

Group therapy allows individuals to realize that they are not alone and others may be facing similar struggles, which can be a beneficial aspect of treatment.

Exercise

It is very important to exercise regularly because it releases feel good hormones called endorphins and raises your serotonin level! Use the five minute rule. Commit to begin an activity for five minutes and add a minute each day until you achieve thirty minutes. In a month's time you will be exercising for a thirty minute session. Getting started can be the biggest step!

Nutrition

It is also important to eat healthy and include nine servings of fruits and vegetables daily. Avoid processed foods and sugar!

Recommendations To Follow

• Do not isolate yourself and be sure to make social contact.

• Do not forget to take time out to do something you enjoy!

• Depression can hurt you and those closest to you, so don't delay in getting the help you need to start feeling better.

Remember, depression is treatable and not your fault or a sign of weakness!

Insomnia

We sleep because our bodies need sleep. Deep restorative sleep is one of the most important factors that contributes to our overall health and well-being.

If you don't sleep then your body doesn't get a chance to refuel itself. This can have an effect on your mood, memory and concentration. As we age our sleep patterns change and *women are twice as likely as men to experience insomnia!*

Insomnia is a sleep disorder characterized by difficulty falling asleep and/or staying asleep. People who have insomnia commonly report experiencing the following:

• Difficulty falling asleep

• Waking up often during the night and having trouble going back to sleep

• Waking up too early in the morning

• Feeling tired upon awakening

Insomnia can vary in how long it lasts and how often it occurs. It can be short-term, called acute insomnia, and can last one night to a few weeks.

It can be long term, which is called chronic insomnia and can last thirty days or more. *Hormones do play a role!*

Researchers see insomnia rise when menstruation begins at puberty and again at the start of perimenopause. Menopause can certainly have a significant effect on sleep too.

Interruptions in normal sleep patterns are common complaints of perimenopausal and menopausal women. Many conditions contribute to sleeplessness during this period of a women's life (no pun intended).

• Night sweats and hot flashes

• Anxiety, when our minds are overactive

• The need to urinate during the night

• Heart palpitations

• Heartburn

• Headaches

• Body aches and pains

How Hormones Can Affect Your Sleep

The powerful role that hormones play in sleep may help you understand why so many women have difficulty falling asleep or staying asleep when their hormones are fluctuating.

Many different hormones influence sleep and when their levels fluctuate or change, sleep is often affected. A hormone deficiency or imbalance can contribute to feeling exhausted and/or waking up feeling tired.

The following hormones can influence your sleep:

Melatonin

This hormone is produced by the pineal gland located in the brain which regulates and promotes good sleep. This hormone lowers body temperature and its production is triggered by darkness. A decrease in the level of melatonin, such as with women experiencing PMS or perimenopause, can lead to:

• Difficulty falling asleep
• Difficulty going back to sleep after waking up
• Feeling anxious and agitated during sleep

Growth Hormone

This hormone is produced by the pituitary gland located in the brain and is essential throughout life for growth, development and repair of body tissues. It is released from the gland early in the evening and at the onset of sleep. Deficiency of growth hormone can lead to the same symptoms as described for melatonin deficiency.

Cortisol

This hormone triggers the type of slow wave, restorative sleep found in stages 3 and 4, as well as the production of growth hormone. Cortisol levels usually rise in the late morning and early afternoon, and then decrease by evening. A deficiency of this hormone can be associated with feeling un-refreshed upon awakening, even if you slept through the night. During sleep, cortisol mobilizes energy stores from the body to be ready for use the following day.

Thyroid Hormone

This hormone regulates your metabolism. A deficiency in thyroid hormones may cause you to awaken with puffy eyes and a swollen face in the morning. The same symptoms that you would see with a melatonin, cortisol and growth hormone deficiency, are found with a thyroid deficiency too. Thyroid replacement has been shown to improve sleep quality. *(Please read Chapter 8 for more detailed information on thyroid disease.)*

Can you now see how closely these hormones work together?

Estrogens

This group of hormones helps to regulate the production of many hormones that are secreted when we sleep, like melatonin, growth hormone and cortisol. When your estrogen levels fluctuate, your sleep can definitely be affected. Estrogens promote REM sleep and declining levels of estrogens can be associated with sleep disturbances, leading to exhaustion.

Progesterone

This hormone has been shown to produce a calming and sedative affect in many sleep studies. Progesterone appears to reduce the amount of time it takes to fall asleep and the number of wakeful disruptions through the night. A decreased level of progesterone may lead to problems falling asleep.

Testosterone

This hormone may help enhance concentration, focus and libido. A testosterone deficiency has been linked to feelings of fatigue, even after a full night of sleep. This may contribute in part as to why women are twice as likely as men to encounter sleep problems.

Common Causes Of Acute Insomnia

- *Significant life stress:* Loss of job, death of a loved one, divorce, or moving
- *Illness:* Acute or chronic
- *Emotional or physical discomfort:* Pain
- *Environmental factors:* Noise, spouse snoring, light, extreme temperatures (hot or cold)
- *Medications:* Over-the-counter preparations used to treat colds and allergies. Prescription medications used to treat depression, high blood pressure and asthma
- *Changes in normal sleep pattern:* Jet lag, travel, having a newborn or switching to a night shift at work

Causes Of Chronic Insomnia

- Depression and/or anxiety
- Chronic stress
- Prolonged pain or discomfort at night
- Persistent hot flashes during perimenopause and menopause

Sleep Deprivation

- Decreases the ability to concentrate
- Decreases reaction time

- Increases memory lapses and forgetfulness
- Increases the likelihood of accidents or injuries to occur
- Increases moodiness and anxiety
- Increases susceptibility to illness
- Can make you feel tired throughout the day

Changes Sleep Deprivation Can Cause

- *Appetite:* Changes in metabolism that produce a state of hunger and how your body handles insulin, which could lead to insulin resistance, weight gain and eventually diabetes.
- *Immune system:* Your immune system can become weakened, increasing your chances of infection.
- *Memory and concentration:* Forgetfulness and inability to focus and concentrate.
- *Mood:* The threshold for depressive symptoms to appear can be lowered and even an acute schizophrenic episode may occur with severe sleep deprivation!

Brief Description Of Other Sleep Disorders

Sleep Apnea
This condition causes you to stop breathing while you are sleeping. This is often associated with snoring, obesity and diabetes. Sleep apnea disrupts your sleep cycle during the night and so you feel sleepy during the day.

Narcolepsy
This condition results in sleep attacks, which are sudden periods of uncontrollable sleep during waking hours.

Restless Legs Syndrome (RLS)
This condition causes prickling or tingling sensations in your legs and feet at night. This sensation is brought on by lying down in bed or from prolonged periods of sitting (driving, flying or sitting in a theatre). Individuals with RLS often want to walk around and shake their legs to help relieve the uncomfortable sensation.

Tips For A Good Nights Sleep

- *Set a Sleep Schedule*
Go to bed at the same time each night and get up at the same time each morning. Try to get up with the sun. Sunlight helps your body

reset its internal clock each day. (For every hour of sleep you receive between the hours of 9:00 PM and 2:00 AM, you may get the benefit of receiving two hours of sleep per hour.)

- *Get Regular Exercise*
Exercise for at least 30 minutes or more every day in the morning if you can. Be sure *not* to exercise at least 5 hours before bedtime. Do gentle stretching at night to direct blood flow to hands and feet, improving circulation.

- *Relax Before Bedtime*
Associate restful activities with sleep and make them a part of your bedtime ritual. Try a warm bath, massage, slow deep breathing exercises, reading or listening to music. You can combine any of the above to enhance the effect.

- *Make It Dark and Cozy*
Be sure it is dark, quiet, and not too warm or too cold. If light is a problem, try a sleeping mask. If noise is a problem, try ear plugs or a fan to cover up the sounds.

- *Take a Hot Bath, Shower or Jacuzzi*
You can trick your body into dropping its temperature, which promotes sleep.

- *Avoid Caffeine, Nicotine and Alcohol Late in the Day*
Caffeine and nicotine are stimulants. Do not consume caffeine in the evening, including coffee, chocolate, soft drinks or teas. Be careful with over-the-counter pain relievers and weight loss supplements because they may contain caffeine. Alcohol can cause waking in the night and can interfere with sleep quality.

- *Don't Just Lie There*
The stress of not being able to fall asleep can actually contribute to insomnia. If you can't sleep, get up and read or do something that is not overly stimulating until you feel sleepy.

- *Don't Eat a Heavy Meal Late in the Day*
A light snack before bedtime may actually help you sleep.

- *Avoid Using Your Bed for Anything Other than Sleep and Sex*
You will then only associate your bed with sleep and intimacy.

Diagnosing Insomnia

If you think you have insomnia, talk to your clinician. An evaluation may include:

- A complete physical exam with blood tests to check for any other medical conditions
- A sleep diary (keeping track of your sleep patterns) and a possible interview with your sleep partner to determine the quality and quantity of your sleep. You can download an app like Fitbit on most cell phones or wear a watch that can track your sleep patterns.
- A referral to a sleep study center

Treatment

Treatment for insomnia usually involves nonmedical therapy such as developing better sleep habits and talk therapy (psychotherapy). Insomnia may not require any further treatment other than just modifying your sleep patterns.

Try warming your feet with thermal socks, providing you're *not* experiencing any hot flashes.

Sleep medications may be needed with certain individuals.

Over-The-Counter Sleep Aids

These medications usually contain an anti-histamine, such as Benadryl and may help if you have *occasional* problems dozing off.

Prescription Sleep Medications

You may require a prescription sleeping pill for a short time, thirty-five days or less. It is possible for you to develop dependence in as little as six weeks, so don't ask for refills!

Commonly prescribed medications that you may recognize are divided into two different families of drugs.

Medications that belong to the *Non-benzodiazipine* family are typically the first medications used to help treat short term insomnia:

Ambien (zolpidem), Sonata (zaleplon) and Lunesta (eszopiclone). An oral spray called Zolpimist contains the same active ingredients found in Ambien and should be used for a short duration only. The FDA now requires manufacturers of this medication to offer lower doses for women because they metabolize the drug more slowly than men.

Another medication called *Rozerem* works differently and is similar to the sleep hormone melatonin. This medication does not cause morning sleepiness and is not addictive.

Belsomra (suvorexant) is a relatively new medication that works by blocking chemicals in the brain that keep you awake, helping to promote sleep. This medication is referred to as an orexin receptor antagonist.

Medications that belong to the **Benzodiazepine** family are:

Restoril (temazepam), Dalmane (flurazepam), ProSom (estazolam), Ativan (lorazepam), Xanax (alprazolam) and Halcion (triazolam). These medications help you fall asleep and/or stay asleep.

WARNING: Most of these medications are addictive with extended use and are dangerous if taken with alcohol and other drugs that depress the central nervous system! They can also cause morning sleepiness.

Side effects in general tend to be less with the non-benzodiazepine group of sleep medications.

In some cases an antidepressant medication may be prescribed to help individuals diagnosed with depression. These medications are currently not approved for treating insomnia.

Silenor (doxepin) is in the family of hypnotic medications and is used to treat insomnia in individuals who have trouble staying asleep.

Your clinician can assess you and determine which and if any prescription therapy is needed.

Meditation
This practice has been used for many years throughout different cultures and can promote relaxation to improve sleep. Yoga and biofeedback can also help reduce tension and promote sleep.

Cognitive Behavioral Therapy (CBT), Relaxation Training And Sleep Restriction Therapy
These behavior approaches may help change behaviors that worsen insomnia and encourage behaviors that promote sleep.

Restriction Therapy: It is important to cut down on the number of hours you stay in bed, no matter how little sleep you actually get during the night.

Relaxation Training: Consider taking a warm bath before bed or practice yoga ending with a corpse pose where you totally relax your mind and all the muscles in your body.

Cognitive Behavioral Therapy: Cognitive behavioral therapy for the treatment of chronic insomnia is a structured program that helps you identify and replace thoughts and behaviors that cause or make sleep problems worse with new habits that promote sound sleep.

Studies have shown that CBT actually works better and for a longer duration than medication in alleviating insomnia. This form of therapy should be considered on a case-by-case basis due to the variability of an individual's motivation, lifestyle and other medical conditions that may be of concern.

Remember reading in Chapter 12 about how CBT was effective in helping change the behaviors associated with eating disorders?

Hormone Replacement Therapy (HRT)
Hormone replacement may be an option to treat hot flashes and related symptoms of menopause that promote ongoing insomnia. Natural progesterone cream may help create a calming effect to promote sleep and should be used in the evening before bedtime.

(Please read Chapter 3 for detailed information on hormone replacement therapy.)

Herbal Remedies
Many herbal remedies have commonly been used to help relieve insomnia:

- **Anise seeds and oil** may have estrogen-like effects promoting sleep.
- **Lemon Balm extract** drops can be dissolved into water and taken 30 minutes before bed.
- **Valerian root** may help promote sleep and decrease stress.
- **Evening Primrose oil** may act as a sedative.
- **L-Trytophan** can promote drowsiness.
- **Melatonin** is the hormone that promotes sleep.
- **Rooibos tea** (an African bush tea, which contains no artificial colors, additives, preservatives or caffeine) promotes relaxation.
- **Somnapure** is a combination natural product that contains Melatonin, L-Theanine, Valerian, Hops and Lemon Balm extracts, as well as Chamomile and Passion flowers. Many of my patients have reported that this supplement really works.

NOTE: *Use caution when taking herbal supplements. Scientific evidence regarding their safety is lacking! (See Chapter 3 for more detailed information on herbal remedies and supplements.)*

Sleep deprivation can be detrimental to your health! It is also very important to identify and treat underlying health conditions or health problems that could be causing the insomnia.

Do not delay in getting the help you need.

Sweet dreams!

Websites for further information on:

Anxiety and Depression

Anxiety Disorders Association of America: **https://www.adaa.org/**

National Institute of Mental Health: **https://www.nimh.nih.gov/**

National Mental health Association: **http://www.mentalhealthamerica.net/**

Office on Women's Health: **https://www.womenshealth.gov/mental-health/illnesses/anxiety-disorders.html**

Office on Women's Health: **https://www.womenshealth.gov/mental-health/illnesses/depression.html**

National Alliance for the Mentally Ill-Mental Health Conditions: **http://www.nami.org/**

National Foundation for Depressive Illnesses: **http://www.depression.org/**

Sleep and Insomnia

American Sleep Association-healthfinder.gov: **https://healthfinder.gov/Find Services/Organizations/Organization.aspx?code=HR3926**

American Sleep Apnea Association: **https://www.sleepapnea.org**

What is Insomnia? National Institutes of Health: **https://www.nhlbi.nih.gov/health/health-topics/topics/inso/**

National Sleep Foundation: **https://sleepfoundation.org/**

Restless Legs Syndrome Foundation: **https://www.rls.org/**

Chapter 14

Brain Health

Your brain can be thought of as the control tower that runs your life. It weighs in at about three pounds and resembles a walnut in shape.

The changes that occur during menopause can affect your health in many ways, and brain function and memory may become altered in some women.

It is thought that female hormones are needed for the brain to function well and some reports show that women have more *memory* and *mood* problems after menopause.

Estrogen And Your Brain

Estrogen influences many functions throughout our body and strongly impacts the parts of the brain that control emotion.

Some of estrogen's positive effects:

• Increases the level of serotonin and the number of serotonin receptors in the brain (serotonin has a positive effect on mood)

- Influences the production of endorphins, the "feel-good" chemicals in the brain

- Protects nerves in the brain against damage and possibly stimulates nerve growth

- Influences dilation of the blood vessels and helps direct blood to parts of your brain that are most active

- Promotes an anti-inflammatory effect on the blood vessel wall, helping to prevent damage from free radicals and plaque formation

How Menopause Impacts The Central Nervous System

The Hot Flash Effect

Hot flashes are known as the classic symptom of menopause and approximately eighty-five percent of perimenopausal women experience them. A hot flash consists of a sudden sensation of heat in the upper body, often followed by sweating and a chill. This sensation originates in the brain as a direct response from a low level of estrogen being detected in the thermoregulatory center of the part of the brain called the hypothalamus.

New evidence suggests that a hot flash is not only a classic symptom of menopause but may also lead to further neurologic problems.

Hot flashes have been directly correlated with memory impairment in women who have undergone surgical removal of their ovaries. The abrupt and severe decline of estrogen after having your ovaries removed can result in cognitive decline as early as two months and commonly occurs within five years after surgery.

Decreased cerebral blood flow to the brain has been documented during a hot flash with the use of single proton emission computed tomography (SPECT) scan in healthy menopausal women. The patterns of decreased cerebral blood flow imaged during a hot flash resembled changes seen in Alzheimer's disease. The greatest change occurred in the part of the brain called the hippocampus, a center for memory and cognition. Great, just what we need? NOT!

NOTE: Studies have shown that estrogen replacement resolved the hot flashes and restored normal patterns of blood flow.

Memory Function

The risk of developing dementia and Alzheimer's disease does increase with age. Postmenopausal women have a greater risk than men for developing this disease.

The brain volume begins to decline even in healthy older women when estrogen levels begin to decline during the perimenopausal period. These cerebral changes identified in women may contribute to the frequently seen perimenopausal complaints of decreased mental clarity, short term and verbal memory problems. A similar loss in brain volume does not occur in men until a decade later (about 60 years of age) due to the gradual loss of male sex hormones.

Studies of the effects of estrogen replacement therapy (ERT) on cognitive symptoms have reported inconsistent results.

According to the Women's Health Initiative (WHI) study:

• Women who take estrogen and progesterone may have an even higher risk of developing cognitive impairment.

• Women who take estrogen alone may be at just a slightly higher risk for developing dementia and mild cognitive impairment.

Other studies have reported weak evidence that estrogen replacement therapy (ERT) improves cognition and helps prevent dementia. However, many researchers have found a significant association between ERT and cognition, particularly with verbal memory.

Another effect of low estrogen and brain function is a slowdown in the speed of brain processing. This contributes to loss of postural stability resulting in an increase number of falls among postmenopausal women. Both brain processing speed and postural stability have been reported to improve with ERT.

Effect On Mood

The neurotransmitter serotonin plays an important role on brain synapses involved in mood regulation. In women of reproductive age, blood levels of estradiol correlate closely with blood levels of serotonin. Studies have shown that blood levels of serotonin are decreased in postmenopausal women.

Estrogen does have many positive effects on the brain, although some women report experiencing an improved mood after menopause when the estrogen levels are very low.

Some women appear to be sensitive to the menstrual cycle's changes in estrogen levels. This roller coaster ride of fluctuating hormone levels throughout the reproductive years may create mood disturbances.

Decreased Brain Function And Depression
A study published on January 14, 2015 in *Neurology* reported that:

Individuals who developed dementia during the study also developed behavioral changes and mood symptoms sooner than individuals who did not develop dementia. Reported behavioral changes included apathy, appetite changes, irritability and depression. Those who developed dementia were more than twice as likely to develop depression sooner than those without dementia; concluding that behavioral changes may precede memory loss.

Modifiable Risk Factors Associated With Alzheimer's Disease

A set of nine potentially modifiable risk factors have been identified in two-thirds of individuals diagnosed with Alzheimer's disease worldwide, according to a study published in the Journal of Neurology, Neurosurgery and Psychiatry published online August 20, 2015.

• Obesity
• Current smoker (in the Asian population)
• Carotid artery narrowing with plaque
• Type 2 Diabetes (in the Asian population)
• Low educational attainment
• High levels of homocysteine
• Depression
• High blood pressure
• Fragility

NOTE: Chronic inflammation, infections and exposure to toxins have also been shown to be associated with cognitive decline.

The researchers suggest that implementing a combination of preventative strategies which address diet, prescription medication use, body chemistry (metabolism), mental health, underlying diseases and lifestyle may help reduce the number of new cases of Alzheimer's disease.

How To Keep Your Brain Healthy

Avoid Stress
Continued stress can damage brain cells and impair your memory. Try yoga, meditation or a walk in the mountains or on the beach, where you can relax your mind!

Eat A Healthy Diet
Eat more lean proteins (salmon, organic chicken, turkey, eggs, tofu, low fat dairy products, beans, nuts such as walnuts and seeds), fruits and vegetables.

Carbohydrates: Choose organic carbohydrates such as blueberries which are one of the richest sources of antioxidants. It is the *anthocyanins* which contribute to the high level of antioxidant activity found in blueberries.

> *A study done by James Joseph, PhD, at the USDA Human Nutrition Research Center, found that aged rats fed one cup of blueberries daily experienced significant improvement in memory and motor function.*

Try chocolate covered blueberries-yum! It's important to eat all other berries, cherries and oranges as well. Oats and whole grains such as whole wheat are also good carbohydrates to consume daily. Avoid processed carbohydrates from a box!

Vegetables: Broccoli, red peppers, spinach, tomatoes and yams.

Fats: Avocados, coconut and olive oil, olives and nut butters, such as almond butter.

Liquids: Water and green or black tea. The substances in green and black tea called polyphenols, especially catechins, may help protect against neurodegenerative diseases like Alzheimer's and Parkinson's, according to a Japanese study published in the American Journal of Clinical Nutrition.

Get Eight To Nine Hours Of Sleep Per Night
Your brain is active when you are asleep and your body is recovering from the stress of the day.

Learn To Keep Your Brain Active
Try a new hobby, write a book, work on the computer/tablet, solve puzzles like Sudoku, play games or even try painting. Be creative!

Take A Nap

It can boost memory and concentration. A midday snooze is more than just an indulgence; it can actually improve performance and mental alertness, according to a Harvard Neuroscience study.

Exercise Regularly

There are studies that show exercise increases circulation to the brain, promotes cell health and balances neurotransmitters (chemical messengers).

Sexual activity also promotes increased circulation to the brain.

Coordination exercises such as dance, learning music, sports and juggling can stimulate cerebellum activity and improve the processing of brain speed and judgment.

Avoid Substances That Stress The Brain

Substances to avoid are:

• Caffeine

• Nicotine

• Drugs

• Alcohol

• Nutrasweet and all other artificial sweeteners

NOTE: These substances actually decrease blood flow to the brain, which can cause damage and premature aging.

Take Supplements

Research shows that *Omega 3 fatty acids (fish oil), vitamin D* and a good *multiple vitamin* can promote brain health.

Recently the natural herb *Turmeric (curcumin root)* has been reported to help boost brain function.

Ginkgo Biloba supplement has been touted as a memory booster. Unfortunately research has not supported this to date.

Resveratrol is part of a group of compounds called polyphenols which are thought to act like antioxidants, protecting the body against damage from toxins. Polyphenols are found in the skin of red grapes, peanuts and berries. Early research suggests it might help protect against inflammation, nerve cell damage and fight plaque build up that can lead to cognitive decline.

A relatively new brain health supplement called *Prevagen* is made from the protein apoaequorin found in certain species of jellyfish. This supplement is available at your local drug stores. A memory study done in Paris, France, published in 2011, showed improvement with short term cognitive function in individuals who were taking 10 mg daily. As with any herb or supplement please discuss with your clinician before taking because it can potentially interfere with prescription medications and be harmful!

Listen To Music

Listening to certain types of music, such as "Mozart's Sonata in D for 2 Pianos," can relax and help heal the brain.

Avoid Negative Thinking

These are involuntary negative thoughts that go through your head throughout the day. When you feel sad, upset or anxious, you should write out what you are thinking. Can you justify these thoughts or are they promoting unnecessary stress? Address and resolve these thoughts before they can have an effect on your mood and cause undue stress.

Cultivate New Friendships

Socializing and making new friends can lead to increased brain stimulation and, of course, having some fun.

NOTE: Try implementing these tips to help preserve and improve brain function.

Memory Markers Can Be Very Helpful

- Keep lists and a diary of important events
- Keep a detailed calendar or use your favorite electronic device to help store information.
- Follow a daily routine.
- Connect things in your mind. Use landmarks to find places and pneumonics to remember names.
- Keep eye glasses and keys in a designated place. Be sure to always put them there and also keep a spare pair handy.
- Use timers or alarm devices when needed.
- Use post-it or sticky notes.
- Take notes and write down information you need to remember.

Remember These Tips To Help Maintain Your Brain

- Read! Read! Read!
- Do crossword puzzles like Sudoku!
- Learn something new! Learning a new language or how to play a new instrument has been proven to grow new brain cells and connections.
- Play chess or scrabble.
- Play table tennis.
- Try a new hobby.
- Move, stay physically active.
- Sleep eight to nine hours a night.
- Avoid watching too much TV or computer overuse.
- Avoid excessive alcohol and caffeine.
- Take an omega-3 fatty acid fish oil and vitamin D supplement daily unless you are on blood thinners. (I discuss supplements in further detail in Chapters 3 and 6.)
- Laugh, laugh, laugh and enjoy life!

Websites for further information on:

Brain Health

Alzheimer's Association: **http://www.alz.org/**

Brain Health & Wellness: **http://www.aarp.org/health/brain-health/**

Eat Smart for a Healthier Brain: **www.webmd.com/diet/features/eat-smart-healthier-brain**

What is Integrative Medicine? Andrew Weil, M.D.-Dr Weil: **https://www.drweil.com/**

The Amen Clinic: **http://danielamenmd.com/**

Chapter 15

MENOPAUSAL HEADACHES

Definition
Headaches that cause persistent pain, pressure and tension in the head due to hormonal imbalances along with their associated symptoms are termed menopausal headaches.

Causes
Headaches can commonly occur for many women approaching menopause around age 50 and women can experience five times more headaches than men during this time period. Women also experience more headaches during puberty, pregnancy and with their monthly menstrual cycles when hormones levels are also fluctuating.

Headaches that occur during this menopausal period can range from mild to debilitating and can even become incapacitating for some who experience them. Women entering the perimenopausal period (the five to ten years leading up to menopause) may begin to experience headaches for many reasons, although the most common reason is due to fluctuating hormone levels.

During perimenopause, a women's estrogen and progesterone levels surge and dip many times before they finally adjust to the constant low levels that occur as one journeys through menopause and beyond. Hormone related headaches can occur when the estrogen level happens to be elevated and also when the estrogen level is declining. Clinicians have reported that some headaches occurring during the perimenopausal period can be even more severe than menstrual headaches, due to the prolonged duration of an increased estrogen level followed by a sudden drop.

Research is still ongoing to determine exactly why hormonal fluctuations cause headaches during the menopausal period. We do know that estrogen and progesterone have an effect on the brain and its blood vessels. Estrogen causes blood vessels to dilate and progesterone causes them to constrict. As these hormones continue to fluctuate the blood vessels are directed to expand and contract, resulting in intense pain in the head. This hormone imbalance can affect the brain in many ways and the onset of headaches can occur frequently.

Types Of Headaches

There are different types of headaches that menopausal women may experience as a result of fluctuating hormone levels. The symptoms may vary depending on the type of headache that occurs. I will outline below the three most common types of headaches you may experience during the menopausal period.

Tension Headaches

Tension headaches are the most common type of headache experienced by almost ninety percent of women at some time in their life.

Signs And Symptoms

A tension headache can produce mild to moderate pain located throughout the entire head.

This type of headache is usually described as "pressure like or a squeezing sensation" that may occur alone or with migraines. This feeling has also been described as "a tight band cinched around your head" similar to wearing a tight fitting swim bathing cap. The pain can sometimes be described as an intense pressure spreading over your entire scalp and your head feels as though it could explode if the headache continues. I am certain that many of you who experience these headaches know exactly what I am talking about. A tension headache may also cause pain in the back of your neck near the base of your skull.

These headaches can also be associated with:

- Neck muscle spasms causing tenderness that usually intensifies as the day goes on
- Anxiety
- Depression
- Perimenopause due to hormonal changes

NOTE: It is important to treat these headaches so they do not become chronic. That is when you have them frequently on more than half the days in a month. This is one of the headache types that can make up a "Chronic daily headache."

Migraine Headaches

Twenty-eight million Americans currently suffer from migraines and seventy percent of these individuals are women. Women are three times more likely than men to suffer from migraines and usually they occur between 15 to 55 years of age.

Many women can relate to having experienced incapacitating headaches in association with their monthly menstrual cycle and hence discovered the association between headaches and hormones. Whether you have found that your headaches are worsening with age or you began experiencing your first migraines in midlife, menopause may be the reason for intense frequent headaches.

Menstrual related migraine (MRM) headaches usually occur on the first or second day of menstruation and subside once the cycle has ended. Since migraine headaches typically start with the onset of your menstrual cycle, one would think they would improve with menopause, although without proper treatment they may continue.

The hormone level fluctuations that occur during perimenopause can certainly trigger a painful migraine headache. A drop in the level of estrogen can be a strong migraine trigger for many women. If a woman experiences heavy menstrual bleeding during perimenopause this can lead to anemia which can also trigger migraine headaches.

Hormone replacement therapy can either intensify the severity and number of migraine headaches or may afford pain relief in some women.

Signs And Symptoms

Migraines may progress through four stages which include a prodrome, aura, headache and postdrome.

Prodrome

One to two days before you develop a migraine you may experience a few subtle changes that will alert you the headache is on its way. These changes include:

- Constipation

- Depressed mood

- Certain food cravings

- Hyperactivity or irritability

- Neck stiffness

- Uncomfortable yawning

Aura

There are two types of migraine headaches, those with an aura and those without an aura.

Migraines with an Aura

Some women will experience a warning sign, called an *aura* just before the headache occurs. This sensory (neurological) phenomenon that signals a headache is coming typically appears about thirty minutes before the headache begins and occurs in about a third of individuals who experience migraine headaches.

An aura usually involves visual changes like flashing lights, blind spots or zigzag (wavy) lines seen at the edges of the field of vision, which may even cause temporary blindness.

Other neurological signs may occur such as:

- A strange sense of smell, taste or touch

- Numbness and tingling (pins and needles) in the hands and arms which can spread to the face

- Mental confusion

Migraines without an Aura

Migraine headaches that occur without an aura are the most common type and a woman may experience all the typical symptoms of a migraine without the sensory symptoms beforehand. Some individuals may feel fatigued or experience mood swings about twenty-four hours before the headache actually begins.

This type of headache can be associated with:

• Nausea and vomiting
• Sensitivity to light (photophobia), sound (phonophobia) and/or an odor
• Sweating of hands and feet

Headache (Attack)

When untreated, a migraine usually lasts from four to seventy-two hours, although the frequency of headaches can vary from individual to individual. If you experience "migraines", you may have them a few times in your life, once or twice a year or as often as every week or even daily. During a migraine, you may experience the following symptoms:

• Pain on one side of the head (unilateral), although can involve both sides of the head in some individuals
• Pain described as a throbbing or pulsating sensation with moderate to severe pain and may be worsened by head movement
• Nausea and vomiting
• Blurred vision
• Lightheadedness and possibly fainting

Postdrome

This is the final phase of a migraine, known as the postdrome which occurs after the attack. During this phase you may feel exhausted, although some individuals report feeling mildly euphoric.

Causes

The causes of migraine headaches are not fully understood although researchers believe they are associated with changes in the levels of brain chemicals. These changes can cause swelling of the blood vessels which may press on nerves (i.e. trigeminal nerve) causing a migraine. Some evidence shows that hormonal headaches are associated with varying levels of the hormone serotonin. When the hormone estrogen declines so does the level of serotonin.

Ninety percent of individuals with migraine headaches have a positive family history.

Physical changes that have been reported during a migraine are:

- The brain is in a state of hyperexcitability, which leads to a reduced threshold for stimuli and every day occurrences can trigger a headache.
- The gut (stomach and intestine) function is slowed down which can delay the absorption of medication and can be a real catch 22 if you are in search of pain relief!
- Anemia caused from heavy menstrual bleeding

Migraine Triggers
- Breathing in smoke
- Sleep disturbances (too little sleep)
- Stress (anxiety)
- Hormonal imbalance, premenstrual and during perimenopause (remember the drop in estrogen mentioned earlier)
- Hormonal changes that occur when taking the birth control pill and/or hormone replacement therapy
- Exposure to bright light (especially fluorescent lights)
- Loud noises and/or sounds
- Missing meals or fasting
- Air travel and time zone changes
- Changes in barometric pressure (altitude) and temperature (especially if the outside temperature is above normal)

Foods and Beverages
- Aged cheeses (Most cheeses are ripened or aged. As cheese ages, bacteria continues to grow, making the cheese firm while also changing its texture and flavor.)
- Alcoholic beverages (especially red wine), artificial sweeteners, food additives such as nitrates (found in lunch meats), caffeine, chocolate, MSG (monosodium glutamate), certain vegetables like avocados, pea pods, lima beans, onions, beans, nuts, peanut butter, raisins and yeast-containing foods like breads and donuts.

I should talk since I am now on a cruise enjoying a warm freshly baked cinnamon roll–yum! I anticipate my headache will begin very soon. Don't worry, after you finish reading the nutrition chapter, you probably won't be eating many breads or donuts.

Migraines can impact your quality of life and family relationships. A survey concluded that individuals who have persistent migraines were:

• More likely to argue with their partner and children

• Less likely to communicate well with others

• Less likely to spend time with their partners and family

• Less likely to be productive at work and more likely to miss work

NOTE: The Women's health study (WHS) results suggest that women who experience migraines with an aura are at an increased risk for developing an ischemic stroke. Women 45 years of age or less who smoke and are using the birth control pill may carry an even greater risk. Please read Chapter 5 for more information on cardiovascular disease and stroke.

Sinus Headaches

The third type of headache most frequently experienced during the menopausal period is a sinus headache. I will first give you a little background on the anatomy of sinuses to help you understand how these headaches may occur.

Your sinuses are air-filled cavities located behind the forehead (frontal), bridge of nose (ethmoid) and cheeks (maxillary). These sinus cavities produce a thin mucus that drains out the nose and down the throat. When one of these cavities becomes swollen due to an allergic reaction or an infection, the inflammation (swelling) can prevent proper mucus drainage, promoting a headache. Therefore, this type of headache is caused from the inflammation, creating a blockage in the sinus cavity or cavities and can also be referred to as a congestion headache.

Signs And Symptoms

• Facial pain around the sinuses located in the forehead, behind the eyes and above the nose

• Pain in upper teeth can be referred from the sinuses

• Nasal congestion (running nose), sore throat and a possible cough

• Facial pain that worsens with movement such as bending over or lying down

• Feeling fatigued (tired)

Prevention And Treatment For Menopausal Headaches

Lifestyle Changes

Stress Reduction

Meditation, aromatherapy, psychotherapy and hypnotherapy can help decrease stress, which can trigger a headache.

Biofeedback, acupuncture, massage and pet therapy have been reported to have helped many women reduce their stress. *Apply gentle pressure when massaging painful areas.*

Cognitive behavior therapy, also referred to as problem solving therapy, has been reported to help reduce the occurrence of tension headaches by dampening the pain pathway.

Rest in a cool dark room and place a cold pack or warm compress on your forehead, neck and/or over your eyes.

Exercise

Do muscle relaxation exercises like yoga or stretching and don't forget to take deep slow breaths.

Exercise regularly five days a week for at least thirty minutes.

Diet

Eat a healthy diet with more fresh fruits and vegetables and decrease your sugar intake.

Foods with soy, apples, alfalfa, cherries, potatoes, rice, wheat and yams may help promote natural estrogen. *(Remember, an apple a day keeps the doctor away.)*

Smoking

If you smoke, quit!

Cefaly Device

A relatively new device approved by the FDA on March 11, 2014 for the prevention of migraine headaches in individuals 18 years of age and older is now available by prescription. This is a portable device that is battery operated and worn like a head band. The Cefaly delivers electrical impulses to the skin over the forehead stimulating the branches of the trigeminal nerve known to be associated with migraines. You can use this device for 20 minutes a day. You will experience a tingling sensation over your forehead when it is working.

Alternative Medicines

Some herbal supplements have been reported to help provide relief from menopausal headaches.

Black Cohosh is a **phytoestrogenic herb** (contains estrogen-like plant products) that may help balance the fluctuating hormone levels, decreasing headache occurrences. The body will naturally decrease its own production of estrogen when it receives hormones from outside the body. Be careful and do not take this supplement more than the recommended amount of time because you may be increasing your susceptibility to develop further headaches.

Vitamin B9 (folic acid) helps to lower the level of the amino acid homocysteine and was also found to help reduce symptoms of migraine headaches.

Other types of supplements do not contain estrogen like products and are called **non-estrogenic herbs.** These herbs work by stimulating the pituitary and endocrine glands to produce hormones on their own, restoring balance and therefore decreasing headaches.

A few of the commonly used supplements are:

Macafem is a popular branded non-estrogenic herbal supplement that has been used by many women and reported to help reduce headache occurrences.

Butterbur is a root extract known as **Petasites hybridus.** This herb can be found throughout Europe and Asia and is known for its anti-inflammatory properties which help provide pain relief.

WARNING: Some butterbur products contain chemicals called pyrrolizidine alkaloids (PAs) which can damage the liver. Look for certified products that are labeled "PA-free" and consult with your clinician before using this supplement.

Feverfew is another herb similar to butterbur although this remedy is made from the leaves of the plant and also has anti-inflammatory effects which promote pain relief.

Gliacin is a branded supplement which contains the herb *boswellia* which comes from the same family of small trees from which frankincense is derived. This supplement has been reported to help reduce inflammation and headaches.

Magnesium is a mineral known for helping afford pain relief from migraine headaches. It may also cause loose stools which could be a benefit in some individuals who experience constipation.

Riboflavin is one of the B vitamins (B2) reported to help reduce the pain associated with a migraine and can also be used for prevention of headaches.

Co-enzyme Q10 is another supplement that has been reported to help improve headaches. This supplement is also commonly recommended to take along with a prescription statin medication (to reduce cholesterol in the blood) which helps protect the liver.

Peppermint oil when rubbed on the temples and tight muscles in your head, neck and shoulders can help relieve tension headaches.

Migravent is a nutritional supplement recommended by neurologists for migraine pain relief which contains a combination of butterbur, riboflavin (B2), Magnesium and Coenzyme Q10.

NOTE: Please read Chapter 3 for further information on herbs and supplements. Use caution when taking herbs and supplements and consult with a herbologist or clinician because dangerous side effects and drug interactions can possibly occur in some individuals.

Over-The-Counter Pain Medications

If you have a *mild migraine, tension or sinus headache,* you may want to try one of the over-the-counter pain medications for relief. Common medications like acetaminophen (Tylenol), aspirin, aspirin-acetaminophen (Excedrin Migraine), ibuprofen (Advil and Motrin) and naproxen sodium (Aleve) have all been reported by many women as helpful in reducing the pain associated with hormonal headaches.

Some women report better relief when they take a NSAID like Advil or Aleve with a caffeinated beverage.

It is a good idea to check in with your clinician if you find that you need to take over-the-counter medications for more than a week. These medications can have many side effects and the potential to interact with other medications.

Sinus headaches may also require allergy medication, a decongestant and/or antibiotics if a sinus infection is present.

Decongestants help open the blocked sinus cavities by reducing the amount of mucus and swelling (inflammation) in your nasal passages.

Do not use nasal decongestants for more than three days and oral decongestants for more than a week without consulting your clinician.

Advil cold and sinus and Tylenol cold and sinus are combination products which have a pain reliever and a decongestant to help clear sinus congestion. Do not use decongestants if you have high blood pressure and consult with your clinician because decongestants can further elevate blood pressure.

Antihistamines can help if your sinus headache is related to allergies.

Nasal steroid sprays can help reduce the swelling in your nasal passages and promote pain relief. Nasacort and Flonase are now available over-the-counter.

Nasal saline sprays can help keep your sinuses moist. Humidifiers, vaporizers and moist heat with a warm towel over your face for a few minutes can also be soothing to your sinuses.

Nasal irrigation with salt water can be achieved by using a bulb syringe or a Neti pot which can help moisten the nasal passages and clear mucus. Be careful when using a nasal irrigation device and keep it clean to prevent further contamination and a possible infection.

Avoid nasal irritants such as perfumes, cigarette smoke and chemicals because they can further irritate your nasal passages.

NOTE: Try to avoid continued use of caffeine compounds such as Excedrin Migraine, as this can often lead to an increased occurrence of headaches over time.

Prescription Medications
If you experience moderate to *severe tension and migraine headaches* that interfere with your daily activities, you may need a prescription medicine. There are many effective medications that may work quickly to relieve the pain and other associated symptoms.

Commonly prescribed medications to stop *migraine headaches* are Non-steroidal medications (NSAIDs), ergotamines, triptans and a few other prescription medications described below. Hormone therapy can also be prescribed to help stop migraine headaches.

Non-Steroidal Medications (NSAIDs)
Prescription strength NSAIDs, such as ibuprofen (Motrin) and naproxen (Naproxen, Anaprox) can be used initially to relieve mi-

graine pain. They help decrease the pain and inflammation associated with the inflammatory phase of a migraine attack. When a migraine attack occurs, prostaglandins are released which sensitize pain sensors and NSAIDs block this process.

Examples of prescription strength NSAIDs used are:

- **Ibuprofen** 400 mg, 600 mg or 800 mg taken with food twice daily
- **Anaprox** DS 550 mg taken twice daily with food.
- **Naproxen** 500 mg twice daily with food
- **Celecoxib (Celebrex)** 200 mg given once daily can be prescribed if you have gastrointestinal discomfort
- **Diclofenac (Cambia)** is a newer NSAID formula that can be dissolved in water and works within 15 minutes to relieve pain. This is an encapsulated liquid preparation that improves the solubility of the drug promoting faster relief.

Ergotamines

A class of drugs called *ergotamines* have been used to treat migraines for many years and work by constricting the blood vessels in the brain. These medicines are available in tablets, nasal spray, suppositories and injections. Names you may recognize are Migranal (dihydroergotamine), Cafergot and Migergot (ergotamine with caffeine).

These medications may not be as effective in stopping migraines as the newer triptans discussed below.

Midrin and Duradrin are names of the oral form of a prescription medication that belong to a class of drugs referred to as vasoconstrictor combinations. This drug combines a pain reliever (acetaminophen) with (isometheptene) which constricts blood vessels along with a mild sedative (dichloralphenazone) to help stop a migraine. This prescription medication should not be taken if you have glaucoma, kidney disease, high blood pressure, heart problems or liver disease. It also reacts with a class of drugs called monoamine oxidase inhibitors (MAOI) which are rarely used these days. Your clinician will determine if Midrin is an appropriate treatment for your headaches.

Triptans

A class of drugs called Triptans (Serotonin Receptor Agonists) which include: Axert (almotriptan), Frova (frovatriptan), Maxalt (rizatriptan), Imitrex and Treximet (sumatriptan), Amerge (naratriptan) and Zomig (zolmitriptan). Triptans work by constricting the blood vessels in the brain and therefore relieve swelling. They also help relieve sensitivity to light and sound and help improve nausea and vomiting found to be associated with migraines.

These medications are all available in tablet form and rizatriptan can be dissolved under the tongue which is good if you are feeling nauseous. Sumatriptan and zolmitriptan can also be administered as a nasal spray.

Sumatriptan also comes in an injection form and usually works within minutes.

Onzetra is a nasal spray now available to be used with the Xsail device (sumatriptan nasal powder) and is approved by the FDA for treatment of acute migraine headache with and without an aura.

Other Prescription Medications
Commonly prescribed preventative medications for persistent *migraine headaches* include:

• *Aimovig (erenumab)*
  This new class of drugs was just released to be administered once-monthly by self-injections for prevention treatment of migraine in adults. This drug works by blocking the activity of calcitonin gene-related peptide, a molecule involved in migraine attacks.

• *Inderal (propranolol) and Toprol (metoprolol)*
  This class of drugs is called beta-blockers and is typically used to treat high blood pressure. They work by relaxing constricted blood vessels, promoting pain relief.

• *Cardizem and Verapamil (diltiazem)*
  This class of drugs called calcium channel blockers are also traditionally used to treat high blood pressure and work by reducing the constriction of blood vessels promoting pain relief.

• *Elavil (amitriptyline) and Nortriptyline*
  This class of drugs belong to the tricyclic antidepressants and have been used traditionally to treat depression and chronic pain. These medicines have been used for many years to help prevent migraine headaches.

• *Depakote (valproic acid) and Topamax (topiramate)*
  This class of drugs are called anticonvulsants and they are tradi-

tionally used to treat seizures and can also be used to treat persistent migraine headaches. These medications can have a lot of side effects and drug interactions so the risks and benefits must be discussed with your clinician and carefully weighed if you have serious persistent headaches.

- *Botox (botulinum toxin)*
This class of medications can be injected in small amounts around the face and scalp and may be repeated in three months to promote headache relief.

- *Nerve Blocks*
A nerve block is the injection of medication onto or near nerves using a small needle to treat pain. Nerve blocks are used to treat migraine pain when other medications or treatments have failed to control the pain or are not tolerated due to side effects. A nerve block works by interfering with the passage of nerve impulses and are most commonly done in the back of the neck near the occipital bone. Other nerves on the scalp may be injected if needed to control the pain.

All of the above listed medications can help prevent and/or reduce the number of migraine headaches. You should discuss with your clinician which medication therapy would be right for you.

NOTE: It is important if you are of childbearing age and could possibly become pregnant to discuss all medications with your clinician. The good news is that your migraines may actually improve during the second and third trimester of pregnancy. A survey reported that one third of pregnant women's headaches improved, one third remained the same and one third progressively worsened.

Hormone Therapy

Progesterone cream has been reported to help with the hormonal imbalance and reduce headaches. Estrogen patches may provide even more relief in women with migraines with an aura. A continuous same low dose (monophasic) birth control pill may be prescribed up through perimenopause to help decrease the incidence of migraine headaches. Although it is important to understand that taking combination birth control pills has been shown to be associated with an increased ischemic stroke risk in individuals who have migraines with an aura! (See Chapter 3 for further information on hormone therapy.)

Summary

It is important for you to keep a headache diary. Once you identify certain triggers, you may be able to reduce the number of headaches you experience.

Chronic daily headaches can lead to depression and problems with your work and social life, so talk to your clinician to determine which treatment is right for you!

New studies suggest that migraine headaches with an aura can be associated with heart disease and stroke. Please read Chapter 5 for more information.

It is important to obtain proper treatment for your headaches so you won't develop a heightened sensitivity to pain and continue to experience headaches throughout the menopausal period and beyond.

The sooner you pursue relief, the sooner you can continue to enjoy life!

> *NOTE: New headaches can also occur during this time period and any new headache should always be brought to the attention of your clinician. If you ever wake up with or experience an intense headache that comes on like a thunder clap, you need to call 911!*

Partner Alert

The next time she tells you, "I am not in the mood because I have a headache," you will understand-right?

Websites for further information on:

Headaches

National Headache Foundation: **http://www.headaches.org/**

National Women's Health Information center: **https://www.womenshealth.gov/publications/our-publications/fact-sheet/migraine.html**

North American Menopause Society: **www.NAMS.org**

The Headache Center-The Neurology Center of Southern CA: **http://www.neurocenter.com/the-headache-center.aspx** (This center has a headache class for patients.)

Migraine Awareness Group: A National Understanding For Migraineurs: **http://www.migraines.org/**

Managing Migraines-Association of Migraine Disorders

http://www.migrainedisorders.org/managing-migraines

Chapter 16

CONFRONTING CANCER

Menopause And Cancer

Menopause does not cause cancer, although the risk of developing cancer increases as a woman ages. Women who have gone through natural menopause have a higher risk of developing cancer because they are older. The incidence of developing cancer does increase with age for both men and women. ***Three out of every four cancer diagnoses are in individuals 55 years and older!***

A woman who experiences menopause after the age of 55 has an increased risk of developing ovarian, breast and uterine cancer. The risk is greater if a woman began her menstrual cycle before the age of twelve. This is because a woman who menstruates longer than normal during her lifetime is exposed to more estrogen and has more ovulations. A longer exposure to estrogen increases a woman's risk of uterine and breast cancers and having more ovulations than normal increases a woman's risk for developing ovarian cancer.

Hormone replacement therapy with estrogen alone should be considered only for women who have had their uterus surgically removed (hysterectomy). Estrogen replacement alone, not balanced with progesterone, can promote growth of the uterine lining, which increases the risk of uterine cancer.

Please read Chapter 3 for more detail on hormone replacement therapy and further information on associated risks.

As a woman, you have a one in three chance of receiving a diagnosis of cancer in your lifetime!

The most common cancers affecting women overall are listed in order below:

1. Breast
2. Lung
3. Colon (colorectal)
4. Uterine (endometrial)

The leading causes of cancer death in women are listed in order below:

1. Lung
2. Breast
3. Colon (colorectal)

In this chapter I will give a brief overview of the different types of cancer that occur in women.

Definition

Cancer is an overgrowth of abnormal cells in the body. Some types of cancer cells can grow in your body for several years before you even become aware that something is wrong.

Causes

Changes we can control:

• Excessive alcohol consumption, greater than 2 glasses per day for men and 1 glass per day for women.
• Chemical exposure
• Radiation exposure
• Infections
• Smoking

NOTE: The longer you have contact with these agents, the greater your risk for developing cancer.

Changes we cannot control:

- Abnormal changes in cells that are inherited
- Uncontrollable factors that alter our immune system. (Our immune system is what helps our body fight disease.)
- Our body's hormones

Research has shown that these following factors may increase your risk of developing cancer:

- Poor diet (nutrition)
- Inactivity
- Obesity
- Prolonged unprotected sun exposure
- Prolonged stress

Weight And Cancer Risks

If you are overweight or obese you may carry an increased risk for developing several different types of cancer. Individuals who are obese have more fat tissue that can produce hormones, such as insulin and estrogen, which may promote cancer cell growth.

How your weight changes throughout your life may also affect your cancer risk.

A higher birth weight is associated with a higher cancer risk. Weight gain during adulthood can be a risk for developing several types of cancer. Weight cycling (losing and gaining weight repeatedly) may also increase the risk of developing cancer.

Research has shown that maintaining a healthy weight is associated with a lower risk for developing cancer and a lower risk for cancer recurrence (when cancer comes back after treatment) in cancer survivors.

Types of cancers linked to obesity:

- Breast cancer (women who have gone through menopause)
- Colon and rectum
- Uterine

- Kidney

- Esophageal

- Pancreatic

- Endometrial (lining of the uterus)

- Thyroid

- Gallbladder

- Ovarian

- Cervical

- Liver

Please see Chapters 3 and 12 for more detail on obesity and body mass index (BMI), which is often how obesity is measured.

Reducing Cancer Risk

Try To Live A Healthy Life In Mind, Body And Spirit!

Nutrition Prevention

Maintain a healthy weight! One third of adults are obese and another third are overweight. Control what goes into your mouth and it just may keep you out of trouble and could even possibly save your life.

Remember to eat 9-13 servings of fresh fruits and vegetables daily. You can also take a whole food supplement, if you are unable to eat all your daily servings. Fresh fruits and vegetables are rich in anti-oxidants which fight cancer and disease.

Choose fresh foods, not processed from a factory in a box. Choose whole grains, brown in color rather than white. Limit fatty foods and avoid hormone fed meats. Choose organic if possible.

Avoid fast food, remember, fresh is best.

(Refer to Chapter 3 for further nutritional information.)

Exercise Prevention

Unfortunately we come from a nation of couch potatoes, so you need to move to reduce your cancer risk! The American Cancer Society recommends exercising 30 minutes a day, 5 days a week for cancer prevention. You can try any of the following:

- Walking has many health benefits and you can walk indoors on a treadmill or outdoors and get some fresh air.

- Yoga is good for your body and a great stress reliever. Don't worry if you are not flexible because you will improve in time.
- Dancing can be a fun form of exercise. You can attend a Zumba class at the gym, dance at home or go out on the town with your friends.
- Rollerblading can be fun and will certainly work on your balance. Make sure you wear protective gear which includes a helmet, and knee and elbow pads.
- Cycling is an exercise that you can do at home on a stationary bike or go outside and explore on a traditional bicycle.
- Hiking is great exercise and depending on where you live, can be quite scenic.
- Swimming is a total body form of exercise where you work all the muscles at the same time. There are also water aerobics classes available at the local gyms that can be very joint friendly.
- Tai Chi is a Chinese martial art that promotes health through slow moving exercises and breathing techniques along with meditation.

(See Chapter 3 for further information on exercise.)

Alcohol Prevention
Limit alcohol use to one drink or less daily. Increased alcohol consumption can lead to an increased cancer risk of the following organs:

- Mouth and oral cavity
- Pharynx (throat)
- Larynx (breathing tube)
- Esophagus
- Pancreas
- Liver

NOTE: The risk is even higher if you smoke.

Tobacco Use And Exposure
Smoking is the most preventable cause of death.

- Smoking cigarettes, cigars, chewing tobacco and second hand smoke can cause lung cancer. The lifetime probability of developing lung cancer is one out of every sixteen for women and one out of every 13 for men. Eighty-five percent of lung cancer deaths are from tobacco use or exposure. Avoid tobacco exposure and quit if you do smoke. Never beginning to smoke is the best prevention method.

Smoking also increases your risk of developing these other cancers:
• Breast
• Mouth
• Pharynx
• Larynx
• Esophagus
• Pancreas
• Cervix
• Kidney
• Bladder

Smoking increases your risk of developing the following diseases:
• Heart disease (# 1 killer of women)
• Strokes
• Lung infections and diseases like bronchitis, pneumonia, emphysema and chronic obstructive pulmonary disease (COPD)
• Gastritis, Gastro-esophageal reflux disease (GERD) and peptic ulcer disease, PUD (stomach ulcers)

NOTE: Lung cancer kills more women every year than any other cancer!

Cancer Screening

Skin Cancer
This is the most common form of cancer in the world. One in five Americans will develop skin cancer during their lifetime. Eighty percent of skin damage occurs before the age of 18. Most forms of skin cancer, if caught early, can be cured.

The most aggressive form of skin cancer is melanoma, which, if diagnosed early, can have a good outcome. Current statistics report that melanoma kills one American every 67 minutes. Two sunburns before the age of 18 can double the lifetime risk of melanoma.

Prevention
• Avoid sun exposure, especially multiple burns before the age of 18.

- Limit sun exposure, especially between the hours of 10 am and 2 pm. (If your shadow is shorter than you are, get out of the sun.) If you tan, your skin will have ultraviolet damage and the body doesn't forget this, so over time skin cancer can develop. A dermatologist once quoted, "Your skin can begin to resemble the paint on a car that has been left out in the sun too long." I am sure you all have seen a vehicle with various layers of peeling paint? How's that for a visual-yikes!
- Wear a broad brimmed hat and sunglasses with ultraviolet protection.
- Use a sunscreen with a sun protection factor (SPF) of at least 30. Reapply generously as needed.
- Be on the alert for any of these skin changes:
    - A mole changing in color, size and appearance.
    - A mole with color variation (not all the same color) and the diameter larger than a pencil eraser.

Remember These ABCs

- A = appearance
- B = border
- C = color
- D = diameter
- E = evolving (change in size or shape)

Be sure to have an annual skin exam with your clinician or dermatologist.

Oral Cancer

Most oral cancers start in the squamous cells, the thin flat cells that line the lips, oral cavity and oropharynx. This type of cancer is referred to as squamous cell carcinoma.

Oral cancers may develop in any of the following areas:

- Lips
- Oral cavity:
    - Front part of the tongue
    - Gingiva (gums)
    - Buccal mucosa (the lining of the inside of the cheeks)
    - Floor (bottom) of the mouth under the tongue

- Hard palate (the front of the roof of the mouth)
- Small area behind the wisdom teeth
- Oropharynx:
  - Middle part of the throat (pharynx) behind the mouth
  - Back part and sides of the tongue
  - Soft palate (the back part of the roof of your mouth)
  - Sides and back walls of the throat
  - Tonsils

Most oral cancers develop in individuals older than 45 years of age. Tobacco and alcohol can increase the risk of developing oral cancer.

Risk Factors For Developing Oral Cancer

- Using tobacco products (cigarettes, cigars, pipes and chewing tobacco)
- Heavy alcohol use
- Being infected with a certain type of human papilloma virus (HPV number 16 in the mouth)
- Exposure to sunlight (lip cancer only)

Oral Cancer Screening

Screening can be done by your dentist or clinician. This screening should be done at least once yearly and preferably twice a year after age 45.

Tests To Determine If You Have Oral Cancer

Toluidine blue stain is a procedure that coats the suspected lesions with a blue dye. The areas that take up the stain are more likely to be or become cancer.

Fluorescence staining is a procedure that looks at lesions in your mouth with a special light. The patient first rinses with a fluorescent mouth wash and the cancerous lesions will look different from the normal cells under a special light.

Exfoliative cytology is a procedure that collects cells from the lips and/or oral cavity with a brush, piece of cotton or a small wooden stick. The cells are then looked at under a microscope to identify any abnormalities.

Brush biopsy is a procedure that collects cells from all layers of a lesion using a brush. The cells are looked at under a microscope to identify any abnormal cells.

NOTE: Early stage oral cancer can usually be cured, unfortunately most oral cancers have spread to the lymph nodes and other areas of the body by the time they are found.

Early prevention is key and don't be afraid to pick up a mirror and take a look inside your mouth.

Have your regular check-ups and routine screenings because it could possibly save your life!

Breast Cancer
Please see Chapter 2 for information on conditions affecting the breast and Chapter 7 for information on breast cancer.

Colon And Rectal Cancers
The third most commonly diagnosed cancer in women is colon cancer. Colorectal cancer can easily be detected by performing a colonoscopy. Having a screening colonoscopy may lead to a lower incidence of developing colorectal cancer and may decrease your chances of dying from it by 50 percent or more, according to a study published on June 16, 2015 in *The JAMA Magazine*.

You should receive a screening colonoscopy at age fifty. You may need to have a colonoscopy before age fifty, if you have a family history of:

• Polyps (these are growths on a stalk in the lining of your colon)

• Colon cancer

Signs Of Possible Colon Cancer
The most common signs of colon cancer are:

• Rectal bleeding or blood in your stools

• New onset of diarrhea or constipation

• New onset of frequent abdominal pains

• Changes in stool, such as stringy or skinny stools

• Weight loss

• Feeling tired (fatigued)

• Anemia (iron poor blood) which means you do not have enough red blood cells to carry oxygen around your body to supply your tissues and organs.

Screening Tests

Digital rectal exam test: (Your clinician inserts a gloved finger into your rectum to check for lumps, growths or other changes in the rectum.)

Guaiac Fecal Occult Blood test (gFOBT): This test is done following the rectal exam. (A sample of your stool on the tip of the glove is placed on a test card and a liquid developer is dropped onto the card. The paper turns blue if any blood is present and the results are read immediately.)

A **fecal immunochemical test (FIT)** is an improved fecal occult blood test ordered by your clinician to screen for colorectal cancer which is collected at home and then sent to the lab. This tests for hidden blood in the stool and detects human hemoglobin in the stool specimen.

A new stool DNA colon cancer screening test called **Cologuard** is now available. This noninvasive test detects colorectal neoplasia (cell changes) associated with DNA markers and also detects hemoglobin (blood) in the stool. It can be done in the privacy of your home and is covered by Medicare. You just collect the stool specimen and return it to the lab via the UPS prepaid shipping envelope.

NOTE: If any of the above tests are positive or a suspicious lump is found during an exam, you should always be referred to a gastroenterologist for additional testing and a colonoscopy!

Procedures

Colonoscopy

You will normally receive a mild sedative for this procedure. Your doctor will insert a scope into your rectum which allows for a careful inspection of the walls of your colon and rectum. Color pictures can be taken with the scope to show you any growths that may be found. If a polyp is seen, it will be removed and sent to the lab to look for any cancer. This procedure is called a biopsy.

Sigmoidoscopy

Your doctor inserts a thin scope about 10 to 12 inches long into your rectum to look for any polyps or suspicious growths and a sample of tissue can be taken if needed for a biopsy. If you have a low risk of developing colorectal cancer you may opt to have a sigmoidoscopy every five years. Discuss your individual risk with your clinician.

Barium Enema

This test is sometimes called a lower GI (gastrointestinal) series. This procedure involves an enema of barium followed by an x-ray tech taking a series of pictures of the colon and rectum. If the barium highlights any suspicious areas or polyps, a colonoscopy will need to be done.

NOTE: Since the advent of the colonoscopy procedure, sigmoidoscopy and barium enemas are typically not recommended for colorectal cancer screening.

Virtual Colonoscopy

This is a relatively new procedure that scans your colon and rectum, although it is not used as a screening test because if a growth is found, you will still need to have a colonoscopy done.

NOTE: This test is less sensitive in detecting polyps than the standard colonoscopy and many insurance companies and Medicare will not pay for this procedure.

Risks For Developing Colon Cancer

Age

Ninety percent of colorectal cancer patients are over age 50 and with each decade after 50, your risk doubles.

I have found colon cancer in a female patient as young as age 27 and in a male at age 42. If you have a positive family history of colon polyps or cancer, you will need to be screened earlier than age 50. Your individual screening colonoscopy recommendation will be determined based on the age of your family member when they received a diagnosis of colon polyps or cancer.

Diet

Eating red meat once a day can double your risk of developing colon cancer. Fat is the culprit here. Animal fat is not only saturated (the unhealthy kind), but exposed to toxic chemicals, like pesticides that you digest. Keep this in mind before making a reservation at your favorite steak house. Remember to eat your fruits and vegetables daily.

Family History

Genetics does play a role in colorectal cancer. If you have one or more family members with colon cancer your individual risk doubles.

NOTE: Be sure to be screened early per your clinician's recommendation if you have a positive family history of colorectal cancer.

Prevention

- Exercise can reduce your risk of colorectal cancer by half, so remember to keep moving! (Please read Chapter 3 for further discussion on exercise.)
- A diet high in fiber can reduce your risk. Try flax or chia seeds, 1-2 tablespoons daily.
- Supplemental calcium may also help lower your risk of developing colorectal cancer.
- Baby aspirin may provide some protection. Discuss with your clinician.

NOTE: A screening colonoscopy could save your life, so be sure to schedule yours today!

Cervical Cancer

Cervical cancer is caused by abnormal changes in the cells of the cervix. A virus known as the human papilloma virus (HPV) can be associated with the development of cervical cancer.

Some other risk factors that may play a role in causing cervical cancer are:
- Having sex before age 16
- Having more than one sex partner and/or having a sex partner who has more than one partner
- Smoking or having previously smoked. Smoking seems to make HPV infections last longer. One study showed that your risk of cervical cellular changes may also increase if you are exposed to second hand smoke (if you are around someone while they smoke).

- Having an impaired immune system, with an illness such as the human immunodeficiency virus (HIV). *(I discuss this virus further in Chapter 1.)*
- Using the birth control pill for more than 5 years may be associated with having an infection with HPV.
- Exposure to diethylstilbestrol (DES), when your mother was pregnant, although this is rare.

Symptoms

Symptoms that may be present are:

- Abnormal vaginal bleeding or a different pattern of bleeding during your menstrual cycle.
- Vaginal bleeding with intercourse or when using a diaphragm. (Any bleeding when something comes in contact with the cervix.)
- Pain with sexual intercourse.
- Abnormal vaginal discharge containing mucus that may be mixed with blood.

Late Findings When Cancer Has Spread:

- Pain in the pelvic region, lower back and legs
- Urinary changes due to possible blockage of a kidney or ureter. *(I discuss the urinary system in Chapter 9.)*
- Leakage of urine or bowel matter into the vagina due to an abnormal opening which has developed between the vagina and the bladder or rectum
- Weight loss
- Anemia due to abnormal vaginal bleeding.

Prevention

Have your routine Pap test and HPV screening done. See list of recommended health screening tests in Chapter 19.

Quit smoking!

Gardasil is the name of the vaccine that can help prevent the development of human papilloma virus (HPV) and protects against many of the strains which can cause cervical cancer. Gardasil also protects against HPV types 6 and 11 that cause genital warts. If the injection is administered before the individual's 15th birthday, two doses will be given at least six months apart. Three doses of this vaccine will be needed if the series is started between 15 and 26 years of age.

Prevent exposure to sexually transmitted diseases.

Remember, the most common cause of cervical cancer is having a persistent infection with the high risk type of human papilloma virus.

Further Testing

The following tests can be performed in the office by a clinician or gynecologist to look for cancer of the cervix:

- Colposcopy and a cervical biopsy are done to look closely at the cells on the surface of the cervix for cancer.

- An endocervical biopsy can be done to look for cancer in the cervical canal.

- A cone biopsy or loop electrosurgical excision procedure (LEEP) can be done to remove cervical tissue and the cells can be examined under a microscope.

NOTE: Be sure to have a pap test done to identify any cervical changes early, before cancer develops! (See Chapter 19, "Promoting Health" for recommended screening tests.)

Ovarian Cancer

Signs And Symptoms

Ovarian cancer originates from cells in the ovary. This includes both the lining of the ovary and the cells which make the eggs. Ovarian cancer is rare but deadly! The symptoms can be very vague and resemble those associated with many different conditions.

The following symptoms usually appear when the disease is in an advanced stage:

- Bloating/abdominal pain

- Nausea

- Vomiting

- Constipation

- Frequent urination

- Flatulence

Some research suggests that ovarian cancer is related to the number of ovulations you experience in your lifetime. Every time you ovulate a small tear occurs in the ovary wall and your body continually repairs it.

Factors That May Decrease The Risk For Developing Ovarian Cancer
Women who have taken the birth control pill may have a lower risk of developing ovarian cancer, due to the decreased number of life-time ovulations.

Women who have had multiple full term pregnancies may have a protective effect as well, due to the decreased number of ovulations.

Factors That May Increase Risk For Developing Ovarian Cancer
• Women with a sister or mother with ovarian cancer

• Women with a sister or mother with breast cancer

• Women who have used fertility drugs in attempt to achieve a pregnancy. (These medications stimulate the ovaries to release multiple eggs during ovulation.)

• Women who are fifty years of age or older

• Women who have never been pregnant

NOTE: If you fall into any of the above categories, you should have an annual pelvic exam and further testing if your clinician determines it is necessary.

Tests That May Be Done To Detect Ovarian Cancer
• A pelvic examination

• A pelvic ultrasound. (A vaginal probe may be inserted into the vagina to better visualize your ovaries.)

• A CA-125 blood test. This test measures an antigen which caus-es the body to fight ovarian cancer. This test is used as a marker to follow cancer and it is not a good screening test. An elevated CA-125 doesn't necessarily mean you have ovarian cancer. The following conditions may also increase the CA-125 test:

  • Endometriosis *(this condition discussed in Chapter 2)*

  • Ovarian Cysts

  • Uterine Fibroids

  • Pregnancy

• A CAT scan commonly referred to as a CT scan, (computerized axial tomography) or a MRI (magnetic resonance imaging). These tests give a clearer picture of your ovaries to check for any tumors (growths).

- A laparoscopy is a minor surgical procedure, where a small incision is made near your belly button and a scope is inserted to give a close up view of your ovaries. Abnormal tissue and growths may also be removed with this procedure and a general anesthesia is used. This procedure can be done as an outpatient and you may go home the same day.

Uterine Cancer (Endometrial Cancer)

Endometrial cancer occurs when abnormal cells (changed cells) grow rapidly.

Too high a level of estrogen for a long period of time causes the cells of the endometrium (lining of the uterus) to grow. This is referred to as "estrogen dominance" and is commonly seen during perimenopause. I discuss this condition in further detail in Chapter 3. Estrogen can fuel abnormal cell growth and lead to cancer!

Factors That May Increase Risk For Developing Endometrial Cancer

- Women who take estrogen replacement without progesterone and still have a uterus. This is referred to as "unopposed estrogen".

- Women over age forty. The risk increases from age 40 to 70 years and then declines around age 80.

- Women who are obese. If you are overweight, your fat tissue produces an estrogen called estrone, especially during perimenopause and menopause. (I discuss the effects of being overweight further in Chapters 3 and 10.) You can calculate your own body mass index (BMI) to determine your risk. A BMI chart can be found in Chapter 3 on page 56 to help you identify your body mass index.

- Women who never have had a baby can carry a greater risk because they haven't experienced a long period of time with a high level of progesterone. (Progesterone is the hormone of pregnancy and remains at a high level throughout the nine months.)

NOTE: Any postmenopausal bleeding warrants a biopsy!

Factors That May Decrease Risk For Developing Endometrial Cancer

Women who have taken the birth control pill may have a lower risk of developing endometrial cancer. If you have taken the pill for at least two years, your risk may be cut in half.

Signs and Symptoms

- **Vaginal bleeding or spotting** which includes bleeding between periods, prolonged bleeding, bleeding after intercourse and especially with vaginal bleeding after having gone through menopause.

- **Abnormal vaginal discharge** can occur, and is described as a watery or bloody discharge. This same type of discharge can occur with a vaginal infection or other non-cancerous conditions. Check in with your clinician when you experience a change in vaginal discharge.

- **Pelvic pain or pressure** during intercourse or at any other time should prompt you to see your clinician or gynecologist.

Types of Uterine Cancer

There are two types of uterine cancer which occur in different parts of the uterus.

- **Endometrial cancer** occurs in the lining of the uterus, referred to as the endometrium. Endometrial cancer is by far the most common form of uterine cancer accounting for about 95% of cases.

- **Uterine Sarcoma** is a rare form of uterine cancer and occurs in the muscles or other tissues of the uterus.

Diagnosis

An **endometrial biopsy** is the most common test used to detect uterine cancer. This test obtains a sample of the endometrial tissue (biopsy) and is very accurate when performed in postmenopausal women.

Another procedure called a **D&C (dilatation and curettage)** can be done if the endometrial biopsy sample does not provide enough tissue or if the results are uncertain.

This outpatient procedure dilates the cervix (opening to the uterus) and a special instrument is used to scrape the tissue from the inside of the uterus.

Treatment

If you should receive a diagnosis of any of the above type of cancers, your clinician will discuss individual treatment options and will refer you to a surgeon and/or an oncologist.

Many times surgery is indicated along with radiation and/or chemo-therapy.

Treatment options can vary depending on the location, type, size and stage of the cancer.

You and your oncology specialist can determine which treatment plan will be best for you.

Prevention
Maintain regular health check-ups and be sure to have your recom-mended health screens done as outlined in Chapter 19.

Be aware of your body, listen and tune in!

Websites for further information on cancer:

Cancer

American Cancer Society-Information and Resources: **https://www.cancer.org/**

American Lung Association: **http://www.lung.org/**

Cancer Treatment & Cancer Research-City of Hope: **https://www.cityofhope.org/**

Cancer Types-Cancer is Not a Single Disease: **https://www.aacrfoundation.org/**

Cancer-Mayo Clinic: **http://www.mayoclinic.org/diseases-conditions/cancer/basics/definition/con-20032378**

National Cancer Institute: Comprehensive Cancer Information: **https://www.cancer.gov/about-cancer/understanding**

The Skin Cancer Foundation: **http://www.skincancer.org/**

Chapter 17

KEEPING YOUR JOINTS HEALTHY

As estrogen declines during the perimenopausal and menopausal years, joint pain can become a common symptom experienced by many women. Estrogen is known for its wonderful anti-oxidant effects and calms inflammation (swelling).

As we "baby boomers" age we can expect to join the joint club. We come from a generation of aerobics, jogging and a lot of high impact sports. Yes, our aching joints will be a constant reminder of the years we have pounded the pavement.

You have probably heard of the term rheumatism, which is a general term used to describe swelling (inflammation) or breakdown of the body's connective tissue, not caused by injury or infection. This term also includes joints, muscles, tendons and other tissues.

Defining Arthritis

Arthritis is one type of rheumatism, which refers specifically to inflammation of one or more joints.

One in three women in the United States will have some type of arthritis, according to the Arthritis Foundation. There are many different disorders that can affect our joints. Osteoarthritis (degenerative joint disease) is the most common.

Pain in your joints should not be ignored and arthritis is not something you just have to live with.

Common Types Of Arthritis Found In Women

Osteoarthritis

Osteoarthritis (OA) is ***more common in women than men after the age of fifty-five*** and is the ***most common form of arthritis*** seen as we age. It can affect the larger and smaller joints in the body to include: hands (base of thumb), feet (big toe), wrists, neck, lower back, hips and knees. Men typically experience OA in their hips and women tend to develop it more commonly in their knees and hands. This disease can develop from long term wear and tear of the joints, previous trauma, excess body weight, heredity and of course from age. Most of us baby boomers either have osteoarthritis or know someone who has it. Some of us may have severe osteoarthritis and be in need of a knee or hip replacement.

Osteoarthritis causes changes in the cartilage and bone of joints. In normal joints, a firm rubbery material called cartilage covers the end of each bone. Cartilage is very much like a protective sponge where bones meet to form a joint and it functions as a shock absorber. When the cartilage breaks down, eventually bone begins to grind against bone and this can lead to swelling and can become very painful.

Risk Factors

- Age
- Family history (heredity)
- Prior joint trauma such as an injury while playing a sport
- Obesity places excess stress on joints, especially in the knees, hips and spine
- Sedentary Lifestyle

Signs And Symptoms

Various levels of pain, stiffness and swelling of joints can occur which can limit your ability to remain active. Pain associated with osteoarthritis tends to occur after exercise, overuse of a joint and later in the day.

When osteoarthritis occurs in the hands, bony growths called spurs can form at the margins of these small joints causing swelling and pain. If these spurs grow at the end of your finger joints they are called *Heberden's nodes* and *Bouchard's nodes* if they are located in the middle joints of the hands.

In advanced osteoarthritis, muscle weakness and limited flexibility can develop from inactivity.

Diagnosis

A **physical examination** will be performed to determine which joints are affected. It is important to identify the pain pattern to help guide further testing that may be needed.

X-rays use low dose radiation to look at bone and visualize cartilage loss. Visualizing bone damage and bone spur formation (a bony outgrowth called an *osteophyte*) can help monitor the disease progression.

A **computerized tomography (CT)** scanner takes many pictures at different angles and creates cross sectional views of internal structures. This type of imaging is used to visualize bone and the surrounding soft tissue.

Magnetic resonance imaging (MRI) combines radio waves along with a strong magnetic field to see more detailed cross-sectional images of soft tissues. This type of imaging may be needed in some cases to visualize cartilage, ligaments and tendons.

Ultrasound uses high frequency sound waves to look at soft tissues, cartilage and fluid-containing structures called bursas, located in a joint. Ultrasound is also used to guide needle placement when a joint aspiration (withdrawal of fluid) or injection is needed.

Prevention

• Make an appointment with your clinician when you first experience joint pain. The goal is to keep your cartilage as healthy as possible and prevent further injury.

• Control your weight to avoid excess stress on your joints. (For every 10 pounds of excess weight, you will add 30 pounds of pressure on the knees.) Yikes!

• Exercise regularly, avoid activities that pound on your knees and hips (like jogging). Yoga, Pilates and swimming can help improve flexibility and strength. Swimming and water aerobics are also great for keeping your weight down and preserving joint function.

• Avoid frequent consumption of foods in the nightshade family such as bell peppers, eggplant, potatoes and tomatoes. These foods may promote inflammation in joints.

Treatment
The goal of treatment for osteoarthritis focuses on relieving symptoms and improving function.

Physical and Occupational Therapy
Physical therapy and occupational therapy can be helpful in many patients. Exercise can improve range of motion and strengthen the muscles surrounding joints.

An important concept for an individual undergoing physical or occupational therapy is to have a good understanding of the Mobility-Stability Model. In your body you have joints that are designed to be more mobile and some that are more stable. If your mobile joints (ankles, hips, mid-back, shoulders, wrists and upper neck joints) are tight, then your stable joints (feet, knees, pelvis, lower back, shoulder blades, elbows and mid-neck joints) are called upon to do jobs or motions they are not built to do, leading to breakdown referred to as osteoarthritis. Limited motion in one mobile joint can also increase stress in one's other mobile joints.

Traditionally occupational therapists would treat hand injuries as their emphasis was placed primarily on helping individuals return to writing, feeding, dressing and other daily living functions. In recent years occupational therapists now treat elbows and in some facilities shoulder injuries as well.

If you should need to have physical or occupational therapy you can expect that your therapist will need to assess and treat the joints above and below the area of your pain. Many areas of pain in your arm can be coming from your neck. For example, carpal tunnel syndrome causes pain in your wrist which can be the result of nerve compression in your neck. Tennis elbow discomfort (pain located on the outside of your elbow) can arise from compression of the lower nerves located at the base of your neck. There are many other areas of pain that can be referred from compression of nerves in your neck or back. Osteoarthritis can cause degenerative changes in the neck and spine which can refer pain to different locations in your body.

To ensure that you receive the best physical and occupational therapy, make sure your therapist is assessing the function of your body and not just treating the site of the pain.

Acupuncture
Acupuncture has been reported to help reduce pain so you can remain active.

Over-The-Counter Supplements:

- **BioAstin (Astaxanthin)** is an antioxidant supplement made in Hawaii that helps reduce inflammation.
- **Boswellia** extract helps reduce inflammation.
- **Bromelain** extract from pineapples can help ease swelling and pain.
- **Coenzyme Q10** can be helpful in reducing muscular pain.
- **DHEA** is sometimes helpful if you are experiencing joint pain and fatigue (See Chapter 3 for further information on DHEA).
- **Ginger root** extract has anti-inflammatory effects that may help osteoarthritis.
- **Glucosamine-Costochondrotin** and **MSM** have both been reported to have helped some individuals. I have found in my practice that you are either a responder or not, there's no in between. Give it a try for about two to three months and see what happens. You can also buy this product in powder form at a feed store (human grade) and it's less expensive and easier on your stomach. Don't take MSM if you have a sulfa allergy! You can purchase these products separately or in combination.
- **Omega-3 fatty acids/fish oil** capsules have been reported as helpful for reducing inflammation and joint pain.
- **Traumeel** is an herbal supplement that contains a combination of diluted plant and mineral extracts and has been used in Germany for many years to treat the inflammation associated with joint injuries. Traumeel is available in tablets, drops, ointment and can be given as an injection directly into the painful joint.

Discuss with your clinician, orthopedist or rheumatologist which form would work best for you.

- **Turmeric** (curcumin root) has also been reported to help reduce inflammation.

- **Relief Factor** is a natural product that contains Turmeric (curcumonoids), Fish oil Omega 3, Japanese fleeceflower (root) and Epimedium (Arerial) and Icariin which in combination help reduce the inflammation associated with muscle and joint pain. **You should not take this product if you have a soy or shell fish allergy!**

- **Calcium supplements** may help reduce joint inflammation too. Some recent studies show that vitamin D may slow the progression of arthritis, so be sure to take your calcium with a vitamin D supplement. You may need to have your vitamin D blood level checked. Please read Chapters 3 and 6 for further information on Vitamin D.

Prescription Medications

Analgesics only reduce pain and have no effect on inflammation. Analgesics combined with narcotics are used commonly for acute and chronic pain.

- Acetaminophen (Tylenol) with codeine and tramadol (Ultram) are commonly used for pain relief.

- Narcotics containing oxycodone (Percocet and OxyContin) or hydrocodone (Vicodin and Norco) may be used for acute and chronic pain. These medications need to be monitored closely due to the possible addiction potential. If you need to be on these medications for a long period of time you should probably be followed by a pain management specialist.

Non-steroidal anti-inflammatory drugs (NSAIDs) reduce pain and inflammation.

- There are many different brand names of prescription strength NSAIDs available such as: Celebrex (celecoxib), Motrin (ibuprofen), Mobic (meloxicam), Naprosyn (naproxen sodium) and Voltaren (diclofenac) to name a few.

- Some prescription strength NSAIDs are available in a cream or gel form and can be rubbed directly on to joints to aide in providing pain relief.

- Over-the counter NSAIDs are available and include ibuprofen (Advil and Motrin IB) and naproxen sodium (Aleve).

NOTE: Be careful because oral NSAIDs can cause stomach irritation, gastrointestinal bleeding, ulceration and perforation of the stomach and intestines. They can also reduce kidney function. **Certain NSAIDs may cause an increased risk of serious cardio-vascular events which include heart attack and stroke.** *Check in with your clinician!*

Corticosteroids are a class of drugs that are known to reduce inflammation and calm the immune system. Common names you may recognize are prednisone and cortisone. Corticosteroids can be taken by mouth or injected directly into a painful joint. Corticosteroids can have many side effects so you should be closely monitored by your clinician.

Joint Injections
Hyaluronic acid and corticosteroid injections are used to help reduce pain and improve mobility. Hyaluronic acid may help regenerate new cartilage. Your primary care clinician, orthopedist or rheumatologist can decide which treatment will be best for you.

Surgery
When traditional treatments have been found to be ineffective for reducing pain or you experience major difficulty moving and using your joints, surgery may be necessary.

Arthroscopy
This procedure can be used in certain cases to diagnose and repair joint damage at the same time. An incision is made near your joint and a small flexible tube called an **arthroscope** is inserted through the skin into the affected joint. The arthroscope transmits images from inside the joint to a video screen.

Joint Replacement
This procedure removes your damaged joint and replaces it with an artificial joint. Hips and knees are the most commonly replaced joints. This type of surgery has proven to be very successful for alleviating joint pain associated with severe osteoarthritis and rheumatoid arthritis.

Take This Test To See If You Are At Risk For Developing Osteoarthritis

- Are you 45 years of age or older?
- Have you ever had an injury to your knee severe enough to keep you in bed, needing to use a walking aide or required surgery?
- Are you more than 10 pounds overweight?
- Do you or have you in the past participated in heavy physical activity for greater than three hours a day?
- Did you have hip or knee problems which caused you to limp as a child?

NOTE: If you answered yes to any of the above questions make an appointment with your clinician, so you can receive treatment early and keep moving!

Gout

Gout is a form of arthritis in which uric acid crystals are deposited in joints and other tissues causing inflammation. This condition causes sudden, severe episodes of pain, tenderness, redness, warmth and swelling of joints. Gout usually affects one joint at a time and the most common joint affected is the big toe. Individuals who develop gout either produce too much uric acid or their bodies have a problem removing it.

Causes

Uric acid is made naturally in our body and the level can increase when we consume a diet rich in purines, found mainly in organ meats and seafood. An increased level of uric acid in the blood can cause sudden severe episodes of pain in certain joints.

Our kidneys attempt to maintain a normal level by filtering out the excess uric acid through our urine. Estrogen stimulates the kidneys to excrete more uric acid in the urine. As we approach menopause, estrogen begins to drop and our kidneys become less efficient at clearing excess uric acid from our body. Gout can then develop over time and is more commonly seen in women during the postmenopausal years.

An attack of gout can also be triggered by:

- Diet: crash dieting or intake of high purine foods

- Alcohol: Consuming too much alcohol, more than two drinks a day (Women should limit to one drink a day)
- Trauma and stress to the body including surgery and a severe illness.
- Medications: especially diuretics (water pills) and chemotherapy agents. Beginning a medication to lower the uric acid level can also trigger a gout attack.

Sign And Symptoms
Gout usually occurs in three phases.

- The first phase is marked by sudden joint pain and swelling that usually lasts about five to ten days. The most common joint affected is the big toe, although women can experience symptoms in their upper body as well. The skin may look shiny and red or have a purplish appearance around the affected joint. The joint is usually extremely tender to touch.
- The second phase is marked by a period of no symptoms followed by new sudden attacks of gout.
- The third phase occurs after many years without treatment. Persistent swelling, stiffness and pain in one or more joints can occur. Crystals of uric acid can form deposits under the skin called *tophi*. Women tend to have more uric acid deposits around their joints and these nodules are usually not painful, although can be very unsightly.

Some individuals may only experience one attack and others may experience numerous attacks. If you do not receive treatment with medication, the attacks of gout may occur more often and even last longer.

NOTE: Women who are obese and those with hypertension (high blood pressure) carry a greater risk for developing gout after menopause.

Prevention
Consume a healthy diet low in purine foods. Reduce the amount of protein intake including seafood (especially shrimp and lobster), since these foods tend to be high in purines.

Try to eat more low fat dairy products and vegetables and limit your portion size when eating red meat and seafood.

Exercise regularly, five days a week for at least 30 minutes.

Diagnosis

- *Joint Aspiration* is the most important test to perform to confirm the diagnosis of gouty arthritis. A needle is inserted into the affected joint to withdraw fluid to be tested. The fluid is then examined under a microscope to look for gout crystals or signs of a bacterial infection. Sometimes gouty arthritis is diagnosed based on physical exam only and a joint aspiration is not performed.

- *Blood Tests* may be ordered to look at your white blood cell count, uric acid level and to assess kidney function. The level of uric acid in your blood may not always be reliable for making the diagnosis of gout. Typically the level of uric acid is lowered during an attack and should be checked after the attack has resolved. *Uric acid levels can be elevated in about eight percent of the general population of individuals who do not have gout, so it is not always a reliable diagnostic test.*

- *X-rays* are taken to look for underlying joint damage in patients who have had several episodes of gouty arthritis.

Treatment

If you experience only a few mild gout attacks, lifestyle modifications may be the only treatment you will need.

If you experience any of the following listed below you need to take medication:

- Frequent gout attacks
- High uric acid levels
- Uric acid kidney stones
- Joint damage and tophi formation

Your clinician can prescribe medicines to lower the uric acid level in your blood, prevent further attacks and treat the inflammation, which will also help treat the pain. Medications for treating gout are divided into the following three categories.

- Uric-acid lowering medications
- Prophylactic medications (These medications are generally used

immune system is working and this testing is also used to
the progression of the disease.

test to assess kidney function to determine if there is any
involvement

lysis to detect blood or protein in the urine

ent

ortant to make an appointment with a rheumatologist as soon
ceive a diagnosis of SLE. There is not a cure for lupus so the
t goal is to provide symptom relief and to slow the progression
ge to your organs. Symptoms can come and go and the treat-
u receive will depend on the symptoms you are experiencing
organs that are affected. Medications are available to help re-
ammation and the activity of the immune system. Proper nutri-
g with appropriate exercise and rest are essential.

yle Changes and Non-Medication Treatments

s reduction is very important, and daily relaxation techniques
elp improve your quality of life. Try meditation, gentle yoga
assage.

so important to **consume a healthy diet** which includes fresh
and vegetables. Avoid eating too much sugar and eliminate
ssed foods.

d sun exposure! Individuals with sun-induced rashes should be
nt about wearing sunscreen, cover-up clothing and a hat while
ors.

cise and rest when needed. Learn to recognize your body's
ing signals of an impending flare. A combination of rest during
along with a supervised exercise plan will help with muscle
oint pain. Exercise as tolerated five times a week for 30 minutes.

ces

cent years, various devices that claim to increase blood flow,
en and energy to your muscles and soft tissues have become
able for purchase. These devices include holograms, magnets,
ive ions and certain minerals and metals. There is very little
rch on these products, although many individuals have reported
iencing decreased pain and fatigue with an increase in strength
nergy when utilizing these devices. Not all these products pro-

along with uric acid lowering medications to decrease the risk of
having another attack within the first 6 months of starting treatment)

• Rescue medications (These medications provide immediate pain
relief)

Uric acid lowering medications are prescribed to help lower the
blood level of uric acid in the body. The goal of treatment is to lower the uric acid level to 6 or below. Names you may recognize are:
Allopurinol (**Zyloprim** and **Aloprim**), febuxostat (**Uloric**), probe-
necid and pegloticase (**Krystexxa).** These medications also help to
decrease the size of tophi and some of the newer medications have
shown promise at resolving tophi formation. Remember tophi are
those nodules that form on your joints.

Prophylactic medications are typically used the first six months
of therapy along with an uric acid lowering medication to help
prevent gout flares and/or to decrease the number and severity of
flares. We use these medications together because any medication
that decreases or increases the level of uric acid can potentially
trigger a gout attack. *Any of the previous mentioned medications
used to lower the uric acid level can potentially trigger an attack.*
Commonly prescribed prophylactic medications are: Colcrys (colchicine), NSAID medications such as Indomethacin (indocin), Diclofenac (voltaren), ibuprofen (Advil) and naproxen sodium (Naprosyn).

Caution: NSAID medications can worsen underlying kidney disease!

Rescue medications are used during an acute gout attack to decrease
the pain and inflammation.

Colchicine (Colcrys) and a non-steroidal medication (NSAIDs) as
mentioned previously can be used to help decrease the pain and inflammation during an acute gout attack.

***Please read potential serious side effects associated with NSAID
medications listed above in the arthritis section.***

Corticosteroid medications referred to as steroids can also be used
during an acute gout attack. Prednisone and methylprednisolone
(Medrol) are typically used for a short duration only, due to potential
side effects such as cataract formation and bone loss.

Arthritis And Systemic Lupus Erythematosus

Systemic Lupus Erythematosus (SLE or Lupus) is one of the autoimmune connective tissue diseases that can cause inflammation, swelling, pain and gradual joint damage. In lupus, the immune system produces antibodies against the body's healthy cells and tissue. (This means the body sees its own connective tissue as foreign.) This disorder is referred to as systemic because it can affect many different body systems including the skin, kidneys, blood vessels, nervous system, heart and other organs.

Different Types Of Lupus:

• **Discoid (cutaneous) lupus** which only affects the skin.

• **Drug-induced lupus** is the least common form of the disease caused by certain drugs that are taken for other medical reasons. In most cases once the medication is stopped the symptoms will disappear.

The Hormonal Factor

• Menstruation, pregnancy and menopause can all trigger lupus.

• About 90 percent of all cases of lupus occur in women.

• Women are 9 times more likely to develop lupus than men.

• SLE commonly occurs in women during the child bearing years, ages 15 to 45.

• Women can also develop lupus during their perimenopausal and menopausal years. (Women who do develop lupus after menopause tend to have milder cases.)

Signs And Symptoms

SLE is known as one of "the great imitator" diseases because it mimics other illnesses. Symptoms can vary from individual to individual and come and go unpredictably. Common symptoms that can occur are:

• 30 to 50% of individuals will have a rash across the nose and cheeks (butterfly rash).

• A scaly disk shaped rash on the face, neck, ears, scalp and /or chest.

• Sensitivity to sunlight, where you can develop a severe rash or become ill from the sun.

• Sores on the tongue, inside the mouth or nose (can be painless)

• Arthritis (pain, stiffness and swelling in the joints)

• Fever, fatigue and muscle aches

• Pain in your chest and/or sides of your do need to seek medical attention imm symptom because it could also be assc

• Dark colored urine which could possib

• Sometimes individuals with SLE may eye inflammation, fevers, weakness, fa sion, hair and weight loss.

• Some individuals may also develop ar called Sjogren's syndrome which caus eyes. This condition can also cause va what you need when you are going thr

NOTE: You need to see a clinician as s op any of the above symptoms. The ear the better the outcome.

Diagnosis

Blood tests are ordered if your clinicial symptoms that you may have SLE.

The following blood tests are usually o the disease.

• An **ANA** test confirms the presence of monly seen in individuals with SLE. test and not necessarily have lupus; th done as well.

• A **CBC** (complete blood count) to det you have a low platelet count, abnorn

• Other blood tests can show if there is system such as: anti-double-strand DI **Smith** (referred to as anti-Sm) or anti false positive blood test for syphilis, that you do not have syphilis.)

The presence of antiphospholipid antib patients can be associated with an incr ory difficulties and blood clots that car damage.

• Complement protein blood testing ma

wel
mo

• A b
kid

• A u

Trea
It is i
as yo
treatn
of da
ment
and t
duce i
tion a

Lif
Str
can
and

It's
fru
pro

Av
vig
out

Exe
war
flar
and

Dev
In r
oxy
avai
neg
rese
exp
and

duce the same results but it would certainly be worth trying some of them to see if they help control your individual symptoms.

One such device is called the *EFX USA* and is available to be worn as a bracelet or necklace. Patients who have used this device have reported excellent results with symptom relief.

Physical and Occupational Therapy

Physical and occupational therapy has been reported to be of great benefit in most patients. A physical or occupational therapist can assess your body's function to make sure that the joint and muscle pain you are experiencing is not just from various orthopedic issues. As discussed earlier in this chapter, the joints in your body have their various jobs and when one joint is not working correctly, the other joints have to work harder to compensate leading to breakdown and pain.

It is important that the physical or occupational therapist that you are working with performs a complete functional evaluation and is not just assessing the area of pain. Once this comprehensive evaluation is completed, then your clinician can recommend a treatment plan that will be right for you.

Medications

Most individuals with lupus will need to take medication as part of their treatment. The type of medication needed will depend on the extent of the disease and how active it is. Different types of medications may be needed over time and with different symptoms that may appear.

Non-steroidal anti-inflammatory drugs (NSAIDs) are used to provide relief from muscle or joint pain. These medications are available over-the-counter and in prescription strength to help decrease swelling, pain and a fever if present. Brand names you may recognize: Motrin IB and Advil (ibuprofen) and Aleve and Naprosyn (naproxen sodium).

CAUTION: Remember, NSAIDs can have serious side effects such as cardiovascular events (stroke and heart attack), stomach bleeding and kidney damage, so check with your clinician before starting these medications.

Prescription Medications

• *Hydroxychloroquine (Plaquenil) and chloroquine* are anti-malarial drugs used to treat lupus when individuals do not respond well to non-steroidal medications. These medicines work well for improving rashes, fatigue, joint and muscle pains. Plaquenil has been shown to help decrease the number of flares in individuals with SLE. *You should have an eye exam with an ophthalmologist before beginning this medication.*

- **Immune Suppressing Agents**

  Some individuals with SLE may require treatment with immune suppressing agents to control their symptoms such as: ***azathioprine (Azasan or Imuran), cyclophosphamide (Cytoxan and Neosar).***

  A relatively new B-cell-suppressing treatment is called ***Belimumab (Benlysta).*** This medication blocks the stimulation of B-cells and is used to treat patients with autoantibody-positive systemic lupus erythematosus in addition to receiving the standard therapy.

- ***Topical steroid creams*** can help lupus-associated rashes when they develop. Be careful when using steroid creams on the face and be sure to be monitored by your clinician because it can cause thinning of the skin.

- ***Steroids*** are used when it becomes necessary to reduce inflammation quickly.

  Prednisone is a common name you may recognize and is the preferred steroid used during pregnancy because it crosses the placenta barrier into the fetus much less than other steroids. Steroids should be used for a short duration of time. They have dangerous side effects such as lowering one's immune system and increasing susceptibility to developing serious infections. If you have to take steroids more than several weeks the dosage should be tapered down slowly. Never stop the medication abruptly! Your clinician will instruct you on how to take your medication properly.

  You may need to take a blood thinner if clots form easily in your blood. Medications such as warfarin (Coumadin) and heparin may be used to prevent blood clots from forming. Heparin is the preferred medication used in pregnancy because warfarin can cause adverse effects to the fetus.

NOTE: It is very important to be closely followed by your rheumatologist so they can monitor your symptoms and the disease, as well as treat any side effects from these medications.

Emotional concerns can surface at any time with a diagnosis of lupus which can be expected with a chronic illness. Joining a support group may help you share your frustrations with others who are experiencing similar problems. Talking with a therapist may also provide emotional support when needed.

Fibromyalgia

This condition is characterized by chronic widespread pain and stiffness in muscles and soft tissues around the joints, which is thought to be associated with hypersensitive nerve fibers. Fibromyalgia, referred to as FMS, means pain in the muscles, tendons and ligaments, which are the fibrous tissues in the body. Women are more likely than men to be diagnosed with fibromyalgia. This ongoing pain can lead to an increased sensitivity in certain areas of the body, as well as feelings of fatigue, sleepiness, memory challenges and mood changes.

Causes

Fibromyalgia is not arthritis per se, because there is no damage to the joints, although it can be found in association with arthritis. No one really knows what causes fibromyalgia. Certain factors such as an infection, physical trauma or *hormonal changes* may trigger the development of this generalized condition which has become the leading cause of musculoskeletal pain in the United States.

Signs And Symptoms

• **Widespread pain:** The pain associated with fibromyalgia is often described as a constant deep muscle ache that has occurred for at least three months. The pain may also be described as throbbing, shooting or stabbing. Most individuals report that they ache all over. They often report that their muscles feel like they have been overworked or pulled and sometimes they may twitch or burn. The pain must occur on both sides of the body and above and below your waist to be considered widespread.

• **Fatigue:** Some individuals say they feel tired all the time and others report feeling incapacitated. The fatigue has been described as "brain fatigue" and individuals feel totally drained of energy. Patients have described the following sensation, *I feel like the muscles in my arms and legs have cement in them.*

• **Sleep disturbances:** Most individuals report waking up and feeling like they have been hit by a Mack truck. The problem is that most patients with FMS can fall asleep but are then awakened several times throughout the night from repeated arousals. Experiencing these repeated arousals prevents you from reaching a deep restorative sleep pattern.

- **Brain Fog:** Many individuals report experiencing trouble concentrating, retaining new information and word-finding. The constant pain may be a contributing factor which can interfere with concentration. These symptoms are also commonly seen during the perimenopausal and menopausal years.

- **Mood:** Changes in mood can be a common symptom of fibromyalgia. Feelings of sadness and being down are often reported and some individuals may have associated depression and anxiety. Many individuals who have a chronic illness may find themselves feeling depressed at times while attempting to cope with their pain and fatigue.

- **Morning stiffness, muscle cramping and weakness:** You may experience muscle stiffness upon awakening in the morning. Some muscles have rope-like knots called *myofascial trigger points* which can lead to muscle weakness and cramping.

- **Digestive disorders:** Constipation, diarrhea, abdominal pain, gas and bloating are reported symptoms in about 50 to 70 percent of individuals with FMS. Heartburn (acid reflux) and slowed digestion are also common. Please refer to Chapter 11 for further information on digestive disturbances.

- **Bladder discomfort:** Some individuals with FMS will experience bladder spasms which can create an increased sensation to urinate and find themselves urinating more frequently.

- **Headaches and Migraines:** Many individuals with FMS report experiencing frequent tension and migraine headaches. The trigger points located in the head, neck and shoulder regions can promote these headaches. Please refer to Chapter 15 for further information on headaches.

- **Temporomandibular Joint Dysfunction:** This condition is referred to as TMJ and causes significant face and head pain in about 25% of individuals with fibromyalgia. The pain is thought to be associated with muscles and ligaments surrounding the joint.

Diagnosis

The diagnosis of fibromyalgia should be suspected if you hurt all over and feel extremely fatigued on most days. Routine lab tests are unable to detect the widespread pain of fibromyalgia and the diagnosis instead is made by a physical examination of tender points on the body. Light pressure is applied to the surface of certain muscle groups throughout the body and if pain is identified at these specific tender point sites, you probably have FMS.

Criteria for receiving a diagnosis of FMS

• You must have widespread pain in all four quadrants of the body for at least three months.

• There are 18 specific tender points on the body used for identifying fibromyalgia and you must have pain elicited in at least 11 of these points. These 18 sites used to make the diagnosis are located around the neck, shoulder, chest, hip, knee and elbow regions.

Treatment

Some individuals may have only mild symptoms and lifestyle changes may be enough to alleviate the discomfort. Other individuals will need a more comprehensive treatment plan to include educational programs, exercise, relaxation techniques and medications. Educational programs and support groups are available to help you understand the symptoms so the appropriate treatment can be obtained.

Lifestyle Modifications

• Consume a diet rich in fresh vegetables, fruits, whole grains and lean protein. Avoid processed sugars and foods.

• Exercise programs that stretch muscles, such as yoga and pilates can help relieve discomfort.

• Try relaxation techniques to ease muscle tension and stress.

• Treat yourself to a weekly or bi-monthly massage.

• Physical therapy to ease pain and improve mobility and physical function. (See osteoarthritis section for further detail.)

Supplements

• *BioAstin (astaxanthin)* is a supplement made in Hawaii that has been reported by many patients to help relieve pain associated with FMS.

- *Fibroplex* is a supplement which contains chelated magnesium, malic acid and B vitamins. This supplement has also been reported by many patients to afford pain relief.

- *Ginger root* is a powerful anti-inflammatory herb and can help relieve muscle spasms. It improves circulation and produces a warming sensation thereby reducing pain.

- *Magnesium* is often found to be depleted in patients with fibromyalgia and it is very important to have your blood level checked and to take a supplement if needed to promote proper muscle and nerve function. (A magnesium deficiency can interfere with normal nerve conduction and muscle contraction.)

- *Traumeel* is an herbal supplement mentioned earlier in the osteoarthritis section that contains diluted plant and mineral extracts. Traumeel has been used in Germany for years to treat inflammation and is available in tablets, drops and an ointment formulation.

- *Turmeric (Curcumin root)* is a natural anti-inflammatory which can help ease muscle tension and discomfort.

These non-drug therapies may be used along with prescription medications to help alleviate pain and improve mobility.

Prescription Medications

Traditional treatments are focused on improving sleep patterns and reducing pain. The sleep disturbances generally found in association with FMS are considered to be a major contributing factor in promoting the symptoms experienced with this syndrome. Stage 4 sleep is so important for many body functions including tissue repair, regulation of neurotransmitters, hormones and the immune system.

Three FDA approved medications are now available for the treatment of fibromyalgia. You may recognize the following prescription medications:

- Cymbalta (duloxetine)
- Savella (milnacipran)
- Lyrica (pregabalin)

Cymbalta and Savella belong to a class of medications called serotonin and norepinephrine reuptake inhibitors (SNRIs), traditionally used to treat depression, anxiety and diabetic peripheral neuropathy. These medications can help boost your body's level of serotonin, a neurotransmitter that regulates sleep, pain, mood and immune system function.

Lyrica (pregabalin) is *not* an antidepressant medication. It has traditionally been used to treat nerve pain associated with shingles and diabetic neuropathy. Lyrica is also used to treat seizures. This medication is a FDA approved treatment to relieve the pain associated with FMS, and works by decreasing the number of nerve signals transmitted, therefore calming oversensitive nerve cells.

Muscle relaxants like Flexeril (cyclobenzaprine) have been used to reduce muscle spasms.

Over-the-Counter medications
Nonsteroidal anti-inflammatory medicines such as Advil (ibuprofen) and Aleve (naproxen sodium) may provide pain relief. Be careful with these medications due to potential cardiovascular events, stomach irritation and kidney damage from usage. Discuss with your clinician.

Trigger point injections can be very helpful for relieving muscle pain. A trigger point injection is an injection that is given directly into the painful tissue area. The injection typically has an anesthetic such as: lidocaine (Xylocaine) or bupivacaine (Marcaine) or a corticosteroid (cortisone medication) alone or mixed with an anesthetic to reduce pain and swelling.

Devices
The ***Avacen medical device,*** approved by the FDA in March of 2014, is used for the treatment of pain associated with arthritis, fibromyalgia and migraine headaches. This machine uses dry heat therapy and has been reported to be beneficial in affording pain relief for many patients.

The ***EFX USA device,*** worn as a necklace or bracelet, has been reported by patients to provide pain and symptom relief associated with arthritis, fibromyalgia and SLE.

See your clinician or rheumatologist to discuss treatment options for you!

Rheumatoid Arthritis (RA)

This is an autoimmune form of arthritis and women with RA outnumber the men three-to-one. Rheumatoid Arthritis (RA) causes inflammation in the lining of the joints, leading to warmth, decreased range of motion, swelling and pain. Typically it affects many different joints on both sides of the body and can cause damage to the cartilage, bone, tendons and ligaments of the joints. The most common joints affected are in the hands, wrists and feet. Ankles, knees, shoulders, hips and elbows can also be involved in the early stages of the disease.

Signs And Symptoms

Initial signs and symptoms of RA usually occur in women between the ages of 25 and 50. These early symptoms of rheumatoid arthritis can mimic many different diseases so it can become a challenge to diagnose in the early stages. Typical symptoms are:

• Stiffness of the affected joints, especially in the mornings.

• Joint pain, tenderness, swelling, redness and warmth

• Many of the joints described above involve both sides of the body (symmetric)

• Fatigue: You may also have a general feeling of sickness and feeling tired within weeks or months after the onset of the disease.

Later stages of the disease can occur if the inflammation persists or does not respond well to treatment. Damage of the nearby cartilage, bone, tendons and ligaments can develop which can lead to joint deformities resulting in possible permanent disability.

In some individuals the symptoms may be mild with intermittent periods of worsening joint inflammation called flares. This disease is continuously active and progresses over time, so it is very important to be tested for rheumatoid arthritis early on when symptoms first appear to prevent joint damage. Osteoarthritis, in contrast, develops over many years.

Diagnosis

There is not a single test per se that would be conclusive for diagnosing RA, so many factors must be considered that would suggest a diagnosis of the disease.

We begin with the *history* of the symptoms. Patients will typically report experiencing morning stiffness in joints on both sides of the body.

A *physical examination* can determine which joints are involved. Your clinician will look for symmetry (involvement of both sides of the body) as well as any bumps or nodules called *rheumatoid nodules*.

Blood testing is done to determine if *rheumatoid-factor (RF) antibody* is present in the individual's blood. RF antibody can also be found in individuals who may not have rheumatoid arthritis. An *antinuclear antibody test (ANA)* is a test which identifies an autoimmune disease and is found to be present in some individuals with rheumatoid arthritis. A newer more specific test is used today called *cyclic citrulline antibody test (anti-CCP),* which can identify a more aggressive form of rheumatoid arthritis. Many individuals with RA will have ongoing anemia (iron deficient blood), so a *complete blood count (CBC)* should be ordered to help monitor the disease process. An *erythrocyte sedimentation rate (ESR)* and a *C-reactive protein (CRP)* blood test can both identify signs of inflammation.

X-rays are ordered to look for changes in the joints that occur with RA and to determine if there is any bone destruction.

Diagnosis Criteria used by the American College of Rheumatology

- Morning stiffness in and around the joints for a least one hour
- Swelling or fluid around three or more joints simultaneously
- At least one swollen area in the wrist, hand, or finger joints
- Arthritis involving the same joint on both sides of the body (symmetrical arthritis)
- Rheumatoid nodules are firm lumps under the skin that you can feel, found in individuals with rheumatoid arthritis. These nodules are usually found on pressure points of the body, most commonly the elbows.
- Abnormal amounts of rheumatoid factor in the blood
- X-ray changes in the hands and wrists can show destruction of bone around the involved joints. (These changes are typical of later-stage RA disease.)

NOTE: Rheumatoid Arthritis is officially diagnosed if four or more of the above listed criteria are present.

Treatment

You need to see a rheumatologist and begin treatment as soon as possible when you receive a diagnosis of rheumatoid arthritis. Several other diseases such as osteoarthritis, gout, fibromyalgia and systemic lupus erythematosus (SLE) as outlined earlier, can all look like RA in the early stages of the disease, which makes the diagnosis even more challenging. RA can sometimes take up to nine months to properly diagnose and can lead to disability and limit your ability to work if you do not receive proper treatment. There are many new effective treatments available which can improve your quality of life.

The goal of treatment in rheumatoid arthritis is to reduce joint inflammation (swelling) and pain, improve joint function and *prevent* joint damage.

The medications used to treat rheumatoid arthritis are divided into two categories:

First-line drugs and slow-acting second-line drugs also called *disease modifying anti-rheumatic drugs (DMARDs)*. Many times a combination of first and second line medications are used to treat rheumatoid arthritis.

First-line drugs
Acetylsalicylate (aspirin), naproxen (Naprosyn), ibuprofen (Advil and Motrin) and diclofenac (Voltaren) are all examples of non-steroidal anti-inflammatory drugs referred to as NSAIDs. These NSAIDs reduce swelling, pain and inflammation. *Remember these medications can have serious side effects, from stomach ulceration to increased risk for having a stroke or heart attack. Discuss all potential side effects with your clinician or rheumatologist.*

Corticosteroid medications, such as *cortisone* and *prednisone* can be given orally or injected directly into the tissues and joints. These medications are more effective at reducing pain and inflammation and can help improve joint function and mobility.

Second-line drugs
Methotrexate (Rheumatrex, Trexall and Otrexup) and hydroxychloroquine (Plaquenil) are used to encourage disease remission and prevent progression of joint destruction. These medications may take weeks to months to become effective and are appropriately termed slow-acting medications. They may need to be used for many years to prevent joint destruction and deformities.

In some individuals with a more aggressive form of the disease, immunosuppressive medications may need to be used to suppress the immune system.

Methotrexate is considered to be an immune suppressive medication but without the same potentially serious side effects that other immune suppressive medications have and for this reason has become the preferred second-line choice for treating RA. Methotrexate is taken once a week in pill, liquid or injectable form.

Azathioprine (Imuran), cyclophosphamide (Cytoxan), chlorambucil (Leukeran) and cyclosporine (Sandimmune) are strong immune suppressive medications that do have serious side effects and need to be closely monitored. These medications can:

• Depress bone marrow function

• Cause anemia, low white blood cell and platelet counts. (A low white blood cell count can lead to infections and a low platelet count can cause bleeding to occur.)

• Cyclosporine can cause kidney damage and high blood pressure.

• Methotrexate does have the potential to harm the liver and must be monitored through blood testing.

NOTE: All the medications described above can have serious side effects, so you and your rheumatologist can discuss which treatment will be best for you.

Exercise, Activity and Rest

Moderate physical activity *(exercise)* on a regular basis can help decrease fatigue (feeling tired), strengthen muscles and bones, increase flexibility and can improve your over all sense of well-being.

Some individuals may need to have some physical therapy to help improve their range of motion in certain joints. (See osteoarthritis section for further detail.)

Rest a joint when it is red, painful and swollen.

Joint Injections may be given to help reduce the inflammation in a joint. The most commonly used anti-inflammatory medications for joint injections are corticosteroids. Methylprednisolone and triamcinolone are powerful steroids used to help reduce the swelling in the joint which provides pain relief.

In contrast, hyaluronic acid injections such as Hyalgan or Synvisc are not used to treat RA because they do not help reduce inflammation and are only approved to treat osteoarthritis.

Joint Replacement may become necessary when you have severe RA with joint erosion and destruction which can develop over time. This type of surgery has been a major breakthrough and an important therapeutic option in the treatment of rheumatoid arthritis.

Summary

Are You At Risk For Joint Pain?

• Have you ever been diagnosed with arthritis?

• During the past twelve months, have you had pain, aching and stiffness or swelling in or around a joint?

• In a typical month are these symptoms present daily or intermittently?

• Do you have pain in your knee or hip when climbing stairs or walking three blocks on a flat surface?

• Do you have daily stiffness in your hand joints?

• Are you limited in any way in activities because of joint symptoms such as pain, aching, stiffness or loss of motion?

If you answered yes to two or more of these questions, you might have symptoms of arthritis. Schedule an appointment with your clinician and then you can be referred to a rheumatologist if needed.

Research has found that chronic pain occurs more often, is more intense and lasts longer in women than in men.

Hormones can certainly play a role and some research suggests that women do respond differently to pain medications. Women may sometimes find themselves focusing on the emotional aspects of their pain, which can actually promote more intense pain. Try to keep a positive attitude! Thinking about your aching joints won't help the pain and may make you feel helpless, stressed and depressed. When you find yourself thinking negatively, stop and write your thoughts down on an index card. Turn the card over and write an honest comeback that is positive and reflect on what you can do to make it better. Patients say this really works!

I encourage all women to take an active role in obtaining a diagnosis, receiving early treatment and implementing relaxation techniques to provide and maintain pain relief.

If you experience joint pain, you need to be evaluated by your clinician so you can begin a treatment plan. The sooner the better to maintain the goal of keeping your joints healthy!

Websites for further information on:

Arthritis

American Academy of Orthopedic Surgeons: **http://www.aaos.org/**

American College of Rheumatology: **http://www.rheumatology.org/**

Arthritis Foundation: **http://www.arthritis.org/**

Arthritis and Musculoskeletal Disease

National Institute of Arthritis and Musculoskeletal and Skin Diseases: **https://www.niams.nih.gov/**

Fibromyalgia

Fibromyalgia-Mayo Clinic: **http://www.mayoclinic.org/diseases-conditions/fibromyalgia/basics/definition/con-20019243**

National Fibromyalgia Association: **http://www.fmaware.org/**

Lupus

Lupus Foundation of America: **http://www.lupus.org/**

Lupus-MayoClinic: **http://www.mayoclinic.org/diseases-conditions/lupus/basics/definition/con-20019676**

Chapter 18

HORMONES AND ORAL HEALTH

Women are at increased risk for developing oral health problems due to the hormonal imbalance.

Hormones influence:

• Blood supply to the gum tissue and can alter the body's response to the toxins that result from plaque build-up.

• Taste and sensations in the mouth.

• Sensitivity to hot and cold foods and beverages.

• The amount of saliva present in your mouth.

Oral Conditions

Dry Mouth
Dry mouth, called xerostomia, is a feeling of abnormal dryness in the mouth caused by a decrease in saliva production.

Dry mouth can be a common occurrence in your menopausal years due to decreased estrogen and the need to take prescription medications for other medical conditions.

Certain over-the-counter medications like antihistamines, decongestants and pain relievers can also cause dry mouth.

Smoking and beverages containing alcohol or caffeine can also promote dry mouth.

Signs and Symptoms
- Dryness and stickiness in the mouth
- Soreness of the mouth and tongue
- Difficulty speaking
- Sore cracked lips
- Bad breath
- Decreased taste

Prolonged dry mouth with decreased saliva can lead to the development of tooth decay and gum disease. Saliva not only moistens and
cleanses the mouth but also neutralizes the acids produced by plaque.

Treatment
Over-the-counter treatments for dry mouth are palliative (provide
relief from discomfort):
- Biotene Dry Mouth Oral Rinse and Moisturizing Oral Rinse
- Biotene Dry Mouth Moisturizing Spray
- Biotene Oral Balance Dry Mouth Moisturizing Gel
- Biotene Toothpaste would be a good choice because it is non-irri-
  tating
- Oasis Moisturizing Mouthwash rinse or Dry Mouth moisturizing
  spray
- Salese with Xylitol lozenges are available in three flavors:
  - Peppermint
  - Wintergreen
  - Mild lemon
- Xylitol Moisturizing Mouth Spray

Prescription treatments to relieve symptoms of dry mouth:
- **Evoxac (cevimeline HCL)** is a prescription medication typically
  used to treat dry mouth in patients with a connective tissue disorder called Sjogren's syndrome, although it may be used for other

purposes. This medication works by stimulating certain nerves to increase the amount of saliva you produce. This drug belongs to a class known as cholinergic agonists and can have serious side effects so your clinician will determine if it would be appropriate treatment for you. This medication is taken by mouth usually three times a day.

- *Salagen (pilocarpine HCL)* is another prescription medication used to treat symptoms of dry mouth associated with Sjogren's syndrome or injury to salivary glands from radiation therapy used to treat head and neck cancers. This drug stimulates the nerves to produce more saliva and also belongs to the class known as cholinergic agonists and can have serious side effects. This medication is also taken by mouth three times a day.

NOTE: If you have a persistent dry mouth, it may be an indication of a more serious medical condition and you need to see your clinician for an exam.

Burning Mouth Syndrome

This condition causes a chronic burning pain described as a "sunburn in the mouth" and affects up to 7% of the general population. Burning mouth syndrome is more commonly seen in menopausal woman 50 to 70 years of age. The pain can be severe, as if you had scalded your mouth.

Signs and Symptoms

- A burning sensation that may affect your tongue, lips, gums, palate, throat or entire mouth
- A tingling or numb sensation in your mouth or on the tip of your tongue
- Mouth pain may worsen as the day progresses
- A sensation of dry mouth
- Increased thirst
- A sore throat
- Loss of taste or taste changes, such as a bitter or metallic taste

The pain pattern associated with burning mouth syndrome may vary, ranging from waking up without pain, to pain that begins slowly and worsens throughout the day, progressing to severe. The pain may come and go with pain free intervals or may last the entire day.

The Role of Saliva

- Saliva lubricates the mouth so our food can be swallowed easily. It would be very difficult to swallow food without saliva. It can sometimes be a challenge just to swallow on command without a glass of water.

- Saliva keeps our mouth clean by washing away food debris. The body produces saliva throughout the day and the rate slows down at night when we are sleeping. Our mouth will typically produce about two to four pints of saliva within a day.

- Saliva helps maintain a neutral pH in the mouth (helps to balance the acid environment).

Treatment

- Hormone replacement therapy in menopausal women has been reported to help afford pain relief.

- A prescription drug called clonazepam (Klonopin) is available in a dissolvable form and can be administered twice daily. This medication has shown some promise for providing pain relief. *Clonazepam is a controlled substance and has an addiction potential so must be closely monitored by your clinician.*

- Hormone replacement taken along with clonazepam has been reported to provide significant pain relief.

- A compounding pharmacy can formulate a pain relief cream which contains benzocaine, lidocaine, tetracaine, olive oil and methyl cellulose to help afford pain relief. They can also include the medication Gabapentin in this cream formula to help calm down the nerves in the mouth if needed. *(Gabapentin is a medication used to treat chronic nerve pain and is used to treat seizures.)*

- Capsaicin oral rinse, artificial saliva products, Carafate liquid, a SSRI or tricyclic antidepressant and cognitive behavioral therapy may be considered to help afford some pain relief.

- A recent report by Dr. Maria A. Nagel, (BMJ Case Reports, April 1, 2015) suggests that the herpes virus (HSV-1) may sometimes be associated with burning mouth syndrome without a breakout of obvious cold sores and an antiviral medication may help treat the symptoms.

NOTE: If you experience a persistent dry mouth and/or burning pain in your mouth you need to see your clinician and your dentist, so they can work together to formulate a treatment plan.

Periodontal Disease (Gum Disease)

Hormonal changes during the menopausal years also increase a woman's risk for developing periodontal disease.

Definition

Periodontal disease is a chronic bacterial infection that affects the gums and bone supporting the teeth. This disease begins when bacteria in plaque (the sticky film that constantly forms on your teeth) causes the gums to become inflamed.

If you do not remove the plaque by brushing and flossing your teeth, it can build up and infect your gums, teeth and the bone supporting them. If you are not treated by a dentist, you can lose your teeth!

Signs and Symptoms

- Gums bleed easily and are red, puffy or swollen
- Gums may have pulled away from your teeth
- Your bite may have changed and your teeth don't fit together properly
- Pus (collection of bacteria) can appear between your teeth and gums
- Constant bad breath or a bad taste in your mouth can occur

Gingivitis

This term is used to describe the early form of periodontal disease. It causes the gums to become red, swollen and bleed easily when brushing your teeth.

This condition can also occur during pregnancy and if you notice any swelling or bleeding when flossing you should check in with your dentist who may recommend:

- Dental cleanings every three to four months
- Vitamin C and B complex supplements

Periodontitis

This condition results when gingivitis is not treated with good oral hygiene and professional care. The plaque can spread and grow below the gum line eventually reaching the roots of the teeth.

The gums become further irritated by a toxin which is produced by the bacteria in the plaque which promotes an inflammatory response. The body turns on itself and the tissue and bone that support the teeth are broken down and destroyed. The gums separate from the teeth, forming pockets (spaces between the teeth and gums) which become infected.

Prevention
You can try a product like Enamelon to help decrease tooth decay, sensitivity and help prevent gingivitis.

Advanced Periodontitis
This condition is the final stage of periodontal disease. When this process progresses deeper pockets are formed destroying more gum tissue and bone. This bone loss is irreversible without bone grafting. Bone, once lost, will not regenerate and grafting is not always a possibility.

Your teeth can begin to shift and loosen which will affect your bite. If treatment by a dentist and periodontist are unable to save your teeth, they will eventually have to be removed.

Medical Conditions Associated with Periodontitis
This condition can be associated with some chronic systemic diseases like heart disease, respiratory disease, diabetes and human immune deficiency virus (HIV), which all suppress the immune system.

Periodontitis is commonly found in association with diabetes mellitus, especially when your blood sugar is poorly controlled. Periodontal disease is listed as the sixth complication that can occur from having a diagnosis of diabetes.

Inflammation and Periodontitis
A study published in the Journal of Periodontology reported on "inflammatory effects from periodontal disease, a chronic bacterial infection of the gums causes oral bacterial by-products to enter the bloodstream and triggers the liver to make proteins such as CRP (C-reactive protein) that inflame arteries and promote clot formation." These effects may cause blood clots to form, clogging arteries, which can result in a heart attack or stroke.

Researchers have known for some time that elevated C-reactive protein (CRP) levels increase the risk for heart disease. The New England Journal of Medicine identified elevated CRP levels as a stronger predictor of heart attacks than elevated cholesterol levels alone. They recommend having both CRP and cholesterol screening done to accurately identify risk for cardiovascular disease. (Refer to Chapter 5 for more information on heart disease.)

Bone Health

The decline in estrogen that occurs with menopause also increases a woman's risk for loss of bone density. Loss of bone density in the jaw can cause you to lose teeth.

If your gums begin to recede this could indicate that you have some bone loss. Receding gums also expose the tooth surface, which increases the potential for further tooth decay.

An acid environment can lower your sodium level and slow the nutritional exchange in and out of your cells, leaching calcium from your bones.

Many postmenopausal women are being treated for bone loss with a class of drugs called "bisphosphonates" which work by decreasing the amount of bone that is being destroyed. Some common names you may recognize are: Actonel (risedronate), Boniva (ibandronate) and Fosamax (alendronate). Always tell your dentist if you have taken or are currently taking any of these bisphosphonates.

There have been reports of a possible link between bisphosphonates and a rare disorder called osteonecrosis (death of the bone involving the jaw). Osteonecrosis can also affect other bones in the body such as the hip and femur.

NOTE: Most of the cases reported were in patients being treated for cancer with chemotherapy and intravenous bisphosphonates to treat cancer that had spread to the bone. There have been only a few cases reported in individuals taking oral bisphosphonates, which was associated with active dental disease or having had a recent dental procedure. Osteonecrosis is very rare and usually only found in individuals with cancer or active dental disease.

Do not stop taking a bisphosphonate without talking to your doctor or clinician!

Prevention Measures For Maintaining Oral Health

Be sure to brush and floss your teeth at least twice a day and three times a day would be even better to prevent tooth decay.

Use an antibacterial toothpaste with fluoride like Colgate Total.

Ask your dentist if you could benefit from using an antibacterial mouth rinse.

See your dentist twice a year for an oral exam, which includes a full mouth inspection and cancer screen. (Most oral cancers occur in people older than 45 years of age. Please see Chapter 16, "Confronting Cancer" for more detail on oral cancer screening.)

See your hygienist for a cleaning twice a year and more frequently if you tend to form plaque easily.

Use a Waterpik or water flosser device to clean in between your teeth and gums.

Some oral surgeons recommend adding one half a teaspoonful of household bleach to approximately 600 milliliters of water before using the Waterpik to help fight bacteria. Be sure to try and spit out all the water in the sink and be careful not to swallow after rinsing. Do another final rinse with just water.

Consume a balanced diet rich in foods that contain adequate Vitamin C, Vitamin D and calcium. (Please read Chapters 3 and 6 for more information on supplements and nutrients.)

Select healthy foods to snack on that do not erode the enamel on your teeth.

Avoid:

- Drinks which contain a high amount of sugar, especially soft drinks and even diet drinks that contain citric acid.
- Candy and especially sticky candies that adhere to your teeth.
- Breakfast cereals with a high sugar content and pastries.
- Starchy processed foods like pastas, rice, breads and potatoes.
- Coffee, tea and red wine also increase the acid in your mouth, weakening the enamel and potentially staining your teeth. *(I have found that mixing one third a teaspoonful of pure coconut oil in your hot coffee or tea creates a light oil slick on the surface and prevents staining of the teeth.)*

NOTE: The bacteria in your mouth break down sugar and starch-es, creating acid which erodes the enamel.

Summary

Good oral health is not just important from a dental standpoint, but is nec-essary for overall health and well-being. Many times we forget to consider that our mouth is part of our body and we need to remember how import-ant it is to keep it healthy. Be sure to make your appointments with your oral healthcare professional and dentist for regular check-ups to maintain oral health!

Websites for further information on:

Oral Health

Mouth Healthy-American Dental Association:
http://www.mouthhealthy.org/en

Gum Disease (Gingivitis and Periodontitis) Symptoms:
http://www.webmd.com/oral-health/guide/gingivitis-periodontal-disease#1

Periodontitis-Mayo Clinic:
http://www.mayoclinic.org/diseases-conditions/periodontitis/home/ovc-20315537

Burning Mouth Syndrome

Burning Mouth Syndrome-American Dental Association:
http://www.ada.org/%7E/media/ADA/Publications/Files/patient_53.ashx

Osteonecrosis of the Jaw

Osteonecrosis of the Jaw (ONJ)-American College of Rheumatology:
http://www.rheumatology.org/I-Am-A/Patient-Caregiver/Diseases-Conditions/Osteonecrosis-of-the-Jaw-ONJ

Chapter 19

SCREENING TESTS - PROMOTING HEALTH FOR WOMEN AT EVERY AGE

The tables on the following pages are recommendations for screening tests and should be used as a guide only. Talk with your clinician about health risks and individual needs to promote health and wellness.

GENERAL HEALTH TESTS

Test	Ages 18-29	Ages 30-39	Ages 40-49	Ages 50+
Complete Checkup	Every 2-3 yrs. or more frequently if problems arise	Every 2-3 yrs. Discuss with your clinician	Every 2-3 yrs. Discuss with your clinician	Every year
Thyroid Test (TSH)	Discuss with clinician	Start at age 35 then every 5 yrs	Every 5 yrs. or sooner if symptoms occur	Every 3-5 yrs. or sooner if symptoms occur. Discuss with your clinician
Hearing Test	Start at age 18, then every 10 yrs.	Every 10 yrs.	Every 10 yrs. or sooner if you notice changes with your hearing	Every 3 yrs. Discuss with clinician if you notice changes
Vision Test	Start between ages 20-29	Every 5 yrs	Baseline age 40 with an ophthalmologist. Discuss with clinician if you notice changes	Every 1-2 yrs. Discuss with clinician if you notice changes
Skin Exam & Mole Check	Start at age 20, then every 3 yrs.	Every 3 years	Every year	Every year

HEART HEALTH

Test	Ages 18-29	Ages 30-39	Ages 40-49	Ages 50+
Blood Pressure Check	Start age 18, then with every office visit.	Every 1-2 yrs and/or with every office visit.	Every 1-2 yrs. and/or with every office visit.	Every year and/or with every office visit.
EKG	If symptoms are present.	If symptoms are present.	Routine baseline EKG at age 40 then every 5 years or sooner if risk factors or symptoms present.	Every 3 to 5 years or sooner if risk factors present or as symptoms arise. Discuss with clinician.
Cholesterol Test (lipid panel)	Start at age 17-21, then every 5 yrs.	Every 5 years if normal.	Every 5 years if normal.	Every 3-5 years. If positive family history or abnormal results, test sooner.

BONE HEALTH

Test	Ages 18-29	Ages 30-39	Ages 40-49	Ages 50+
Bone Mineral Density Test (DEXA scan)			Discuss with clinician if you are at risk.	Baseline bone density test when you have reached age 65, then every 5 yrs. if normal. Every 2 yrs if abnormal & receiving treatment. In women younger than age 65 discuss with clinician to determine fracture risk.

DIABETES

Test	Ages 18-29	Ages 30-39	Ages 40-49	Ages 50+
Blood Sugar Test	Baseline fasting blood sugar (glucose) if you are overweight or have risk factors for diabetes	Discuss with clinician if you are overweight or have risk factors for diabetes	Start at age 45 with baseline, then every 3-5 years if you are not at risk for diabetes or overweight	Every 2-3 years if you are not at risk for diabetes or overweight. Every year after age 60.

BREAST HEALTH

Test	Ages 18-29	Ages 30-39	Ages 40-49	Ages 50+
Breast Self-Exam	Monthly	Monthly	Monthly	Monthly
Clinical Exam	Every year	Every year or if you feel a palpable lump, have breast nipple discharge or see a change in breast shape	Every year or sooner if symptoms appear	Every year or sooner if symptoms appear
Mammogram	Discuss individual risks with clinician	Your clinician may recommend a mammogram if you are at high risk or have symptoms	Annual mammogram for women 40 and older. Discuss with clinician	Annual or discuss with clinician

REPRODUCTIVE HEALTH

Test	Ages 18-29	Ages 30-39	Ages 40-49	Ages 50+
Pap Test	Start at age 21 and then every 3 years if test results normal	Every 3 yrs if previous pap tests normal. Option to extend to 5 year pap testing with HPV (co-testing) if results normal and depending on individual risk.	Every 3 yrs if previous pap tests normal. Option to extend to 5 year pap testing with HPV (co-testing) if results normal and depending on individual risk.	Every 3 yrs if previous pap tests normal. Option to extend to 5 year pap testing with HPV (co-testing) if results normal and depending on individual risk. After age 65 discuss with clinician
HPV	Not recommended if you are younger than 30 years of age, unless pap smear is abnormal	Option to test every 5 years (co-testing with pap) is preferred method if results normal and depending on individual risk.	Every 5 years (co-testing with pap) is preferred method if results normal and depending on individual risk.	Every 5 years (co-testing with pap) is preferred method if results normal and depending on individual risk. After age 65 discuss with clinician
Pelvic Exam	Yearly beginning age 21	Yearly	Yearly	Yearly
Sexually Transmitted Disease (STD)	Screening test every year if you are younger than 25 and sexually active. Test annually in individuals older than 25 if you have risk factors: such as a new partner or multiple partners or a partner with a sexually transmitted disease.	Discuss with your clinician.	Discuss with your clinician.	Discuss with your clinician.

REPRODUCTIVE HEALTH (continued)

Test	Ages 18-29	Ages 30-39	Ages 40-49	Ages 50+
Gonorrhea & Chlamydia	Screening test every year if you are younger than 25 years old and sexually active. Test annually in individuals 25 years of age and older if you have risk factors: such as a new partner or multiple partners or a partner with a sexually transmitted disease.	Discuss with your clinician	Discuss with your clinician	Discuss with your clinician
HIV Testing	Baseline test at least once and/or before the start of sexual activity	Baseline test and/or if you have unsafe sex or share any injection drug equipment. Annually if you are at high risk.	Baseline test and/or if you have unsafe sex or share any injection drug equipment. Annually if you are at high risk.	Baseline test and/or if you have unsafe sex or share any injection drug equipment. Annually if you are at high risk.

NOTE: High Risk = History of a blood transfusion or history of I.V. drug use.

COLORECTAL HEALTH SCREENING

Test	Ages 18-29	Ages 30-39	Ages 40-49	Ages 50+
Guaiac Fecal Occult Blood Test (gFOBT)	If symptoms present, discuss with clinician	Discuss your individual risk with your clinician to determine which test would be appropriate.	Yearly testing for blood in stool.	Yearly testing or sooner if symptoms present.
Fecal immune-chemical test (FIT)		If symptoms present, discuss with clinician	Discuss your individual risk with your clinician to determine which test would be appropriate.	Yearly
Stool DNA test (Co-loguard). NOTE: If any of the above tests come out positive you need to have a colonoscopy!	If symptoms present. Discuss with clinician	Discuss your individual risk with your clinician to determine which test would be appropriate.	Every 3 years if results are negative and no symptoms arise.	Every three years if you are low risk for developing colon cancer and no symptoms arise. Colonoscopy is preferred baseline test.
Digital Rectal Exam		If symptoms present, discuss with clinician	Yearly. Discuss with your clinician if you have a positive family history of colon cancer and/or polyps	Yearly

COLORECTAL HEALTH SCREENING (continued)

Test	Ages 18-29	Ages 30-39	Ages 40-49	Ages 50+
Colonoscopy		If you are at increased risk, discuss with your clinician	If you have blood in your stool or are at high risk due to a family history of colon polyps or cancer you should be tested sooner than age 50. Typically you should be tested 10 years sooner than the age your family member was diagnosed with colorectal cancer.	Regular baseline screening colonoscopy at age 50 and then every 10 years if normal. If abnormal every 3-5 years depending on what type and how many polyps are found during your colonoscopy. Discuss further with your clinician. You may opt to have a sigmoidoscopy every 5 years if you have a decreased risk for developing cancer or polyps. Discuss with clinician.

MENTAL HEALTH

Test	Ages 18-29	Ages 30-39	Ages 40-49	Ages 50+
Depression Screening	Discuss with your clinician if you have symptoms and/or a positive family history	Discuss with your clinician if you have symptoms and/or a positive family history	Discuss with your clinician if you have symptoms and/or a positive family history	Annually per new recommendation. Discuss with your clinician as needed should symptoms arise.

Websites for further information:

American Cancer Society: **https://www.cancer.org/**

American Heart Association: **http://www.heart.org/**

Centers for Disease Control and Prevention: **https://www.cdc.gov/**

Kaiser Permanente: **https://healthy.kaiserpermanente.org/**

Sharp Health Care, Sharp Community Health Group: **https://www.sharp.com/**

National Institutes of Health: **https://www.nih.gov/**

National Women's Health Information Center: **https://www.womenshealth.gov/**

U.S. Department of Health and Human Services: **https://www.hhs.gov/**

U.S. Preventive Services Task Force (USPSTF): **https://www.uspreventiveservicestaskforce.org/**

Chapter 20

51 Recommendations To Help You Enjoy Midlife

1. Be happy you have friends and make time to enjoy them.

2. Keep cheerful friendships alive and try to help the cranky ones feel better.

3. Take the opportunity to tell the people you love just how much they mean to you.

4. Enjoy the simple things in life.

5. Surround yourself with what you love, whether it's family, pets, music or flowers.

6. Listen to your favorite songs, a trickling waterfall, ocean waves, a crackling fire or birds singing in the trees.

7. Keep learning and never let your brain idle. Learn more about electronic devices, gardening, cooking or even try a new hobby.

8. Be alive when you are alive!

9. Laugh every day and you will feel better and maybe even live longer.

10. Accept the beauty that comes from within and be comfortable in your own skin.

11. Try giving of yourself and help someone out. It makes you feel good to know that you have made a difference.

12. Appreciate the knowledge you have gained over the years and be comfortable and proud of who you are.

13. Wisdom comes with age which can help you enjoy:
    - More confidence in your relationships
    - More control in your life
    - Greater security in your career

14. Avoid guilt trips. Take a trip to the mall and go shopping or to a place you have always longed to go instead.

15. Go for a ride topless, in a convertible, that is and take in some fresh air and sunshine. Feel free to crank up the tunes and sing along. (Don't forget to wear a hat and put on your sunscreen.)

16. Head to the mountains and breathe in the fresh air while you go for a hike.

17. Since you are headed over the hill, put on those hiking shoes and enjoy the view.

18. If you live on the West Coast, take in a sunset near the water and allow yourself to relax.

19. If you live on the East Coast, get up early to watch the sunrise over the water.

20. Go for a walk in the snow or go skiing, if you have the opportunity and that's what you enjoy.

21. Dance as if nothing hurts!

22. Express your attitude without inhibition.

23. Express your sexual freedom and creativity.

24. Cherish each new day as a gift.

25. Be grateful you wake up breathing, it's another new day.

26. Take a moment to take in a deep breath and it will calm your mind.

27. Make peace with your past so you can embrace the future.

28. Embrace the tears and move forward learning from the experience.

29. It's not too late to have a happy childhood and the second one is up to you.

30. Be grateful for your health.

31. Be grateful you can exercise.

32. Go ahead and take a swim, your hair will dry.

33. Practice your faith and enhance your spirituality.

34. Verbalize each day three things you are grateful for and this can help you maintain a positive attitude.

35. Acknowledge your gifts and thank God each day for your blessings.

36. Take time to relax:
    • Schedule a massage with some aromatherapy
    • Lie down in a hammock and take in the fresh air and scenery.

37. Remember today is special, go ahead and use the nice sheets and lingerie.

38. Schedule twenty minutes a day just for you.

39. Be happy that now you:
    • No longer need to pack another tampon or Kotex pad for the trip.
    • Can buy sexy underwear and keep it that way.
    • No longer have to take the monthly hormonal roller coaster ride.
    • Can fit into your jeans because your hips are smaller
    • No longer need to use birth control and worry about pregnancy.
    • Less chin hairs to pluck and less hair on your legs to shave.
      (You can no longer see what hair is left without your glasses on anyway.)

40. If the grass looks greener on the other side, try mowing your own lawn and then take another look. (You don't know what their monthly water bill is either!)

41. Take charge of your own happiness.

42. Don't take things too seriously and allow yourself to stress out, in ten years from now you will never know the difference. (That is what my mother always told me and she was right.)

43. Each day that passes is gone forever, so live each one to the fullest.

44. When you crave chocolate, go ahead and eat it! (Dark chocolate is best for you.)

45. Don't pass judgments because you never know what battles someone is fighting. Try to see the beauty in each individual.

46. Forgive those that hurt you and pursue happiness.

47. Take a day off because you can and accept that your inbox will always be full.

48. Life is way too short, let go of the stress and smile.

49. Write out your bucket list and start making plans now!

50. Believe the best is yet to come!

51. Believe in miracles and await your dreams.
    "I did and became a mom at age 51!"

(May not be for everyone but turned out to be the best thing I have ever done!)

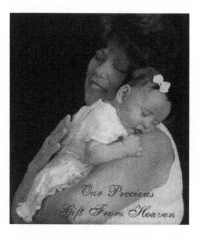

Our Precious
Gift From Heaven

Chapter 21

51 PAGES OF PERSONAL TESTIMONIALS

Autoimmune Disease:
Hypothyroidism/Mixed Connective Tissue Disorder

Patient T. C.

Nineteen years ago, I worked as a registered nurse, providing evening, night and weekend call coverage for Palomar-Pomerado Health Care providers. During my three years of service in this role, I got to know both the health care providers and their patients. One provider who impressed me more than any other was Kay Smith. What I found out quickly was that Kay knew her patients, medically and personally. Along with displaying incredible knowledge in her field, Kay was empathetic, and she under-stood each person's needs as a whole person. I could hear how Kay's patients loved her, in their time of need and when speaking with them on their follow-up calls. I knew then that it was Kay whom I wanted as my primary care provider, and it has been my good fortune to be Kay's patient and friend since then.

As a new patient, Kay helped me make adjustments as needed with my HRT, moving to bioidenticals to augment my body's natural hormone levels, and with my thyroid hormone replacement therapy, which took time but eventually we found the dosage and form of therapy that worked best for me.

Five years ago was when I was in my greatest time of need. It was then that I developed symptoms of generalized pain and fatigue, insomnia, Raynaud's, and swelling and stiffness in my hands.

Kay examined me and referred me to a rheumatologist who confirmed that I had mixed connective tissue disorder, including lupus, scleroderma and thyroid disease. According to the rheumatologist, my prognosis was poor. Plaquenil, methotrexate and steroids were discussed.

I continued this discussion with Kay at my next appointment. Kay did not appear overly alarmed about my status. Her manner was the same, cheerful and straightforward. I shared with Kay my desire to address my health opportunity in a holistic manner, trying first alternative treatments and lifestyle changes. Kay knew that this had already been my path and she supported my choice to research and work toward healing my body without pharmaceuticals.

My journey took me first to Orange County, where I was treated by Drs. Devi Nambudripad and Roy Nambudripad over a course of nine months using Nambudripad's Allergy Elimination Techniques (NAET) a non-invasive, drug free, natural solution to alleviate allergies of all types and sensitivities using energy balancing, acupuncture/acupressure, nutritional, and kinesiological disciplines of medicine. As I regained more strength, I began working out at the gym on a regular basis and have increased my workout routines to approximately two hours, at least three times a week. I refined my diet to almost exclusively non-GMO organic foods and as little sugar as possible, and I began drinking Carlsbad Alkaline Spring Water. For the next nine months, I was under the care of Dr. Chen who had me drinking a detox and immunity building tea. Dr. Toby Campian provided me with three sessions of emotional treatments to help me release significant emotional traumas. For six months, I was treated by Dr. Dan Spinato, Chiropractor/Upper Cervical-Cranial Specialist. Along with Dr. Spinato's adjustments, I underwent the non-invasive treatment of MRS2000+ Pulsating Magnetic Response Stimulation, Biomeridian Sensitivity Clearing, and six treatments of Oasis Synergy Vibration Sound and Light healing.

For the past two years, I have been under the care of Dr. Dan Harper, Naturopath, receiving homeopathic treatments, monthly ozone injections (autohemotherapy) and nutritional supplements based on my lab work. Essential oils are another modality that I partake in to support every system of my body. I receive massage therapy once a month, which enhances the immune system by stimulating lymph flow—the body's natural defense system, releases endorphins-amino acids that work as the body's natural painkiller and increases flexibility, among many other benefits.

I have brought everything alternative and helpful to me to the attention of Kay Smith. Kay can see that I am healthy and thriving. Kay is an advocate for living life in a way that avoids disease and promotes health and wellness, and she knows that I have a great respect for Western medicine. Staying healthy in today's environment is challenging. Kay promotes what she feels is best for her patients, including an optimistic and hopeful outlook on life. I truly love everything about Kay, and am beyond grateful for her as my physician and my friend.

Hypothyroidism (Underactive Thyroid)

Patient M. S.

I am so very thankful for Kay, she changed my life. Before finding her I suffered for many years, knowing that something was just not right with me and my hormones. I was in a very desperate place. I had previously visited many doctors and even suggested that they check my thyroid levels. They continued to tell me that I was fine all around, however I knew better than anyone that I was not OK! I went to see Kay for something completely different and she suggested that I have a complete physical. It was from the blood work that she found I had an underactive thyroid (an elevated TSH) and INDEED I had HYPOTHYROIDISM. She started me on thyroid replacement medication and my life was forever changed. No more anxiety, depression, heart palpitations and no more noise in my head. Because of Kay, I can see clearly now and am forever grateful and she will be my forever Angel!

Hypothyroidism, Menopause and Osteoarthritis

Patient A. M.

I now have been taking thyroid replacement for over thirty years. At the age of 38, the thyroid hormone in my body was only a "measurable trace" and the replacement dosage quickly rose to 200 mcgs of Synthroid daily within a few months. Shortly thereafter the Synthroid was replaced with Levothyroxine, the generic equivalent, and the replacement dosage was changed to 175 mcgs daily. Over time I eventually gained 50 pounds but attributed it to menopause and a sedentary job.

In the past six years I also developed osteoarthritis in my neck, shoulders, hands and right hip. Since retiring, in addition to nutritional changes I had made in recent years, I have become much more active. I now have a personal trainer who recommended four to five workouts weekly at a fitness center and I also include weekly yoga and dance classes. This increased physical activity resulted in a 25 pound weight loss. In the past three months when Kay switched me back to Synthroid I lost an additional 12 pounds. My BMI (body mass index) is now in the normal range for my age. In addition my arthritis symptoms and joint pain have lessened significantly, especially the MCP (metacarpal phalangeal) joint in my right hand. Thus, I believe my improved well-being is attributable to taking Synthroid in addition to the dietary and lifestyle changes I have made.

Hypothyroidism and Systemic Lupus Erythematosus (SLE)

Patient R. S.

As with any autoimmune disease my story is not a short one. Currently I am 51 years old and have been a physical therapist for 29 years working for and owning outpatient/sports medicine facilities including serving as Director of Rehabilitation at San Diego State University Sports Medicine Center, in charge of the student athlete injury rehabilitation. I was diagnosed with SLE (Systemic Lupus Erythematosus) 15 years ago at the age of 36 after having my gallbladder removed, but I believe my lupus symptoms started when I was very young.

In my teens, I had a very difficult time eating foods with fat in them. During high school the pizza after our basketball games was not something that would set well with my stomach, or what I thought was my stomach. For years I had many episodes of what the physicians thought to be gallbladder issues. I was told that I was too young to have any gallbladder issues and the ultrasound testing would always show it to be normal. Later, after having my gallbladder removed, the pathology report stated that my gallbladder had a significant amount of scar tissue in it. My colleagues who practice eastern medicine described it as "the lupus was living in my gallbladder." Even though the gallbladder is not typically known to be associated with SLE, like damage to the kidneys, heart or brain are commonly found to be, I don't think your antibodies with lupus discriminate against any organ.

The second set of my SLE symptoms started in high school when I was diagnosed with having an overactive thyroid (hyperthyroidism), which was controlled with medication up until my first year in college when I received the diagnosis of having an underactive thyroid (hypothyroidism). Thinking that the physicians had over-medicated me, I quickly learned about Hashimoto's Disease. I've been on some type of thyroid hormone ever since. My TSH (thyroid stimulating hormone) was found to be over 400 (normal being 0.45 to 4.5) after my gallbladder surgery, which turned out to be instrumental in leading to my SLE diagnosis.

Again in high school, I experienced the third SLE symptom, a skin rash. This story is actually quite funny as it relates to the Virgin Islands and Pusser's Rum. I was fortunate to be able to spend a few different times down in the Virgin Islands on my parents' sailboat. The first time down, two days into the week, I developed a severe rash all over my body, including my face. Traveling, my parents would allow us to try different local beers, wines and drinks. We attributed the rash to the fruity rum drinks I was having as when I got home the rash went away. I grew up in San Diego; played tennis, golf, softball, water skied, surfed a little, had a sailboat and would go to the Colorado River and Mexico and would never get a rash like I had in the Virgin Islands, so sun exposure was never a second thought. I will say that I was not one to "lie out in the sun" and we also used a lot of sunscreen, so again the sun exposure I had in the Virgin Islands was not considered to be the problem. Back then they didn't have any UV ray clothing available, so men's pajamas were what I used to block some of the sun on our return trips back from Saint Thomas. Now my closet is full of UV ray blocking clothing and I stay out of the sun as much as possible. When I have an episode of the cheek rash, everyone assumes I've been out in the sun, but if you look at my white arms and legs, you will know that I haven't been. I was lucky when my boys took up roller and ice hockey, allowing me to be indoors to watch them compete. During the baseball, football and soccer sports sessions when they did play, I would certainly wear my UV protection clothing and find the nearest shade. The good news is it was not Pusser's Rum to blame, but since my SLE diagnosis and the years of auto-immune suppressants (oral chemotherapy), prednisone and adjunct medications, I made the decision to not drink alcohol to support my kidneys and liver. I know these organs have already taken a beating over the last 15 years. A sip from my husband's different micro-brewery beers is my treat! On a side note, for years I had a horrible "bruise" on my shins and finally my dermatologist told me it was "Plaquenil graying." The good news is that within only a few weeks after stopping the Plaquenil, the bruising on my shins went away.

Joint pain was and has always been a part of my life. I played numerous sports growing up and sustained multiple bone fractures, which may have been related to my diagnosis of SLE.

My biggest and most challenging lupus symptom is "chest pain." The first episode of my chest pain was while I was at SDSU, long hours and lots of stress with caring for NCAA Division 1 athletes, but it was the best job I have ever had. I experienced two different episodes of chest pain that both were diagnosed as costochondritis and treated with high doses of steroids, which helped improve the symptoms. My recurring minor chest pains, along with my history of broken ribs and the costochondritis, again were never thought to be associated with my SLE. It was not until I experienced a number of severe cases of chest pain, along with receiving a diagnosis of pleurisy two weeks after my gallbladder surgery, which landed me in the hospital emergency room twice, was my chest pain finally related to my lupus. To this day, people ask if I'm in remission. I don't think that I have reached total remission. I believe that if I push myself physically and mentally, then left sided chest pain and the cheek rash can easily reappear.

A low platelet count and recurring chest pain have certainly been the symptoms that have caused me the most concern and mental stress. With the chest pain, you do not know if it is just the SLE symptoms or a cardiology issue. Knowing now that I have been incredibly fortunate to have been able to carry and give birth to two sons while having SLE and low platelet counts made for a tense situation at the end of my pregnancies, especially my second one. My platelet count had dropped down well below 80,000 and I needed another C-section delivery. My OB/GYN at the time questioned the low platelets and mentioned preeclampsia, but I did not have any of the other signs or symptoms. Not until my SLE diagnosis did the low platelets make sense and the fact that my OB/GYN said she would not have been my physician knowing I had SLE, did I really understand how blessed I was to have two healthy sons.

Because I live in warm Southern California, Raynaud's disease has not been one of my major SLE symptoms. However, I have had a number of episodes of Raynaud's when I was in colder weather and really feel for those who have regular episodes of this incredibly painful symptom. As with many of the other SLE symptoms I have experienced, I learned to just try and control them with extra layers of clothes, socks and gloves when I am in colder weather.

The most common symptom of SLE is fatigue, yet it is the one that you can control the best. I know that when I have had long weeks, treating up to 75 plus patient visits and have not given myself enough rest and sleep, fatigue will hit me hard. Those days, you can't fight it; you just need to give yourself the rest and sleep that your body is asking for. With that said, I find the more active I can be physically and mentally, the better I feel with the right nutrition and rest.

Even with having all these different symptom episodes and a medical background, I was shocked with the diagnosis of SLE. In physical therapy school we had learned about auto-immune diseases and in my mind, all of the "crazy women" health complaints were just being wrapped up into a few garbage can diagnoses. I will tell you that with my history of injuries, symptoms and knowledge of my body, during those initial years of receiving my SLE diagnosis, I thought I was crazy. At times, I still think some of the pain and symptoms I experience can't be happening, but I've learned to control them, not fight them. You cannot fight SLE, believe me, I tried and it knocked me down.

With all the years of symptoms and continued SLE symptoms, I know I'm one of the lucky ones with SLE. When I was first diagnosed with SLE, as I mentioned my thoughts were "OK let's fight this thing." I really wasn't afraid of SLE until within the first 6 months of my diagnosis, I met a number of people who had relatives or someone they knew that had died as a result of lupus, and then I said, "WHAT!" SLE became more real to me, especially after treating a few patients who have had heart and kidney transplants. As I said, I'm one of the lucky ones with no significant heart or kidney disease. I'm also blessed that I'm able to control my symptoms enough to lead a productive life.

I had two young children and previously owned a 4,500 square foot physical therapy practice with up to twenty employees for seven years back in the mid-nineties, when you had to have a prescription from a physician to see a physical therapist. The physicians were also starting to open up their own physical therapy clinics at that time and stress was certainly at a premium. I tried to fight the lupus, maxing out on my medications including my immune suppressant, prednisone and anti-malaria medications, not to mention all the other medications I had to take to control the side effects of the lupus medications. I would think to myself, "I wish I had a disease I could fight." I think my friends and family would say I have a strong will and you hear about people fighting and beating diseases, but SLE is not one of those.

I decided to sell my business in 1996 knowing I had to make a change. I continued taking the immune suppressants and developed a serious infection in 1997 which confirmed that I had made the right decision.

In the past, I tried multiple different elixirs, medications from multiple rheumatologists, supplements, massage therapy and acupuncture which all helped, but as I know now, were not going to be a cure. Currently, I am off all medications except my thyroid hormone, vitamins, various supplements (including increased calcium and vitamin D), and cinnamon in my protein shakes, and I wear an EFX hologram bracelet daily. I used to have to take an Aleve as part of my daily vitamin pack.

I have now utilized the hologram technology for 8 years with significant reduction in my SLE symptoms. I have only missed wearing it a dozen times and usually paid the price with increase chest pain, fatigue and joint pain. I know there are studies that say this technology does not work, but whether it is physical or mental, I feel better when I wear my hologram technology.

I'm currently making it through menopause, have my "bad lupus days," but I still get "you look so good," even though my SLE symptoms can be active. I know when I was first diagnosed, I sought out many medical opinions and because I was still working, was able to function with having a family and putting up a good front even when I felt like I was dying inside, "you look good" or "you look too good to be sick" were not the words I wanted to hear. Not until I read my first few books on lupus and most authors would describe the "you look good" syndrome as I like to call it, did I realize that is just part of living with SLE.

I am certainly not looking for sympathy sharing my story, as I learned early on with my SLE and again it was confirmed in the books I read about lupus, that when most people ask how you are doing and you start to answer, then you see they have turned their attention to another place. My standard answer just became "I'm fine." I am sharing my SLE path in hope that if it can help even one young person who may be going through similar symptoms to continue to seek out a medical professional like Kay who has her advanced knowledge, incredible intuition and spiritual gift. Kay's continued friendship and my incredible family have really helped me to continue my path in controlling my SLE symptoms.

Birth Control and Eating Disorder

Patient T. M.

For years I had been struggling to find a birth control that worked for me and it seems like I had tried almost everything and I then went to see Kay. She prescribed the Ortho-Evra patch and it has been the best birth control method for my body.

Since I was a little girl I have had eating problems with my weight fluctuating up and down at unhealthy numbers. I changed primary care doctors to Kay Smith, P.A.C. and she has been monitoring my weight and provides me with proper dietary tips and has recommended some lifestyle modifications. My eating disorder with Kay's guidance is now under control and I am happy to report that I have maintained a healthy weight for over two years now. She is the best physician assistant ever and I won't see anyone else! I am currently working with Kay as a medical assistant and plan on furthering my education to become a registered nurse.

Cancer Survivors:

Breast Cancer

Patient S. F.

April 28, 2014 is a day I remember very clearly. I was sitting in Kay's office and she told me the biopsy was positive for cancer. This was a total shock. How could this be? I was healthy and there was no evidence of breast cancer in my family. I knew other women who had been diagnosed with breast cancer, but never considered that I would be joining them as a fighter and survivor. The previous year was the year of change for me. I dropped 30 pounds, changed my eating habits and exercised. Having tried different types of exercise over the years, I discovered Jazzercise and fell in love with it. I became a Jazzercise instructor in 2007. I was strong with a healthy heart, muscular and felt good. I also had yearly mammograms.

Having very dense breast tissue, I was often called back for additional pictures. Each time the pictures turned out OK. One morning in April, I discovered a lump in my right breast. I panicked a bit and called for a doctor's appointment right away. I was worried, but I had so many factors in my favor that I was very hopeful for good news. I had a diagnostic mammogram and ultrasound the following week. I then got the call back for an ultrasound guided biopsy. Everyone was so nice to me and it went smoothly, although the technician doing the biopsy couldn't pull the needle back out. I was pretty certain I was going to have to go home with this needle sticking out of me. (Lesson 1 for the journey: Find humor wherever you can.) The needle was finally removed and I was sent home with an ice pack inside my bra (yep—it was cold). It took a few days to recover from the biopsy, and I then anxiously awaited the results. I continued my daily routine, keeping busy while I waited. I work full-time, teaching 5 Jazzercise classes a week, and am the organist and accompanist for our choir at church. (Lesson 2: Keep busy doing what you love to do.) I kept the news to myself at this time, only telling my family (who all live out of state), my close friends and the people I worked for. I immediately felt the love and support of everyone. Prayers were offered up and I felt reassured that everything would be OK, regardless of the diagnosis. My doctor is Catholic and goes to the same church I do. It was so reassuring to have her remind me during a doctor visit to trust in God. And then bang...at the age of 53, my world as I knew it changed forever with the words I had always feared. The tests were positive for cancer. My very first thought was "as long as I don't have to go through chemo and lose my hair, it will be OK." It was originally thought I could have a lumpectomy and radiation...no big deal. If only that was the case. After getting the pathology report, I didn't know what to do. I left the doctor's office feeling quite numb (clutching a chocolate bunny they thought I deserved – and yes, I ate the whole thing!)

It was 10:30 a.m. on a Monday morning. I knew I couldn't go to work, at least not yet. After shedding some tears, I called Mary, a friend who had just finished all of her treatment for breast cancer. And then Chuck, my husband, called to see how my appointment went. I asked him to join Mary and me for lunch. I found it very hard to tell Chuck, but in doing so found myself telling him it would all be ok. I think reassuring others was a way of convincing myself everything would be all right. Having finished treatment, Mary was a source of information, answered questions and gave me advice, along with a wonderful book called "What Cancer Cannot Do". Her advice was to take it one day at a time.

The next people I told were our very best friends whom I needed to pick up from the airport that evening. I got a text message asking how my doctor's appointment went. It was hard to tell them because I didn't want it to be true. I told them I would still pick them up from the airport, but we would need to stop and have margaritas on the way home. We hugged, shed a few tears and laughed a lot. (Lesson 3: Surround yourself with good friends and spend time with them. Drink margaritas.)

I think telling my kids was the hardest. They both took it pretty hard, and seemed very nervous and scared about the whole thing. We had recently lost a family friend to breast cancer, so I understood their fear. As a mom, I always want to be there for them, and I found myself reassuring them, even though there were many uncertainties.

Next was a visit to the surgeon. On the form under reason for visit I wrote 'pathology results positive'. I met the surgeon and genuinely liked the surgeon. After he did his exam, we talked. The surgeon used the 'M' word. Mastectomy. What?? And he had a lymph node concern. And he was sorry I had been diagnosed with breast cancer. I was in shock. So much changed in that 90 minute appointment. I was not a candidate for a lumpectomy. It was based on location, location, location. I had to have a mastectomy with removal of lymph nodes that felt swollen. And this was when I fully realized I had breast cancer. I had never admitted it before or said those words. The surgeon also suggested I was a candidate for immediate reconstruction, which gave me something else to think about.

Leaving the surgeon's office, we drove to Las Vegas where my sister was getting married that weekend. Honestly, I cried half the way there and cherished the hugs I got upon arriving. It was so good to see family at this time. I sought out a local Jazzercise class in Las Vegas, where I could workout, lose myself in the music and dance. It felt good to move and made me feel alive, even though I had so many fears inside.

I considered and pondered reconstruction. My mom told me I was young and to go for it. I decided that one surgery would be better than two, so I made a phone call and scheduled a consultation with a plastic surgeon. I saw him and we discussed my reconstruction options. We also discussed the pros and cons of a single mastectomy versus a double mastectomy. He indicated I would have the best results with reconstruction if I had a bilateral mastectomy. I started feeling overwhelmed again because there were more decisions to make, more research to do, and there were no wrong or right answers. I wondered what the chances were of me getting cancer in the other breast. I remember talking to Kay, my doctor, and telling her how I felt. She suggested I also have a consultation with an oncologist, so that was my next step.

I met my oncologist, and we discussed the type of breast cancer I had, the risk of getting cancer on the other side, and treatment options. I learned that the mammogram I had AFTER finding the lump came back showing NO abnormalities. That was shocking news and made my husband ask the oncologist why I was having mammograms every year. So that information, combined with the fact there was a 20% risk of getting cancer on the left side helped me decide to have a bilateral mastectomy. I did get good news that the hormone receptor test came back positive which meant I was eligible for hormone therapy. It also meant the cells were still responding and acting like breast cells (as opposed to cancer cells) and the cancer was not as aggressive.

I found it very hard telling people I had cancer. First, it took me awhile to say those words. I would say "the test results were positive" or biopsy results showed I had cancer. But it took some time to say the words "I have cancer." I didn't want people feeling sorry for me. I didn't want to have cancer. Saying it made it more real and I was afraid of everything that was to come.

On May 21st, I got word they had finally scheduled my surgery for June 20th. One month away. Yes, the date was later than I wanted, but there was coordination required between the general surgeon, the plastic surgeon, and the operating room for a 4 hour surgery. I was scheduled for a modified radical mastectomy on the right, meaning they would also remove 12 lymph nodes. On the left, I would be having a simple mastectomy with no lymph node removal. We would do reconstruction at the same time, which I was told would be the most painful part of the recovery.

I had a month to prepare, wait, worry, and get things together. It was a busy time. Now that I had a date, I expanded the list of people I told. I told my team at work and had to make arrangements for backup since I would be out for 6 weeks. I told my Jazzercise classes, and had to arrange for subs to cover my classes while I was out. I told the staff at church and had to make arrangements for a substitute organist. I filed for medical leave and disability at work. All of the arrangements kept me busy. As the time drew closer I became more nervous, but also anxious to just get it done. The love, support, and encouragement from everyone was instrumental in helping me prepare mentally for surgery. A lot of people were praying for me and my battle against cancer. Multiple prayer groups, churches, friends, family, all were lifting me up in prayer. It gave me strength I needed for the days ahead.

I had my pre-op appointments with both surgeons and signed paperwork. I was counting down the days. My Jazzercise classes held Pink Parties for me. Fellow Jazzercise instructors and customers were all dressed in pink, working out and giving me encouragement. Some were customers I had not met before, including 2 breast cancer survivors. They were there to show their support. I received cards, hugs, well wishes, flowers, and gifts from the most amazing Jazzercise customers. Their send-off was amazing and I went home feeling so loved! My Jazzercise family really showed their love for me.

The day of surgery arrived. My husband and I left for the hospital and I was admitted and prepped for surgery. Every doctor, nurse and hospital employee was so nice. While in surgery, I knew in the waiting room would be my husband, children, and many friends. After I came out of surgery, I was taken to a room feeling very groggy. My kids and our friends played cards while I dozed on and off. I woke up and we took pictures (I have no idea why, because I looked very, very drugged.) I was very nauseous from the anesthesia and nothing tasted good. (Lesson 4: Just say no to Salmon and broccoli after surgery followed by Lesson 5: Don't be embarrassed to throw up in front of your friends.)

After two nights in the hospital (I got a bonus second night since I couldn't keep food down at first) I was glad to be home. I discovered naps are good and slept a lot. I saw faith in action, as friends brought flowers, food, sent cards, and came to visit. (Lesson 6: Let friends help.) I had follow-up appointments with the plastic surgeon and then the regular surgeon. I was given the news that the lymph nodes were cancerous and I would definitely need chemo. I had heard such terrible stories of people going through chemo and it scared me very much. My husband and I were both upset by the news, and once again, friends were there to help us cope with the news. (Review Lesson 3: Laugh with friends.)

And then there was a set-back. Recovery from surgery was going well until I developed an infection. I was put on antibiotics which did not help, so I was sent to the ER. Saturday night emergency room provides a lot of entertainment. On July 20, I was admitted to the hospital and had a second surgery the next day. The infected wound was cleaned and because the implants were infected, they were removed. I was heartbroken, not because I needed breasts, but because it felt like a step backwards. And now I had to deal with my self-image and how I looked. Once again, friends were there to cheer me on and be with me. I loved that someone from the Catholic Church stopped by to visit me, pray with me and offer me communion. It reminded me to continue to draw on my faith for support.

My husband and I attended "chemo-training" where we discovered the Caring Bridge, an awesome way to share how I was doing with friends and family. I set up a Caring Bridge account and wrote regular journal entries, allowing an easy way for people to know what was going on. We met with our nurse practitioner who went over all the side effects and we left with a list of vitamins, medicines, and treatments to help me get through chemo. All I could say was "wow". I had no idea. I was scheduled to have a port put in for chemo, another procedure I hope to never have to do again.

On August 1, I felt quite brave. I went to the San Diego Vascular Center to have a port implanted in my chest near the collar bone. This isn't just any ordinary port. It is a 'power' port and able to receive fluid at a high rate. And it comes with a bracelet for me to wear and a key ring card to carry as reminders I have a PowerPort implanted. I am pretty sure I won't be forgetting. This was done as an outpatient procedure with local anesthet-

ic. This is where I get points for being brave because I will be the first to admit I don't do well in these types of situations. The doctor was fabulous and made sure I was comfortable. And it was over before I knew it. I had a lovely gauze pressure bandage on my chest. My daughter told me it looked sexy. :-) There was some discomfort and I could feel it when I swallowed which is weird. Supposedly in a week or so I would no longer notice it being there. That was never the case. It protruded out from my skin and I noticed it the entire time I had it.

Another follow-up appointment with the surgeon and finally -- Six weeks and 3 days after my first surgery, I was finally "drain and tube" free. What a wonderful feeling to no longer have drain tubes! Surely a cause for cele-bration! (Lesson 7: Celebrate everything!) I was cleared to return to work and even though additional healing needed to take place, I was ready.

I attended my first Jazzercise class and it was awesome. Legs felt great, but lots of stiffness in the upper body and my arm movements were still limited. No overhead reaches for me yet. But it felt great to move, dance and see my Jazzercise friends.

While preparing for chemo, I met and had a consultation with my radia-tion oncologist. There, I learned that the chance of cancer coming back on the right side is 30% if I don't do radiation and 5% if I do. For me this was a no brainer. I was to have radiation treatment every day, Monday through Friday, for 5 weeks after finishing chemo.

I started back teaching my Jazzercise classes!!! So exciting to be onstage again dancing with my fellow Jazzercise friends. My goal was to get every-thing back to normal. Return to work, start teaching Jazzercise again and start playing the piano and organ. The entire choir at church was praying for me and supporting me. I wasn't going to let cancer run my life. I was going to fight and win.

And then the chemo began....I was very nervous. I started the day with an awesome Jazzercise class, shower, and a big healthy breakfast. I packed my chemo bag (blanket, snacks, mints, socks, magazine, iPod, water, etc.) and had a friend take me and spend the day with me. I had 4 chemo treat-ments and did not go to any of them alone. My husband bought me beau-tiful bouquets of flowers after each chemo treatment. I took a friend each time and we played cards, read magazines, talked and laughed. We made the most of the situation. I had no idea how I would react to chemo. The steroids they had me take made my face flushed and I felt like I was running a fever, even though I wasn't. I felt pretty good for the 2 days after chemo, but then the unsettled stomach hit me. I never got sick, but just didn't feel good. I ate comfort foods and teased that I was on the mashed potato and ice cream diet, foods that tasted good and didn't bother my stomach. I developed a metallic, chemical taste in my mouth and some foods just did not taste good. I was told to expect to lose my hair about 2 weeks after the first chemo treatment. I attended a class sponsored by the American Cancer Society called "Look Good - Feel Better". It is a free session for women going through treatment and deals with make-up, skin care, loss of hair issues, etc. The most fun was trying on different wigs to see what I looked like. We had lots of laughs over some of those.

One of the fun things about any medical issue is dealing with insurance, so there were times we had to wait for tests to be approved. My insurance company finally approved the CT scan that my oncologist had requested. I had a CT scan with iodine contrast of the chest, abdomen and pelvis area. When I met with the oncologist he had really good news for me. The scan showed no evidence of cancer in the abdomen or pelvis. The report said I was post-surgical and there was scar tissue. Both Chuck and I were so relieved. Time for the Happy Dance! :-) Since cancer had been detected in 6 of the lymph nodes removed, we felt so much better having the clean scan. The appointment was also exactly 1 week after my first chemo treatment. Lab work showed white cell counts were already up above normal. The oncologist was happy to hear I was back exercising regularly and healing progressed.

But now it was time to face the one thing most women fear when going through chemotherapy - hair loss. We spend a lot of money on haircuts and colors, shampoo, conditioners, and styling products. And even though I knew hair loss was a side effect, it was still very hard dealing with the hair falling out. It first started 13 days post chemo....just a few strands but way more than normal. I was pretty depressed and my daughter and I spent an hour looking at my options. I have a couple of stocking caps and a few scarves we practiced tying. The next evening when I showered there was more hair loss and if I ran my fingers through my hair I could easily pull more hair out. So I just didn't do that. Friday morning was not good. The amount of hair coming out during my shower was more than I could deal with. There was hair everywhere and I knew this was it. I cried as I mourned my loss but knew I had no option but to face it. I made it through the work day afraid hair would fall out at work. Or worse yet, a gust of wind would come up and blow it across the parking lot. :-) It was holding on by a thread. A dear friend came up with scissors and clippers. We were both very brave and I so appreciated her willingness to do this for me. I did tell her it was a haircut she couldn't mess up. I taught Jazzercise wearing a baseball cap and my class all showed up wearing hats in support. So fun! This was another part of my journey that I had feared.

My final chemo treatments were uneventful and follow-up visits with the oncologist were good. I just felt a little sluggish and not as energetic. We decided to hire someone to clean our house every other week (highly recommended), and I loved not having to spend my energy cleaning bathrooms, dusting, and vacuuming. I kept on Jazzercising (way more fun than house cleaning) and returned to playing piano/organ at church. The doctor told me that patients who exercise during chemo really do much better. Personally, it makes me feel better physically, emotionally and mentally.

Many people told me I was an inspiration, or that they thought I was brave. I had a hard time accepting those compliments, partly because I didn't feel particularly brave. I was just dealing with the hand that was dealt to me. I talked with my oncologist about it and he said that I am facing head on, with grace, what every woman fears could happen to her. I pondered that and it helped me understand their comments better. I was determined to keep moving forward, with strength and humor each day.

The next phase for me was radiation and hormone therapy. I was told by some that radiation would be a piece of cake. That sounded encouraging and I figured it couldn't be any worse than chemo.

And besides, I like cake. I met my radiation oncologist and was told I would be having radiation on the chest wall, under the arm (armpit area) and on part of the lower neck. And I got my first tattoos!!!!! I had three small dot-like tattoos to help with positioning during each of 25 treatments. The side effects of radiation were nothing like a piece of cake. My skin turned red and got swollen. Wearing shirts became difficult and I bought the extra-large tub of Aquaphor. Symptoms peaked about 7 days after my final radiation treatment. The area by the neck and collar became very pink, itchy and tender to the touch. The other two areas were much worse. They used a bolus across the chest wall and under the arm, which intensifies the radiation at the skin level. There was concern about the cancer coming back in the skin. The skin there was very, very red, almost purple and multiple layers of skin peeled off. The area became very swollen and generally hurt like a burn would.

It was December and I was preparing to participate in an annual cookie baking day with one of my best friends. I was preparing for the day by mixing up several batches of cookies. It became apparent that even though I had been exercising and my arm was getting stronger, I had not yet built up enough strength in my right arm to mix cookies. I was kind of frustrated but quickly came up with a solution for the future. Buy a Kitchen Aid Mixer. (Lesson 7: Look outside the box for solutions and don't dwell on what you can't do.) My new red Kitchen Aid mixer is beautiful!

I finished my last radiation treatment 3 days before Christmas! It was wonderful to be done and start the overall healing. I started taking Tamoxifen December 1 and am on the 5 year plan with that. I dedicated 2015 to year of healing, friends, family, and fun!

I was told by the plastic surgeon I would need to wait about 6 months after radiation to even consider reconstruction. This would allow time for the skin to heal and soften. In the meantime, moving forward meant checking into getting prosthesis. I had no idea what this entailed and was very hesitant as I approached my appointment. I met a wonderful woman who was so helpful, calm and supportive. By now, I was used to getting dressed and undressed in front of others, so trying on mastectomy bras with prosthesis was no big deal. While the bras were not very cute, they were paid for by my insurance company. Really?!?! My medical insurance covered the prosthesis and several bras! I had no idea there were several types and shapes and it was kind of fun trying on the different models. And I could be any size I wanted to be (A, B, C, etc.). The prosthesis arrived in its own little pink carrying case that zipped shut, and kind of reminded me of a hat box. Having the prosthesis has resulted in several mixed feelings. It feels normal to wear a bra and my shirts fit the way they should. My silhouette is normal and I have a "shape" again. But there have been moments of frustration with them. I bought additional bras with built in pockets to wear to my Jazzercise classes. These sport bras are impossible to get off after a workout when I am all sweaty. Not only does the bra come off over your head, but the fake girls come with it, and I feel like a contortionist by the time I am done. And there are times I am in the locker room changing and I wish I didn't have to move prosthesis from one bra to another. I just want my own boobs back. While I know that's not a reality, it is how I feel at times. Another plus is that when it is hot and humid outside (we don't have AC at home), I don't need to wear my prosthesis. It is so much cooler to just wear a tank top and not worry about how I look. But overall, the prosthesis have been a way to look more normal and feel better about the way I look standing in front of the mirror.

In January I got the best news ever when I was told there was no evidence of cancer! I was starting to feel really good, the skin had healed and my hair was starting to grow back. I have continued to improve the flexibility and strength in my arm. I teach 5 Jazzercise classes and can now reach overhead! I started back at the gym, lifting weights to rebuild muscle I had lost during treatment. I am living life, taking it one day at a time, getting used to the new normal. I am loving life and laughing often! I am not the same person I was before my cancer diagnosis. Small things aren't as important anymore. Life is about friendships, relationships with people, and spending time with those who love and care about you.

Breast Cancer and Depression

Patient K. P.

A short time ago, I was diagnosed with aggressive Stage III Invasive Ductal Carcinoma. I thought breast cancer was just for older women and at age 37 could not believe this was happening to me. Being a healthy, active, vegetarian, non-smoker and normal weight individual my entire life left everyone puzzled. In less than a month, I began six rounds of chemotherapy every three weeks. After the initial shock, I had to face the reality that my life would never be the same again. My long blonde hair fell out and I replaced it with every color and style of wig I could get my hands on. I knew that I looked ridiculous but at least I could make myself smile.

Following chemotherapy, a bilateral mastectomy removed the remaining cancer. After eight hours in surgery, I was in remission and started the reconstruction process. Healing went slowly and lifting my arms above my head became a serious achievement.

After a month of rest from the surgery, then came two months of daily radiation therapy. It was a full time job leaving me exhausted! Our sweet little four year old daughter could not understand why mommy was always so tired. Slowly my energy started to come back but the four additional recon-structive surgeries definitely came with a mental toll of depression. I know I am lucky to be alive and have such a supportive group of family and friends.

Among those friends is Kay. Not only medically speaking but also she has a family history of breast cancer. When Kay first found out about what I was to face, she was encouraging and simply explained what was going on. What I didn't realize at the time was the treatment was the easy part of my situation. The treatment was about a year and the reconstruction is a long slow process. Kay has been a shoulder to cry on when the depression just seemed to have no end in sight. Picking up the pieces of routine and coming back to "normal" life has been almost an overwhelming chal-lenge. I keep feeling that I stumble and fall but it can be hard to get back up and keep walking.

Genuine people that care for you mentally and physically are the ones needed for support. This is the way Kay feels not only about me but for all of her patients. I thank God for giving me a second chance on life. Every day I am grateful. Life is short!

Breast Cancer, Depression, Elevated Cholesterol Levels, High Blood Pressure, Hypothyroidism and Pre-diabetes

Patient B. W.

Despite being a breast cancer survivor, I feel I have been blessed with a generally healthy body all my life. I am a large woman, reaching my full adult height of six feet when I was just a pre-teen. My bone structure is large as well. I don't have a willowy frame. I am what some would call Zoftig. Of course I saw it as a reason to go from one diet to the next through adulthood, but I am curvy enough that I have been regularly reas-sured by others that I am not fat. A colleague of mine once told me I looked like a Nazi pin-up girl! Ha!

While being statuesque can have its advantages (except finding available men in the standard American 5'10" market), I have come to realize that it can also stress the body systems. While my sturdy frame did not make me a candidate for osteoporosis, I was not wiry or fast enough to be com-petitively athletic.

Now at 62, I feel healthy and strong, but I battle with some health concerns and red flags. None of them irreversible, many are typical complaints of getting older in a world confronted with a buffet of unhealthy choices.

Breast cancer caught me blind-sided. When I walked in the 3-day breast cancer walk in 2004, I didn't know anyone who had had the disease. I walked because it was a good cause. A short two years later I was diagnosed myself. We still don't have a definitive answer about why this happens, but some common tendencies are offered as theories. Was it because I never breastfed my children? Is carrying extra weight a precursor? What about those years of hormone therapy? Sugar? Alcohol? I needed the care and consultation of another woman I could confide in and who would give it to me straight. I found that in Kay Smith. The relationship I have with this sensitive health care professional could not have been possible with another doctor, let alone a male doctor. As women, our needs as we age are so gender specific and personal. If you cannot sit down and talk to your doctor like a trusted friend, you are seeing the wrong person. Regardless of what happens with the price of health care, for me it is critical to have a continuum of care with Kay. Her knowledge base and insistence of staying up with all things happening in science and medicine makes her my secret weapon for good health.

Kay has seen me though breast cancer, hypothyroidism, pre-diabetes, elevated cholesterol levels, worrisome blood pressure and the depression that comes from the life changes of a woman who has had many challenges in her life, including divorce and estrangement from a child.

I couldn't have predicted the hidden gifts that come with getting a diagnosis like breast cancer, but I feel that I am better informed and have an ally that can help me get through anything. I do not fear what inevitable health challenges I face next with Kay Smith on my team.

Breast Cancer, Diabetes and Osteoarthritis with Knee Replacement

Patient L. G.

I have been fortunate enough to have this wonderful woman help me through my health issues for over 20 years. The time since menopause has been especially challenging. Initially I took hormone replacement therapy (HRT) which worked quite well to reduce the symptoms.

I will always remember the day I went for my annual mammogram and there was a problem. I was very lucky. It was stage one estrogen sensitive breast cancer. My gynecologist informed me that I would not have "felt" this for at least three years and it would probably have been stage 3 or 4 by then. Don't let anyone ever tell you mammograms don't save lives. They saved mine.

I am old enough that I grew up during a time when cancer was a death sentence. Naturally I was depressed. But I quickly realized that I needed to fight this. I did it by being very vocal about my condition. I decided that if just one woman got a mammogram and found her cancer early because of me – my cancer would make sense. I know that this is not something everyone can do – quite frankly I surprised myself – but it has worked for me.

I was treated with surgery, radiation, Tamoxifen and then Arimidex, which are both chemotherapy drugs. I am now almost 13 years cancer free, and consider myself very lucky. However, the treatment has caused its own problems. The radiation left me with substantial scarring under my breast.

The Tamoxifen put me in the throes of menopause again – even though I had made my way though it the first time and had suffered only minor discomfort due to the HRT. It wasn't until a few months after my surgery that they came out with the warning not to use it. This was now out of the question. On the Tamoxifen I suffered hot flashes and could not sleep well. After being on it for over two years they discovered a fibroid tumor that was 8 cm. My gynecologist sent me for a uterine biopsy that was clear, and she said I may have had it for years and it had gone unnoticed because it was unattached to other organs. As a result she was taking a wait and see approach. Then I remembered the CT scan Kay had ordered two years before because of some stomach problems. There was no fibroid on it. I was having a hysterectomy within a month. Even though the biopsy had been clean – 3 months later they found precancerous cells in my uterus. I consider myself very lucky that Kay did that CT scan.

My oncologist switched me to Arimidex as soon as she found out about the fibroid. This drug was fairly new at the time. It helped considerably with the menopause symptoms. I still had some problems but it was much better. After about a year my knees were hurting and it was getting difficult to climb stairs. I went to see a rheumatologist and was diagnosed with osteoarthritis in my knees. Kay had me on Celebrex for arthritis in my back, and they tried Synvisc shots for my knees, which helped a little. My sugar also seemed to be rising at this time and I got on the internet to see if it could be due to medication I was taking. While I didn't find a connection to my sugar problems, I found that Arimidex can cause major joint pain. When I spoke with my oncologist she agreed that it could be causing the problem. She offered to switch me to another medication but by that time I had less than a year left of the 5 years they recommended you take the medication so I decided to stick it out. I was sure that every medication would have some side effect, and at least I knew what this one was. A few months after I stopped the Arimidex the knees were showing great improvement.

The one "side effect" of all of this that no one talks about is the continuous effect that all of the treatment has on your body – long after you have stopped it. The Tamoxifen and Arimidex are chemo drugs – even if they are not given like traditional chemotherapy. The radiation and drugs take a toll on your system. You are sapped of energy and your immune system is weak. When the radiation and medication was completed I started to feel better, but I have never gained it all back. I still find I tire out before others in my age group. I just don't have the stamina that I used to.

My sugar levels continued to be higher than normal. I could not seem to get them down with diet, and exercise was difficult because of my knees. Finally Kay added some medication called Metformin and my blood sugar numbers are doing much better.

The knees, however, continued to get progressively worse. We tried a few bouts of therapy over the years, but it was beginning to affect my back. Kay had found that I had osteoarthritis of the spine when I was in my late 40's, but we had managed to control it quite well with medication. Suddenly it wasn't working too well, and I began to think that my knee problems might be contributing to it, so Kay sent me to a very good orthopedic surgeon. When I asked if he could "clean out" my knee, he laughed. Both knees were bone on bone, and my right knee was angling outward. It was time for the knee replacement that I always knew would someday come.

I was very pleased with the outcome. I had a relatively quick recovery – but part of that was because we didn't wait until it was so bad I couldn't walk. After a year the only thing I have issues with is going up steps. I had not done a full flight of steps in about two years before my surgery. You can replace the joint – but if the muscles haven't been used it takes a long time to get them back in shape. That is why it is so important to get it done before you get to the point you can't walk. I know when it is time for the left knee I will get it done when it needs to be done!

I have been very lucky to go through this with Kay. She has always been proactive and has taught me to be proactive about my health also. She has sent me to some very good specialists, which has made many of the outcomes bright.

Breast Cancer and Heart Attack

Patient P.G.

I must say that going through menopause has been the most difficult time of my life. I recall my older friends and co-workers complaining about hot flashes and other symptoms they were experiencing, but I really couldn't relate and didn't give it much thought. That has all since changed.

I was around 45 when I started experiencing hot flashes, irregular periods, moods swings, anxiety, panic attacks, and trouble sleeping. Kay diagnosed my symptoms as being related to menopause. We discussed treatment options, but initially I didn't decide on any treatments and started reading information on menopause, and spoke to other women. My choice of treatment was to do nothing and to just deal with it as many other women choose to do. As these symptoms intensified, I continued thinking they would all end soon, and I experimented with over-the-counter products and went to a few holistic doctors, but the symptoms only worsened and became more unbearable. I seriously thought about taking estrogen, but feared all side effects, especially, breast cancer.

At the age of 51, I was diagnosed with a form of breast cancer called ductal carcinoma in situ (DCIS). I received the news from Kay. I was blindsided and in denial. I just couldn't grapple with the fact I had breast cancer. Fear set in and I began to obsess and have panic attacks. With the love of God, my husband, friends, family, and doctors, I was able to endure. I had various treatment options to choose from. Keeping in mind that each individual situation is different, my choice of treatment was to have a double mastectomy.

Having a double mastectomy seemed to be the best choice for me; especially as this option didn't require radiation and hormone therapy. After meeting with the radiation oncologist and discussing the area of the cal-

cifications, and potential side effects, I feared the radiation would damage my heart and other organs. My last breast reconstruction surgery was on October 9, 2013. I continued struggling with the classic menopausal symptoms.

On October 30, 2013, I had an appointment with Kay for a checkup and examination. All of my vitals were good and so then we talked about menopause and my continued night sweats, hot flashes, panic attacks, and now painful and excruciating intercourse. Kay discussed using estrogen hormone therapy, but in view of the breast cancer, didn't feel it was in my best interest. What was amazing during that visit is that Kay did instruct me to call 911 should I ever experience chest pain because it could be my heart and NOT just a panic attack!

After my appointment with Kay, I had some errands to run. Around 4:30 p.m., I started experiencing pain in my chest and across my collarbone. The night before, I had felt the same pain for around a minute or so, but it went away. I never mentioned it to Kay during my examination, as I didn't think it was of any importance.

The pain I was feeling at the time was identical to the pain I had the night before, but only more intense and constant. In addition to this pain, I had a terrible shooting pain down my arm and fingers, then a tingling and numbness sensation. It was difficult to breathe and I felt an enormous pressure on my chest. My intuition was telling me "heart attack." I quickly felt ill, but was able to make it back to my car. I yelled for help from a passerby and they called 911. My intuition was right on. I was having a heart attack and was experiencing the classic male symptoms. I was blessed that day. I'm alive and sustained no damage. I praise God every day and thank him for his love. I'm so grateful to have a wonderful loving God, husband, family, friends and doctors. A week prior to my heart attack I noticed pain in my jaws. It started on the left side of my jaw and moved to the right side. I had no other symptoms that I can recall and I didn't have high blood pressure, shortness of breath, or any heart related issues other than border-line cholesterol. Heart problems do run in my family. My father died at the age of seventy-four from a heart attack and my mother recently had a heart attack at the age of seventy-nine. She also sustained no damage.

In 2004, I moved from Northern Virginia, to Poway, CA. I picked Kay Smith from a list of participating doctors. What a wonderful doctor she has been. During the past eleven years, Kay has always stressed the importance of not smoking, a healthy diet and adopting a healthier lifestyle. I finally quit smoking cold turkey when I was diagnosed with the breast cancer, and after my heart attack, I totally changed my lifestyle and eating habits, and started exercising. Although most of the doctors attributed my heart attack to just smoking, I also contend with Kay that menopause was a big factor too.

Ovarian cancer

Patient D. S.

Memorial Day weekend 2012 is one I will never forget and will be ingrained in my brain, foggy or not, forever.

Saturday morning May 26th, 2012 I woke up at my boyfriend Tim's house just not feeling right. It wasn't the flu or a cold, I felt "off." I felt bloated and uncomfortable, full and blah and slightly constipated.

We had plans for a BBQ on Sunday so Tim said we could cancel and I said, "No, let's see how I feel and if not great, I will take it easy."

Sunday May 27th, 2012 I felt the same: Full, bloated, uncomfortable and just not right. Monday I was still not feeling any better.

Side note... Tim is Italian and loves to cook. I had put on a few pounds around my middle, which is where I always gain weight first, being that I had a C-section years ago. So, the weight I had gained over a few months time didn't concern me other than needing to lay off the pasta and wine a bit. Hence this was one of the warning signs I did not see.

Tuesday, May 28th, 2012 I called my doctors office - Kay Smith and Maureen Fleming-Mullins at North County Internists. I described my symptoms to the nurse who relayed them to Kay. Being that both Kay and Maureen are very proactive in their care of their patients, I was seen that day.

Kay had an intern working with her then and had her do the work up on me. The intern (I forget her name) asked a couple questions and said I should do an enema as I was most likely constipated. The intern then went and filled Kay in on my symptoms and Kay told her to think about my age, the symptoms and complaints, etc. The intern realized what Kay was asking and apparently I am a topic of discussion in her medical school. I don't think she will ever forget me or Kay telling her to ask more about the situation! I will forever be grateful to Kay for her diligence, compassion, knowledge and care.

Both a pelvic and an abdominal ultrasound were ordered and, needing to fast for the one, I scheduled to have them done the next morning, May 29th, 2012.

Wednesday morning I had both ultrasounds done and something in the tech reaction tipped me off that she saw something, that and the fact that she said she would get the images over to Kay STAT.

Along with having the two ultrasounds done, I had some blood work done, too. The next day, since it was Kay's day off, I received a call from Maureen Fleming-Mullins, Kay's partner and sister who is a breast cancer survivor... I must say I thought it was significant and I also appreciated that Maureen was the one that called me with my CA125 blood work count and results from the ultrasounds.

My count was 240, yep 240, mind you, ideally it should to be under 30. Being told by a cancer survivor helped, but that was a crushing moment and I remember taking the call at work out in the hallway and just needing to sit down and absorb it for a moment.

The pelvic ultrasound showed a spot on my left ovary. This needed to be viewed in greater detail, so a CT scan was done to verify the spot. The scan came back verifying the spot.

The next step was scheduling an appointment with an oncologist and I got lucky in getting Dr. Bahador. I had a consult with Dr. Bahador and was in surgery two weeks later.

Interestingly my surgery was scheduled for June 18th, 2012. The weekend before this I was at one of my son's volleyball tournaments in Anaheim and all of a sudden my lower back started hurting significantly. I took some Advil to no avail and it hurt all the way up my spine. I think it was my ovary bursting that had my lower back in pain, as when they opened me up they saw that it had burst. Had it not, I may not have had to have the 6 months of chemotherapy I went through. Alas, it did, as Dr. Bahador also saw some dark spots on my intestines. I ended up having 6 inches of my large and 6 inches of my small intestines removed thinking it was perhaps more cancer. Thankfully it wasn't, it was endometriosis (thank you for removing it), but I did have to have a full hysterectomy. I was in surgery for over 7 hours and in the hospital for 6 days. The pathology report came back with me having Stage 1C3.

Once I healed enough to handle pumping poison into me via chemotherapy, I started 6 months of chemo with the first week being a heavy dose, two weeks of lighter, then one week off. My last chemotherapy was January 4, 2013. I celebrate both June 18th and January 4th as my cancer free days! Live life, have love in your life. Give back when you can. I am a 49 year old woman back in school getting my bachelors in business administration with a concentration in operations management because my strengths are customer service and great people skills! I really want and hope to one day work with or around cancer patients in some way, giving some type of help. I now randomly will be asked by different people for my thoughts, advice, experience, outlook and knowledge on what I went through. My outlook on life has certainly changed and mostly for the better. Unless you have gone through something similar it is so very hard to explain exactly. But what I do know is that I appreciate the little things so much more, let many things roll off me as not important in the big scheme and to be thankful and grateful. Thank you Kay, for listening to that voice inside you that said to ask more. In the words of Gandhi, "Be the change you want to see in the world." I hope to be making little impacts now and look forward to making even bigger ones in the near future.

UPDATE: This patient came in yesterday for a follow-up visit and was very excited to inform me that at the age of 51 she just accepted an internship at the Moore's Cancer Center in San Diego and will be working in the radiation-oncology department helping patients. I am so proud of her!

Melanoma and Rectal Cancer

Patient B. L., Co Founder GIST Cancer Awareness Foundation

Kay is my hero! I am a two time cancer survivor (rectal and melanoma) in great part because of Kay. Her proactive approach to my care caught my cancer immediately and got me the treatments I needed. I call her my angel because she, along with God, saved my life. She has taught me to listen to my body and to be my own advocate when it comes to my medical care. Kay is more knowledgeable than any physician I have ever encountered. I count myself truly blessed to have her as my medical care giver.

She has inspired me to reach out to other cancer patients and teach them what I have learned from her about being an active participant in my own medical care. I am forever grateful to Kay!

Uterine Cancer, Hypothyroidism and Menopause

Patient I. S.

I would like to share my experience with you. I was 59 years old and 2 years post menopausal when I was diagnosed with endometrial cancer.

A little background information: I suffered for many years with major menopausal symptoms, not getting any help from my regular doctors. I decided to go to a doctor not covered by my insurance to have my hormones tested and hopefully find some relief. I had just started treatment which wasn't helping me at all when fortunately, I met Kay at a seminar she was holding on menopause. I was surprised to find that she would be able to do the testing and treat me with bio-identical hormones through my health insurance. The medication would be out of pocket but through mail order not too expensive. I also have Hashimoto's thyroid disease, which is an auto immune disease and quite difficult to keep in check. Kay was shocked to see the prescription doses that the other "very expensive" doctor had prescribed for me. The thyroid medication alone was double the amount I needed to be on. Kay started me off on low doses of estrogen, progesterone & testosterone as well as the correct thyroid medication. This helped me to get through a very difficult time. I was free of most of my menopause symptoms although the hot flashes and night sweats were difficult to control. Usually with adjustment of the medication I would get relief but it was quite a roller coaster. I was very thankful to have met Kay, finally to find a doctor that was very knowledgeable on women's issues and who really cared for her patients.

I had been using the bio-identical hormones for around 5 years when I was diagnosed with cancer. In April, I had my yearly physical and my Pap smear was normal. In May, I had an MRI on my hip which had been bothering me, the results showed there was nothing wrong with my hip but there was a thickening in the lining of my uterus. The orthopedic doctor immediately informed Kay, who sent me for a pelvic ultrasound. I was then referred to a gynecologist who did a biopsy followed by a D&C which confirmed that I had Stage 1 endometrial cancer. I was so shocked with the diagnosis, almost disbelief. I have no family history, am in great shape, exercise regularly and eat healthy. How could this be happening to me! I was then referred to a gynecologic oncologist, Dr. Bahador. I felt more at ease after my first appointment with him, all the tests were showing Stage 1 and he was hopeful that it was contained inside the uterus. He performed a total hysterectomy by robot assisted laparoscopic surgery. He also removed lymph nodes to test to make sure the cancer had not spread. He is a very talented and amazing surgeon and everyone in his office were the most kind and compassionate care givers. I was totally relieved when the final biopsy reports confirmed that the cancer was contained, completely removed and my prognosis good. No more treatment was necessary.

My message to everyone is, be very vigilant whether you are taking hormones or not. I did have a small amount of spotting, just one time for a couple of days. The only other symptoms I had were lower back ache, fatigue and just a general feeling of not feeling great which I put down to age and being post menopausal. If you think things are not quite right get checked out immediately. I feel very fortunate that my cancer was caught early; I can only imagine what I would have had to deal with if it had progressed.

Now here I am a year later. Just had my routine physical only to find that my thyroid is not functioning as well as it should be. It has been pretty stable for the past five years, maybe it's from the trauma my body went through last year. Kay has adjusted my meds so hopefully I will be back on track soon. Just a reminder of how important those routine checks are! And yes, I am still dealing with the dreaded hot flashes and sweats and trying every natural remedy to get some relief, but I would rather deal with this than the alternative.

My testimony of healing from uterine cancer, January 2015

Patient J. J.

I enjoy travel – especially when it involves visiting dear friends and family. But visiting the doctor? Well...not so much! So, at the age of 64, when I began to notice some occasional spots of blood on my underwear, I ignored it, excused it away, and kept going with my full-time job and busy life. Then a couple of other problems surfaced, and I knew I had to summon the courage to make an appointment with a physician's assistant whom I had seen sporadically for a few years.

In a very calm and caring way, Maureen (the physician's assistant) explained that it would be best if I saw a gynecologist since the spotting at my age was "something we don't like to see." She already knew I had uterine fibroids; it would be a good idea to see if those had grown, she said. Now might be the time for a hysterectomy. Reluctantly, I made an appointment with Dr. Helen Chang.

About this time I was meeting with a friend from my church on a regular basis, an experience that has greatly enriched my life. Brenda had been through hysterectomy surgery, not due to uterine fibroids, but never-the-less, she knew what to expect. She promised to pray for me.

At my initial visit with Dr. Chang, an in-office ultrasound confirmed that the uterine fibroids had not shrunk after I went through menopause, but were, in fact, growing larger. She recommended an abdominal hysterectomy. I was about to begin teaching a Bible study at my church, so I asked if we could put it off until the Thanksgiving-Christmas holidays. She said that would be fine unless I began having problems with bleeding.

On Thursday, September 11, 2014, I went to the bathroom at work, only to discover a significant problem with bleeding. I hurried home and called Dr. Chang. By then the bleeding had decreased so she advised me to come to her office on Monday unless the bleeding got worse.

That was one of the most nerve-wracking weekends of my life. One minute I would feel fine with no significant bleeding; the next I was rushing to the bathroom to expel the most ominous blood clots I had ever seen. By Monday I was back in Dr. Chang's office, only to hear her say she was going to be away for the next two weeks, so I called another local gynecologist. He, too, was going on vacation the next day. I decided to wait on Dr. Chang and take my chances in the emergency room if the bleeding got worse. Almost miraculously, the bleeding became manageable. But before Dr. Chang left on her trip we put a day and time on the calendar for me to have a hysterectomy. After sixty-four years of never having major surgery (except for a knee injury in high school), I was going to the operating room.

I alerted the pastors and staff where I work and asked for prayer from all my friends. The Tuesday before the surgery they all gathered around me for a special "laying on of hands" with prayers for healing for me, for wisdom and skill for my surgical team, and for the peace of Christ to rule in my heart.

My friend Lois alerted friends that my husband and I would appreciate meals a couple of times a week while I recovered. The schedule was filled in minutes. The pastors announced my name at church on Sunday and asked for prayers for me. It seemed like the entire congregation was pulling for me!

On a Friday morning in October the surgery went off without a hitch! Dr. Chang reported to my husband Steve (a cancer researcher) that everything looked normal. She promised to get back in touch once she got the official pathology report. After two days in the hospital – with wonderful care and support from the hospital staff, I went home to begin a few weeks of recovery.

Get well cards began to pour in at our home, with many church members and friends saying they were praying every day for me. When friends brought meals they stayed and chatted. I took naps and listened to relaxing music. The Lord was a very present friend, gently restoring my health and sense of well-being.

The next time I heard from Dr. Chang it was a different story. She hadn't heard from the Pathology Department so she had called them. They were "passing your slides around the lab," she said, adding that she would get back to me when she heard anything more definite. I thought it was strange, but everything was going so well that I didn't overly stress out about it. Then she called again on Tuesday.

This time Dr. Chang wasted no time in telling me the pathology report indicated cancer. Even living with a husband who has spent years in cancer research, I wasn't prepared to hear the words as they pertained to my life! I felt the rush of adrenaline go through my body! Then Dr. Chang said the words that immediately brought a measure of comfort. She said, "But I've got an appointment for you tomorrow with a specialist, a gynecologic oncologist who I know is very good. His name is Dr. Bahador."

"How do you spell that?" I replied, grabbing for a pen and paper as if they were lifelines!

One of the hardest things about hearing that you have cancer at my age is that you already know too many friends who have wrestled with or died *from the disease. You wonder, "Am I next?" You want the magic formula, one that won't totally wreck the person you know you are in spite of the diagnosis!! What you get, at best, is a great oncologist (like mine!). At worst, there's worry and uncertainty, new tests and procedures, and days of waiting. You develop an immediate appreciation and understanding that your body is "fearfully and wonderfully made." The kindness and compassion of friends means everything; encouraging words are gems that keep you strong. Reading scriptures helped grow my faith for whatever was ahead. My favorite verse became: "A heart at peace gives life to the body…" (Proverbs 14:30). My husband began to rattle off 16-letter words pertaining to my immune system, my type of cancer (uterine sarcoma) and my possible treatment - with such proficiency that all I could do was laugh. I told my oncologist, "He's having way too much fun with this." Dr. Bahador had to agree, but I think he also came to admire Steve's interest and expertise. (Cancer researchers are notoriously passionate about finding a cure!) My husband also prayed, and repeatedly told me, "God is going to heal you. I believe that and am asking God for that." Many, many others in my church were asking God for the same thing.*

Dr. Bahador sent me for a PET scan and to an oncologist for an opinion regarding hormone therapy. And then the day came when the PET scan results came, showing some activity in the lymph nodes on my left side. The cancer-carrying uterus had been removed, but the cancer might have spread and metastasized. Dr. Bahador advised robotic assisted surgery (The Da Vinci Method) to remove those and other lymph nodes. "I can get in there and clean this up," he said. With heavy hearts at having to cancel our Christmas plans in Chicago with our daughter and her family, Steve and I prepared for more surgery.

The Da Vinci Surgical Robot – with its multiple robotic arms - is a huge machine! Blurry though it was without my glasses (I'm very near-sighted), I couldn't help but marvel at this new technology as I waited for the procedure to begin. The surgery lasted three hours, during which Dr. Bahador removed lymph nodes from my left and right sides to send to pathology. He reported to my husband that he was able to remove the lymph nodes on my left side by placing them in surgical pouches, and took seventeen lymph nodes from my right side with no complications. It was time for recovery - and more waiting.

My family and church (and my new Physician's Assistant Kay) continued to pray faithfully for my healing and recovery, and to wait for the results with me. Because the robotic surgery is much less invasive, I was able to go four days after the surgery with my husband and friends to see the Lamb's Players' Christmas Show in Coronado, a yearly event I always look forward to. My daughter Laura began to talk about coming to San Diego to see me in January. Then my friend and co-worker Lois put action to Laura's words, inviting her to be one of the speakers at our church's Women's One-Day Retreat. I was overjoyed!

Two weeks later I was back in Dr. Bahador's office for follow-up. The day was December 24, Christmas Eve. The waiting room was busy. The nurse showed my husband and I into an examination room, informing us that the office was scheduled to close at noon, but they were running a little behind, so Dr. Bahador might be a while. Five more patients were waiting behind us!

In his usual brisk fashion, Dr. Bahador came into the examination room about twenty minutes later, a big smile on his face. "I have good news," he said. "The pathology report was negative for any more cancer in all of the lymph nodes I removed!"

"Yes!" I whooped and pumped my fist. My husband laughed as we both tried to focus on the rest of what Dr. Bahador was trying to tell us.

"I'm your Christmas miracle," I finally got out as we prepared to leave. Five more patients were waiting to see Dr. Bahador, each wanting news about their own health crisis. I felt God's presence as I took the doctor's hand to say goodbye. "And I pray God will bless you with many, many more Christmas miracles to come." Just as with cancer researchers, I'm sure that's the hope of every oncologist in the field.

The true miracle of Christmas, of course, is that God left his throne in heaven to enter our world! My husband has often told me that if a person lives long enough they are very likely to get cancer. But he and I both know that our God is bigger than any disease known to man. God is still – and always will be - in the business of healing body, soul and spirit. And better still, he is always only a prayer away. "... He who watches over you will not slumber." (Ps. 121:3)

Fibromyalgia

Patient J. M., San Diego, California
My Experience with Fibromyalgia and the AVACEN Heat Therapy Device

Whenever possible, I seek out ways to treat my health issues with herbal supplements, acupuncture and other methods, rather than taking chemically based drugs. Kay Smith, PAC, has supported me in this whenever possible. About 10 years ago, after a growing number of seemingly unrelated health problems, she diagnosed me with fibromyalgia and referred me to a rheumatologist for further treatment. Over the next 5 years, I took a variety of prescription drugs, but found that while my symptoms diminished somewhat, they didn't rid me of the "fibro fog," fatigue, and much of the pain which debilitated me. Traditional treatment was not working for me.

Then a friend asked if I'd like to try a new heat therapy device that increases micro-vascular circulation. It was being tested to determine if it might alleviate muscle pains, among other problems. I was skeptical but was willing to try anything which would get me off the medications.

I used the non-invasive AVACEN Medical heat therapy device for 20 minutes once or twice a day, simply putting my hand into the small chamber which created a slight vacuum while heating the palm of my hand. Avacen is an acronym for Advanced Vascular Circulation Enhancement and initially was studied to help patients who suffered from chronic migraine headaches. I continued to take my fibro pills. Six weeks later, I went on vacation and forgot to pack my pills; surprisingly, I found I didn't need them! In fact, I felt better than I had in many years of taking the medications. After that, I never took another fibro drug. It's been 5 years since then, and my fibromyalgia is controlled just by using the AVACEN Medical device on a regular basis. It is now an FDA cleared Class II medical device available to everyone without a prescription for temporary relief from joint pain associated with arthritis, minor muscle and joint pain and stiffness, muscle spasms, minor strains and sprains. This device can also be used to help relax tense muscles. More information is available at https://avacen.com/

Indigestion and Acid Reflux

Patient K. B.

One of the common symptoms of pregnancy along with morning sickness is heartburn as the baby continues to grow. For me, during my second pregnancy, my heartburn was pretty bad. Luckily, after my daughter was born when I was 32, the burning stopped. When I turned 34 years of age the heartburn returned and progressed to acid reflux. I was spitting up acid which felt like I was breathing fire and the pain in my stomach went through to my back. I tried several medications in an attempt to control the symptoms - Zantac, Pepcid, Prevacid and finally, Prilosec. At that time, there were not any TV commercials warning you about possible side effects from taking these drugs, especially from Prilosec. With prolonged use, I began to experience severe stomach pain accompanied with constant diarrhea. My doctor at the time did not realize that this could be a side effect of the drug, so I continued taking it for more than a year, which was way past the recommended use time. It wasn't until I did some research that I became aware of the damage this pill was causing and I stopped immediately! Surprise, the heartburn was gone and YES, I did change doctors!

Unfortunately, that was not that last time I experienced acid reflux. The symptoms returned again between the ages of 36 and 44. I believe I experienced three more rounds of it. This time a relatively new medication called Aciphex was prescribed by Kay and it worked like a miracle.

At age 50, I still experience some bouts of heartburn like most human beings, although I only need to take a few days of a generic acid reliever and my symptoms are gone!

Irritable Bowel Syndrome

Patient C. P.

My symptoms began when I was in my late 30's. Overnight, I went from having two to three bowel movements daily to having two a week, sometimes less. I was constantly bloated. I was a fitness instructor then, so looking like I was nine months pregnant every day wasn't exactly inspiring to my clients or myself. Even more frustrating, I had absolutely no control over my symptoms. I had problems when I was stressed and when I was calm, eating small meals or large, eating gluten, not eating gluten, eating meat or not eating meat, etc... I removed all dairy from my diet for nearly two years and the symptoms did not abate. I drank kefir, ate Activia and brewed strong ginger tea with no effect. High doses of fiber made things even worse. Laxatives and enemas didn't always work. I went the probiotic supplement route with Align and it helped for only a short duration and the symptoms returned. I had a colonoscopy performed and a few precancerous polyps were removed and my symptoms remained unchanged.

By this time, it seemed that my entire life revolved around my digestion and bowel issues. I experienced constant discomfort and pain. I was nauseous and always felt full, even when my stomach was empty. I had burning abdominal pain and difficulty fully evacuating my bowels when I was lucky enough to go at all. On top of all that, I was dealing with an unhelpful, unsympathetic doctor and some increasingly serious menstrual problems.

I changed doctors and was fortunate to find my current medical provider, Kay Smith, P.A.C. She listened to my symptoms and suggested we treat them with two medications, Buspar and Amitiza. The combination worked! We adjusted the dosage until it suited me, which ended up being 5 mg twice a day of Buspar and 24 mcg of Amitiza in the evening and 8 mcg in the morning. I am currently on this same dosage and though I am not completely symptom free, I feel better now than I have in five years. In fact, there are days when I don't even think about my IBS at all, something I could not have imagined would happen after suffering with this condition for six years.

Prediabetes

Patient J. S.

What would you do if you were told you were pre-diabetic? That is what I was told and ...well, I panicked!

I was terrified about what it all meant. I was a few pounds overweight and yes, I ate too much sugar but it still came as a shock to me. I decided I was going to have to make a drastic change. I was going to try and reverse it. I learned as much as I could online and I went to work.

I cut all processed sugar and snacks out of my diet. ALL SUGAR! I went cold turkey. I was very strict about the amount of food I ate. I cut calories and began running a couple of days a week. I bought a really good diabetic cookbook and started my journey. I had always thought about losing a few pounds but I was surprised about what happened next. It was amazing how easy and fast it was, once I made up my mind.

In about a three month period I had lost 25 pounds! I am currently no longer a pre-diabetic and I feel great. Not eating sugar has made such a difference in my whole body. My skin looks better, my hair healthier and my nails are stronger. My sleep has improved as well. I wish I could have done this a long time ago. This is my new life and I am glad.

Prediabetes, High Blood Pressure, Hypothyroidism and Elevated Cholesterol

Patient J. F.

My husband was an exceptional family practice physician and I am a registered nurse. As we worked together over the years, the importance of the annual complete physical exam and lab work was an integral part of our practice. Many physical changes, when identified early, can be successfully treated. Examples are: high blood pressure, diabetes, heart disease, thyroid disease, cancer, various blood disorders, etc. When my husband passed away I needed to find "exceptional" health care for myself. Kay Smith, P.A.C. is exactly the right person. She has a brilliant, inquiring mind-always searching for the latest knowledge to better serve her patients.

She found me to be "just barely pre-diabetic" and immediately started medication and diet to protect my body's ability to process carbohydrates.

She found me to be hypothyroid (unexpected) and immediately treated me before difficult symptoms appeared.

When the new LDL particle (identifies bad cholesterol associated with heart disease and stroke) test became available she immediately included it in her patient evaluation. She found that, even though I have a very high HDL (good cholesterol), my LDL particle number is borderline high so she changed my diet. Kay gives me clear advice on diet, exercise and reasonable supplementation to maintain my active lifestyle.

Prediabetes and High Cholesterol

Patient C. M.

Kay has been my doctor for over a decade now and I am proud to say that I have been a pretty healthy specimen for being 55 years old. I teach tennis for a career and have always been quite active. I never smoked or drank much alcohol and try to eat relatively healthy as well. My ethnic background is Middle Eastern descent (Armenian) and elevated cholesterol runs in my family so always something for me to watch out for.

Not too long ago after my routine blood work was taken, Kay walked into the exam room and said, "I think I may have saved your life today!" Of course, I was somewhat shocked. The week prior to Kay seeing me, she had been at a cardiology conference and was well versed on what an impact having too many bad cholesterol particles in your blood can have on your health. My bad cholesterol particle number (LDL-P) was over 2,000 and off the chart as being way too high! The healthy range is less than 1,000. She explained to me that measuring the particle numbers can help identify if you have too much bad (artery clogging) cholesterol in individuals with a strong family history and can identify a higher cardiac risk sooner. That day I started taking Lipitor to help lower my cholesterol along with continuing my healthy diet and regular exercise. I guess I was predisposed to having high cholesterol. God's timing is always perfect!

I was also informed that my blood sugar was elevated and I am now considered to be a "pre-diabetic!" The test she ordered was called a hemoglobin A1c which measures your average blood sugar over a three to four month period so is very accurate. I now follow a low carbohydrate diet and eat small little meals every three hours to help keep my blood sugar in balance.

I trust Kay with my life! Nobody likes to start taking medications, unless they can help save your life. I trust Kay knows what is best for me. I have been doing great and following her advice. Not only does Kay care about her patients, I believe she has a special gift from God to sense what people need and that is definitely good enough for me!

Heart Disease

Patient P. H.
Locating to a new city can become overwhelming with so many changes all at once. I was given a card for Kay Smith, P.A.C. by my previous physician when I was in search for a good medical practitioner in my new location that could continue my medical care.

On my first visit I found this woman with a warm smile asking questions which put me at ease, taking time to listen to my answers and concerns with professionalism and a caring manner. Her infectious laughter was delightful and as we were finishing up she asked if she could hug me since she was a hugger. As she did so, I knew that she would become the one that no matter what life's twists and turns came about, she would be there to guide me through it all.

Through the years I have found that Kay has this keen ability to listen to you and somehow knows exactly what could be the cause and takes instant action to test and solve the problem. She never hesitates to refer me to a specialist when the need arises that would serve me best.

On one occasion I remember well, when we were finishing up the visit, she asked me if there was anything else that I wanted to discuss. I mentioned that I had experienced a few odd moments that I thought were nothing to worry about. As she listened to my heart it was as if a light bulb when off in her head and she ordered a few tests and suggested I see my cardiologist. Both she and the cardiologist felt it was a good idea to have an angiogram. She was right and the small arteries in my heart were clogged and I had to have stents placed to keep the arteries open. When I reflect back on that visit, if she hadn't asked me if there was anything else I could have ended up in serious trouble.

I tell my family and friends that she is my "Earth Angel." Kay is gifted and dedicated and I am happy to share her with others.

Transient Ischemic Attack (TIA) and Hormone Replacement

Patient S. W.
After years of heavy periods, fibroids and ovarian cysts, in 2002 at the age of 43, my OB/GYN decided that a total hysterectomy was the best option for me. Afterwards I was put on a synthetic hormone and remained on it for a few years. During that time I still had hot flashes and when I talked to my doctor he basically told me that there was nothing else he could do. I decided to change doctors and started seeing Kay Smith, a physician's assistant who was very knowledgeable in menopausal issues. For the first time a health care provider took the time to take a thorough history, and based on that she did a fractionated estrogen as well as a progesterone test and was then able to prescribe a bio-identical estrogen and progesterone combination that was the perfect dosage for me based

on those tests. Prior to that the only test I was told that was available was the standard FSH test for hormones. I was on these medications for about 5 years and I felt great especially knowing that what I was putting in my body was natural and not synthetic and seemed to have fewer side effects.

Sadly, due to a job and insurance change I had to pick a different doctor who wouldn't prescribe anything other than synthetic HRT. I was nervous about taking the synthetic hormone replacement so I made the decision to go off HRT altogether but after a year of night sweats, mood swings, depression, anxiety and a constant feeling of, "I'm ready to jump out of my skin," I went back on the synthetic HRT. I had an elevated cholesterol level and was unable to control it with my diet so I began taking a statin medication, which I took until July of 2014. I was nervous about the side effects of the statins and was going to begin a weight loss program and wanted to try and reduce my cholesterol through diet and exercise. My blood pressure has always been low and the HRT didn't seem to affect that. In January 2015 I was worried about the side effects of being on a synthetic HRT for so many years and feeling like "by now I should be able to wean myself off of this" so I spoke with my doctor. She said to go ahead and begin weaning myself off of the HRT and see how I feel. I hadn't started doing this yet when on 1-26-2015 I had a TIA with the inability to speak and blurred vision and was taken to the hospital. After multiple cat scans and going over my history, it was determined that being on an HRT for so long is what more than likely caused the TIA and I was immediately taken off of it and put back on the statin medication and a daily 81 mg dose of aspirin. I was fine for a month or so with little or no symptoms, but then I began to experience night sweats and would occasionally wake up with pounding headaches. Since beginning the weight loss program in July of 2014 I have lost 50 pounds and went from a very sedentary lifestyle to a very active one which I believe helps in managing the night sweats.

Stroke, High Blood Pressure and High Cholesterol

Patient P. C.

It was a typical Monday morning-so I thought. I woke up from a good night's sleep and went in to use the bathroom. It was 6:00 a.m.

All of a sudden, my left arm shot out in a 90 degree angle. I screamed bloody murder which shocked me because I didn't know I could scream so loud. You see, I didn't think it was my arm because I couldn't feel it. I thought it came out of the toilet.

I proceeded to finish in the bathroom and then walked out my bedroom door halfway down our wood floor hallway. It was then I saw my left arm swinging aimlessly, reaching for it and found it to be completely numb! I called out frantically to my husband who came running. By the time he got to me which was about 10 seconds, I became weak and was slurring my speech. I knew I was having a stroke!

He sat me down, went and woke up our youngest daughter, then tried to dress me or at least get a sweater on. These things didn't matter at that point. He moved his car out of the garage as our daughter watched me and came in, picked me up and carried me to the car.

We were at the hospital within 15 minutes. What I recall was the rush to get me in the emergency room, giving me a shot in my stomach and wheeling me emergently in for a CT scan.

I remember just praying for God to forgive me of my sins. I didn't know what just happened to me. I wanted to be cleansed. I amazingly felt peace and a presence of angels, light and spirit with me in the CT scanner. As the technician pulled me out of the machine, I could feel my left arm and now speak without slurring my words. Everyone was amazed saying, "She is already healing!"

I was taken back in the room where the cardiologist was waiting and he leaned over and said, "What is happening?" I told him what had happened in the CT scan machine and he patted my arm and said, "That's it, your faith." He stood up and looked like he was thinking. It was then he said, "We are not going to give her a beta blocker because she is already healing."

Things started to settle down and I was in the hospital for four days. The first day I was in the intensive care unit (ICU) because my blood pressure was so high. I still couldn't believe that I had had a stroke. I am a fitness instructor and have a healthy lifestyle. My morning routine six to seven days a week at the age of 61 is: Yoga postures, meditation, journaling/gratitude and a walk/sprint workout on the treadmill. I had just stopped teaching high energy aerobics two months prior due to experiencing increased knee pain. My morning breakfast is my biggest meal which consists of oatmeal and berries. I try to have fish every week, vegetables for sure and had cut out bread,

Diet Coke and chips two years ago after learning my cholesterol particle numbers were high from Kay.

Yes, I had a major stress situation a month prior to my stroke but thought I was addressing it with positive habits. My family history is quite sprinkled with heart, stroke and high blood pressure issues. I had none of the symptoms of high blood pressure, cholesterol, etc. prior to menopause. All of these started creeping up after menopause.

Some might say it was an "eye opener, life changer, wake up call or family history." And who knows? It may have been all or none of these?

What I do know is that the stroke doesn't define "who" I am. I still feel healthy, strong and blessed. But if I can help anyone take a closer look at your whole body, mind and spirit by definitely including your doctor's report of your blood pressure readings, cholesterol, etc.. DO SO!

P.C's lab results as follows:

Elevated cholesterol and particle numbers in June of 2015:

Total cholesterol 277, triglycerides 242, LDL-C 182, LDL-P (LDL particle number) 2,447 and normal should be between 1,000 and 1,299 depending on your individual risk. Small LDL-P 1,316 and normal should be less than 527. LDL size 20.8 (Please read Chapter 5 for further detail on cholesterol and particle numbers.)

Stroke and Migraine Headaches

Patient C. E.

A few years back I learned that I had suffered a stroke back when I was in my fifties (no, not a mini one) during the previous six months. This came as a result from an MRI I had done for a condition that turned out to be unrelated.

I was able to track it back to a time when I was celebrating with friends and drinking champagne and had experienced difficulty talking. Fortunately, I had no lingering side effects and am now taking preventative measures like a daily aspirin and watching my diet. I am also being treated with a statin medication to lower my cholesterol. I have now also learned that there is a direct correlation between migraine headaches and strokes, so my migraines are now being treated as well. I am now super aware of stroke symptoms and know to call 911 immediately!

Migraines

Patient K. B.

I have had migraine headaches intermittently since the age of 18 and usually no more than one a year until I reached the age of 39. By then, I would experience maybe 5 to 8 migraines a month, with sensitivity to light, sound and nausea without an aura. Kay referred me to a neurologist who prescribed a very low dose of Topamax (one pill a day) in attempt to prevent the headaches and Imitrex to relieve them. After three months of taking the Topamax with no change, I stopped using the drug. My triggers were hay fever and changes in air (barometric) pressure, particularly when it rained in early spring. Also, I found that whenever I had my period, I would get migraines probably due to the one week break at the end of the pill cycle (when I was not taking the supplemental estrogen). Eventually, spring ended, I ceased having periods by taking the birth control pills without the break and my migraines slowed down to once or twice a month.

Then, when I turned 41 and the allergy/rainy season started, something changed in my head. Now, when I got migraines, my face would tingle and I was experiencing headaches almost daily. A month into this cycle, the tingling went down my arms and legs and I got very weak and found it difficult to speak. Panicking, I ended up going to the hospital thinking that I was having a stroke. There I was observed for several hours and eventually gained my ability to walk again, only my gait tilted to the left. I felt off balance. I was once again sent to a neurologist, who found nothing wrong in my MRI, but I did have some unexplained weakness in my right hand. Further testing did show a loss of the nerve signal from my neck to my hand, but without an explanation.

This time I was prescribed Elavil, an antidepressant, to try and calm the nerves in my brain. It took four months of basically living on my couch hidden under a blanket to block the light. I eventually did regain my balance, the migraines slowed down and the tingling stopped. The side effect from this medication that I did not like was the weight gain of 10 pounds, although luckily the weight came off after the drug was stopped.

My migraines still persisted several times a month and flared a little more when I turned 47 with the associated tingling sensation. This time I tried the Topamax again at a higher dosage, two pills in the morning and two pills at night. Luckily the Topamax worked and I was moderately pain-free for two years. Then, on October 10, 2013, something in my brain changed again. I experienced an intense migraine with all the tingling and some weakness once more. Now the migraines were occurring daily. Imitrex would only relieve the pain for about half a day before the next headache hit. The constant pain made me wish I could just live without my head. I wasn't suicidal, but so very frustrated that they would not stop. Finally, I was able to see another neurologist who recommended Botox injections. Within a few days after receiving the first treatment, my migraines gave me a break. Instead of every day, for the first three months they slowed down to about 15 a month and after the second treatment down to 10 a month. I am now a year into the Botox treatment and in the past three months I have only had 9 migraines. I still have another 6 months of injections to complete with the hope of becoming migraine free at that point. For this, I am eternally grateful! Update in 2016: I can now report that after completing the series of Botox injections I am headache free!

Mood Changes

Patient C. S.

I consider myself to be a "type A" personality filled with energy and always on the go. I began to experience lethargy in my late forties which continued into my fifties and I became concerned because this was so out of character for me. I felt as though I had hit rock bottom and could not "will" myself out of this funk, no matter what I tried. I have certainly had some bad times in my life but this was something totally different and was difficult to explain. I knew I had to make an appointment with Kay since all these changes were going on with me and it was hard to even think about bringing it up let alone discuss it at the visit. I am so glad I did tell Kay what was going on with me.

When Kay explained how fluctuating hormones can affect your brain I then felt relieved that how I was feeling mentally was directly related to my changing hormone levels. She also explained to me how the drop in estrogen has a direct effect on temperature regulation and that is why I was feeling so "hot" all the time. Now it all made sense to me! Kay suggested starting me on a low dose of Sertraline 25 mg to help me through the perimenopausal period.

What a relief it was just to know that I wasn't losing my mind and that my mind was truly being altered by my changing hormones. The Sertraline was just what I needed and I feel back in balance. I feel like myself again. Thank you Kay!

Anxiety, Depression, Obsessive Compulsive Disorder, Osteoarthritis, Osteoporosis and Urinary Incontinence

Patient L. D.

When I turned age fifty-five my body parts seemed to have reached their expiration date!

I suddenly began to suffer from relentless pain due to osteoarthritis, became incontinent due to an overactive bladder and was diagnosed with osteoporosis of both my spine and hips. I also developed a trigger finger and had to have reconstructive surgery on my right knee because of the osteoarthritis. I lead a very active life, always running in high gear up to that point, fueled by my obsessive compulsive disorder and the anxiety I experienced from thinking that I always had to finish all my tasks to the ultimate of my ability. I then tried even harder in attempt to conquer my challenges and found myself becoming more and more depressed having to accept my relatively new physical limitations.

As manager of a horse boarding stable with an average of 60 to 70 horses to care for, the reality of performing the necessary physical labor to meet my own standards was becoming almost impossible.

Horses are my passion and I loved the work involved but in my struggle to thwart off the aging process I just dove in even deeper and tried harder rather than gracefully accepting the fact that I needed to be kinder to my body to prolong its usefulness. I continued to self-medicate the pain in my joints and my heart and spirit had to work harder and longer to compensate for my body. I felt that if I drowned myself in work I wouldn't have time to focus on my body's feeble attempt to draw attention to my new ailments. Little did I know that it wasn't until my body literally said, "No," that I had to listen! I had endured the increasing pain in silence for fear of being viewed as unable to perform my duties and the possibility of losing my job! I did not want the company to view me as a liability rather than an asset.

I found that I was riding my beloved horse less and less because frankly, it hurt! What was I going to do now? Would the knowledge of horses and horse care be enough to deem me still useful to the ranch without my other abilities present?

I finally sought medical help for my physical issues but in the process was given even more helpful and useful treatment in the form of advice from Kay Smith, P.A.C. She was the first medical practitioner that actually took the time to "listen" to my concerns. She heard "me" above all and immediately recognized that I was suffering from depression that was related to having had a hysterectomy at the age of 18. I was not taking hormone replacement, which ultimately lead to my diagnosis of osteoporosis. The lack of estrogen also contributed somewhat to my increasing facial wrinkles and age spots which seemed impossible to conceal, furthering my resentment of the aging process. My usual happy demeanor changed to being on the verge of tears on most days. I am happy to report that after trying several different antidepressants, one that was chosen for me is now working the best and I am feeling better.

Vesicare was prescribed to help with my urinary urge incontinence. It is working well restoring my self-confidence and has improved my quality of life.

Most of all, learning to be mindful of "moderation with all things" has become my mantra! Fortunately, I was blessed with a very capable and caring physician. I always feel better after I leave her office. Thank you doctor Kay and I feel very fortunate to have you as my doctor!

Osteoporosis

Patient L. M.
I work in the medical field as an occupational therapist and was shocked when I was told at the age of only 42 that I had severe osteoporosis. I didn't have any symptoms and if Kay had not convinced me to have a Dexa scan done (bone density test) I would never have known that I had it. Yes, I have small bones and a small stature but never dreamed I would receive this news. I previously was treated with Fosamax and am now receiving the Prolia injection every six months. My most recent follow-up bone density test showed only a modest improvement. I also take supplemental calcium along with vitamin D daily and try to do weight bearing exercises when I can.

Menopause and Natural Hormone Replacement

Patient P. F.

Going through menopause was very difficult for me. I had all the symptoms: fatigue, anxiety, hot flashes and always felt on the verge of tears.

I thought eventually my hormones would adjust and I would feel like my normal self again and that never happened.

Kay suggested that I try bio-identical hormone therapy. It was one of the best decisions I ever made. I took progesterone and estriol. I applied the estriol to my skin and within a half hour I could feel my mood change. It was great to have the feeling of well-being again.

Patient P. K.

For three years, I struggled with many symptoms of perimenopause. I had terrible insomnia, mood swings, foggy thoughts, warm flushes (somehow I escaped the perils of all out hot flashes), hair loss, decreased elasticity in my skin, low libido along with vaginal dryness and many urinary tract infections. I began using progesterone about a year and a half ago which greatly reduced the insomnia and warm flushes but found true relief when I began wearing the estrogen patch six months ago. Almost all of my symptoms disappeared and my life returned to normal and I no longer had to worry, which personally I was waking up worried with each new day. Just before I began taking estrogen replacement, I seriously began to doubt my marriage and the relationship I had been in with my husband for over 25 years and was no longer happy! It wasn't my marriage but turned out to be my hormones. Now that my hormones are back in sync with my body, I can truly say that I am the person I used to be. I have found my relationship with my husband to be stronger than ever. I am happy again and I can focus and think, even multi-task again. It is amazing how hormones can affect someone's life so intensely. I hear friends my age often complain about their relationships and life; I now suggest to them that they should have their hormones checked. Your quality of life can be transformed through hormone replacement, which is absolutely amazing!

Patient G. B.

Bio-identical hormones became part of my daily life about ten years ago. I felt, to my dismay, that my libido was dwindling and for no reason that I could understand. With the help of my physician I began to realize that my body did not produce enough of the hormones needed to maintain a healthy libido.

The solution for me was to choose bio-identical hormone replacement. These hormones are identical to the body's natural chemistry. I now use estriol, estradiol, progesterone and testosterone and with this regimen my libido has returned to a healthy state. To my surprise these hormones have also helped me in unexpected ways. I no longer suffer from vaginal dryness. My sleep has improved and energy increased. Weight control has become easier and I have a definite sense of improved overall health. Along with continued annual check-ups, I plan to continue bio-identical hormones for many more years.

Patient G. E.

One day I found myself in my fifties looking back on a magical life of traveling the world. I was so grateful to also have had a successful business for twenty-six years which I loved.

I had always considered myself to be a happy and healthy person. I just could not understand why I felt so terrible? I wondered if this is what happens when you get older? I was tired, irritable and my joints hurt. Each day it became more difficult to do my job, so I sadly decided to sell my business.

Luckily in the next year I discovered bioidentical hormones and my life drastically changed. I couldn't believe it, I felt like I was thirty years old again! I was dancing and celebrating life. I felt so great that I opened a new business. After enjoying five wonderful years, I just signed another five year lease, not just with the business but also on my new life.

Thanks to bioidentical hormones. Also, a special thanks to Kay for all her help!

Menopause, Burning Mouth Syndrome and Hormone Replacement

Patient P. S.

I had my final menstrual period when I turned 50 years old. I suffered with night sweats, mood swings and loss of sex drive.

When my vaginal dryness became more of a problem at the age of 53, I went to the doctor and was prescribed a vaginal estrogen called Vagifem which helped relieved some discomfort.

Between the ages of 53 and 57, my hair started to thin on my head and moved to my chin. Sleeping became a real problem and my bladder seemed to have an eye for every bathroom. I would see a toilet and couldn't get there and get my pants down fast enough.

At age 57, the skin on my arms and legs began to look like crepe paper!

At age 58, my tongue started to burn and it seemed to feel very stiff, making it difficult to talk at times. I became quite frightened as I have aunts that died from ALS and the symptoms started out exactly the same. I went to see my dentist and an allergist and finally googled my symptoms and came upon, "Burning Mouth" symptoms that can be relieved with hormone replacement therapy.

I am now taking natural hormone replacement under Kay's guidance and am feeling much better. The symptoms have definitely improved and I am hopeful that hormone replacement will also help with my dry eyes.

Urinary Tract Infection Prevention

Patient T. C.

For my FINAL URINARY TRACT INFECTION (UTI) EVER, it was again KAY TO THE RESCUE!

On Wednesday May 20, 2015 near the end of my shift in the NICU (neonatal intensive care unit), I was hit with urinary frequency, abdominal pain and noted bright red blood in my urine. A like-minded co-worker offered me some doTerra Peppermint oil which I gladly accepted and rubbed onto my abdomen and lower back. This helped with the pain so I was able to complete my 30 minute drive back home. Shortly after arriving home, I sent my husband to the store to purchase some D-Mannose per Kay's recommendation and I began taking the supplement immediately and continued around the clock for two days. The second day I suffered with persistent abdominal and back pain and even worse, a headache (I never get headaches). I believe that this horrible headache was the result of the huge E. coli die-off. The bleeding with urination stopped by the end of second day and the headache continued strong until the third day, at which time I experienced a definite decrease in abdominal and back pain. It was still painful to urinate. On the third day I changed to UT Answer D-Mannose & Cranberry Concentrate by Nature's Answer. I began taking one tablespoon (4 grams of D-Mannose) after each meal and continued with this dose for two additional days after all the symptoms subsided. By the fourth day I actually felt human again and continued to hydrate well with water. I did have my urine checked and it was clear without any evidence of an infection.

In Conclusion

I hope reading these personal patient testimonies helped clarify some of the information presented in this book and illustrated how important it is to obtain your recommended health examinations. You should address all concerns with your clinician and never be afraid to talk about what you may consider as being just minor symptoms. It could very well save your life! I know these patients were happy to share their experiences with the hope they could help provide coping suggestions and support should you ever be diagnosed with any of these medical conditions.—*K. S., P.A.C.*

BIBLIOGRAPHY

CHAPTER 1

Amy JJ, Tripathi V. "Contraception for Women: An Evidence Based Overview," *BMJ* (2009); 339: 2895.

"Avoiding the Pap Trap." *Advance for Physician Assistants, Women's Health Issue* (2007, October); volume 15 (10):26-31.

Babcock, O'Connell, C., MPH, PA-C & Zarbock, S. F. PA-C. *A Comprehensive Review for the Certification and Recertification Examinations for Physician Assistants, Fourth Edition,* (2010):273-275, 278-282. Philadelphia, PA: Lippincott Williams & Wilkins.

Baeten, J.M., Palanee-Phillips T., Brown E.R., et al., "Use of Vaginal Ring Containing Dapirivine for HIV-1 Prevention in Women," *New England Journal of Medicine* (2016); doi: 10.1056/NEJMoa150611.

Beauman, Maj, M.C., J. G. "Genital Herpes: A Review," *American Family Physician* (October 15, 2005); 72(8):1527-1534.

"Birth Control Guide Online," accessed May 11, 2012, https://www.fda.gov/downloads/ForConsumers/ByAudience/ForWomen/FreePublications/UCM517406.pdf and https://www.cdc.gov/reproductivehealth/contraception/contraception_guidance.htm

"Chlamydia, Gonorrhea Top List of STDs," *Clinical Advisor Magazine* (2009, April):12.

"Could You Have Herpes? Web MD Guide to Herpes," *Web MD the Magazine* (January/February 2008):63.

"Clinical Management Guidelines for Obstetrician-Gynecologists," *ACOG practice bulletin* (2004, November): number 57.

Eisinger, S.H., Smith, E.A. Emergency Contraception, In: Pfenninger JL, Fowlder GC, eds. *Pfenninger and Fowler's Procedures for Primary Care,* 3rd edition. Philadelphia, PA: Elsevier Mosby; 2011; chapter 129.

"Gynecologic Herpes Simplex Virus Infections," *Obstetrics and Gynecology* (2004); 104 (5): 1111-1118.

"HIV and AIDS," accessed April 9, 2011, https://www.aidsinfo.nih.gov/

"HIV and AIDS," accessed September 25, 2015, https://www.cdc.gov/

Hoppel, Ann M. "HIV: Still Epidemic after 30 Years," *Clinician Reviews* (December 2015):20-25.

Hull, Claire E., MHS, P.A.C and Alison R. McLellan, MMS, P.A.C. "Acute and Recurrent Vaginosis," *Clinical Reviews* (January 2016); 26(1):43-48.

Jensen, J.T., Mishell Dr. "Family Planning, Contraception, Sterilization and Pregnancy Termination." In: Lentz GM, Lobo RA, Gershenson DM, Katz VL, eds. *Comprehensive Gynecology,* 6th Edition, Philadelphia, PA: Mosby Elsevier;2012:chapter 13.

Kimberlin, D.W & Rouse, D.J. "Genital Herpes." *Clinical Practice, New England Journal of Medicine* (2004):350, (19), 1970-1977.

Moodley, P., Wilkinson D., Connolly C., Moodley, J., & Sturm AW. "Trichomonas Vaginalis is Associated with Pelvic Inflammatory Disease in Women Infected with Human Immunodeficiency Virus." *Clinical Infectious Disease* (2002); 34:519-522.

Neblett Fanfair, Robyn, M.D., Ph. D., and Kimberly A. Workowski, M.D. "Clinical Update in Sexually Transmitted Diseases-2014." *Cleveland Clinic Journal of Medicine* (February 2014); 81(2):91-100.

"Postmenopausal Vulvovaginal Atrophy: Communication and Care." *The Clinical Advisor* (October, 2013):59-65.

"Sexually Transmitted Diseases Treatment Guidelines," *Centers for Disease Control and Prevention,* MMWR (2002); 51, (RR6):1-82.

"Sexually Transmitted Diseases Treatment Guidelines," *Centers for Disease Control and Prevention*, MMWR (2006); 55, (RR11):1-95.

Snell, R. S., M.D., PhD. *Clinical Anatomy for Medical Students,* (1973): 303-312. Boston: Little Brown and Company.

"Targeting the Urogenital Health of Postmenopausal Women: A Spotlight on Vaginal Atrophy." *The Monitor, Association of Physician Assistants in Obstetrics and Gynecology, Vaginal Atrophy Supplement* (2009, Autum):1-4.

"The New HPV Vaccine-Be Sure You Know the Facts." *JAAPA, Clinical Journal of the American Academy of Physician Assistants* (2006, September); 19 (9):14-15.

"The Virus that Causes Cervical Cancer," *Health Monitor* (2006, September –October):31.

Thompson, J. S., M.D. *Core Textbook of Anatomy,* (1977):352-354. Philadelphia: JB Lippincott Company.

"Trichomoniasis Fact Sheet," Centers for Disease Control and Prevention, accessed January 6, 2011. https://www.cdc.gov/std/trichomonas/STDFact-Trichomoniasis.htm

Understanding Genital Herpes, Glaxo Welcome Inc. Handout (December 2000)

"Understanding Your Genitalia," *Every Woman, The Essential Guide for Healthy Living, The Nutritional Issue* (2004, July):115-121.

CHAPTER 2

Ahlgrimm, M. R., Ph.D & Kells, John M. *The HRT Solution,* (2003):25-28, 36-43, 48-51. New York: Avery Books.

Dalton, Katharina, M.D. *Once a Month: Understanding and Treating PMS,* (1999):7-12, 29-34. Alameda, California: Hunter House Publishers.

Jones, Marcia L., PhD & Eichenwald, Theresa, M.D. *Menopause for Dummies,* (2003):20-27. New York: Wiley Publishing, Inc.

Kosir, Mary Ann, M.D., FACS, Chism, Lisa DNP, APRN, BC, NCMP, FAANP, Bland, Kelva, M.D., FACS, Chol, Lydia, M.D., Gorski, David, PhD, M.D., FACS and Simon, Michael S., M.D., MPH. "Common Breast Symptoms," *Advance for NPs and PAs* (October 2013):12-15.

Lee, John R., M.D. *What Your Doctor May Not Tell You About Menopause.* (1996):6-8, 11-14, 47-50, 85-91, 139-145, 166-168, 310-314, 331-332. New York: Warner Books, Inc.

Massai, R., Diaz, S., Jackaniez, T., & Croxatto, H.B. "Vaginal Rings for Contraception in Lactating Women," *Steroids* (October/November 2000); 65(10-11):703-707.

Najera, Deanna Bridge, MPAS, MS, PA-C. "An Update on Long-Term Contraceptive Methods," *The Clinical Advisor* (August 2014):41-48.

Northrup, Christiane, M.D. *The Wisdom of Menopause.* (2001):240-247. New York: Bantam Books.

Shulman, L.P. "Contraception 2000: Lunelle, An Injectable Combination Contraceptive Option," *Journal Women's Health Gender Based Medicine* (September 2000):725-729.

Sohn, Emily, "New Secrets for PMS," *Health Looks Good on You* (September 2006):102.

"Testosterone and Belly Fat in Women," *Clinical Advisor* (October 2013):70-71.

Watring, Nicole, M.D., and Mason, Jon D., M.D. "Deciphering Dysuria, Causes of Vaginitis," *Emergency Medicine Update, Clinical Reviews* (December 2008):18(12), 19.

"Women to Women: Choosing Birth Control–Options for Women by Marcia Holmes On-line. Women's Health N.P., accessed September 23, 2006, updated March, 2017, https://www.womentowomen.com/sex-fertility/choosing-birth-control/

"Women to Women: What You Should Know About Endometriosis by Marcella Pick, OB/GYN N.P. and Marcy Holmes, N.P., accessed September 23, 2006, updated March, 2017, https://www.womentowomen.com/sex-fertility/endometriosis-start-with-a-natural-approach/

Yates, Janelle. "Endometriosis," *Clinical Reviews* (November 2015)25 (11):20-28.

Yates, Janelle. "Endometriosis and Pain," *Clinical Reviews* (December 2015); 25(12):36-40.

CHAPTER 3

American College of Obstetricians and Gynecologists. ACOG Practice Bulletin Number 141. "Management of Menopausal Symptoms," *Obstetrics and Gynecology* (2014); 123 (1):202-216.

Agnvall, Elizabeth. "Battling Belly Fat," *AARP Bulletin* (July/August 2012); 53, (6):8-13.

Ahlgrimm, Marla R. Ph., & John M. Kells. *The HRT Solution,* (2003): 33-51. New York: Avery Books.

Apovian, Caroline, M.D. and Gordon, Debra M.S. "Lifestyle Interventions for Obesity and Weight-Related Complications," *The Clinical Advisor Magazine* (September, 2014):47-52.

Archer, David F., M.D. "The Estro-Gel Study Group. Menopause." *The Journal of the North American Menopause Society,* (2003); 10, (6): 516-521.

Basch, Ethan M. and Catherine E. Ulbricht. *Natural Standard, Herbs & Supplement Handbook.* Mosby, Inc., St Louis, Missouri (2005): 75-79, 102-105, 162-165, 197-202, 211-217, 258-262, 275-285, 299-306, 324-332, 419-424, 431-436, 453-468, 550-555, 578-588, 624-627, 636-640.

"Beat the Heat. The American College of Obstetricians and Gynecologists Complete Guide to Midlife Health," *Pause* (2007 Fall/Winter): 31-32.

Beckham, Nancy. "Natural Therapies for Menopause and Osteoporosis," accessed September 28, 2013, http://www.tldp.com/issue/184/Natural%20Therapies.htm

"BMI as A Vital Sign," *The Clinical Advisor* (2014):67-68.

Crandell, Susan. "Living Longer, Exercise." *AARP Magazine* (September/October) 2006:84-87.

Dalton, Katharina, M.D. *Once a Month,* (1999): 192-209. Alameda, California: Hunter House Publishers.

Elkind-Hirsch, K. "Effect of Dietary Phytoestrogens on Hot Flushes: Can Soy-Based Proteins Substitute for Traditional Estrogen Replacement Therapy," *Menopause* (2001); 8(3): 154-156.

Fugh-Berman, Adriane and Fredi Kronenberg. "Red Clover for Menopausal Women: Current State of Knowledge," *Menopause* (2001); 8: 333-337.

Goldstein, Steven, R. M.D., and Laurie Ashner, *The Estrogen Alternative: What Every Woman Needs to Know About Hormone Replacement Therapy and Serms, The New Estrogen.* (1998): 139-152. G.P. Putnam's Sons: New York.

"Herbal Medicine: Black Cohosh—The Woman's Herb," *Harvard Women's Health Watch* (2000); 7 (8):6.

"Hormone Therapy Undergoes 10-Year Review," *The Clinical Advisor* (July 2012):20.

Howard, B.V., J. E. Manson, M. I. Stefanick, et al., "Low-Fat Dietary Pattern Change Over 7 Years: The Women's Health Initiative Dietary Modification Trial," *JAMA* (January 4, 2006); 295(1):39-49.

Hulley, S., et al., "Randomized Trial of Estrogen Plus Progestin for Secondary Prevention of Coronary Heart Disease in Post-menopausal Women. Heart and Estrogen/Progestin Replacement Study (HERS) Research Group," *JAMA* (1998); 280(7):605-613.

"Research on the Effects of Progesterone," *International Journal of Pharmaceutical Compounding* (July/August 2002); 6(4A Review of Current): 245-248.

Lee, John R. M.D., *What Your Doctor May Not Tell You About Menopause,* (1996): 353-381.Warner Books: New York.

Joan Raymond. "Hormone Therapy: Is it Safe?" *Health Looks Good On You* (September 2006): page 100.

Richard Laliberte. "Which Herbs Really Work," *New Choices, Living Even Better After 50* (December 2000/January 2001): pages 22-27.

"Straight Talk on Losing Weight," *Health Monitor Magazine* (September-October 2006):8 and 11.

"The Estrogen Question. The American College of Obstetricians and Gynecologists Complete Guide to Midlife Health," *Pause* (Fall-Winter 2007): pages 33-39.

John R. Lee, M.D. *What Your Doctor May Not Tell You About Premenopause,* (1999): 3-16. Warner Books: New York.

Kaunitz, Andrew, M., M.D. "Update on Menopause," *Clinical Reviews* (August 2015); 25 (8):46-48.

Katz, Anne. "Next Stop Mid-Life, The Roller Coaster Ride through Menopause," *Every Woman, The Essential Guide for Healthy Living* (Winter 2004): pages 125-130.

Jackson Nakazawa, Donna. "Live Longer Diet," *AARP Magazine* (September/October 2006):78-82.

Jones, Marcia L., PhD and Theresa Eichenwald, M.D. *Menopause for Dummies,* (2003): 129-148. Wiley Publishing: New York.

Maresh, Dr Timothy, Gynecologist. Interview by author on March 10, 2012 in Poway, CA discussing an overview of menopause and hormone replacement.

Michele M. Roth-Kauffman, JD, MPAS, PA-C. "Endometriosis," *Clinical Reviews* (July 2009); 19(7):25-30.

Minkin, Mary Jane, M.D., FACOG, NCMP. "Postmenopausal Vulvovaginal Atrophy: Communication and Care," *The Clinical Advisor* (2013):59-64.

"National Institute on Aging: Menopause," accessed January 20, 2007 and August 18, 2015, http://www.nia.nih.gov/health/publication/menopause, and "National Institutes of Health: Menopause Hormone Therapy Information," accessed February 12, 2006 and July 22, 2015, https://www.nih.gov/health-information/menopausal-hormone-therapy-information.

Northrup, Christiane, M.D. *The Wisdom of Menopause,* (2001): 134-154. Bantam Books: New York.

Parch, Lorie, "The Nine Best Herbs for Women," *Natural Health* (September 2006): pages 74-79.

Seibel, Machelle, M.D. *The Estrogen Alternative, the Soy Solution for Menopause.* Pg 80-81. Simon & Schuster: New York.

Taubes, Gary. *Why We Get Fat and What to Do About It,* (2010):8-10. Anchor Books: New York.

"The Buzz on Bioidenticals. Why You Should Choose FDA-Approved Menopausal Hormone Therapy Products Over Compounded Drug and What You Need to Know About Menopause and Hormone Therapy," *A supplement to The Female Patient* (July 2009):8-9, 10-12.

"UCSF-led study on November 29, 2004 suggests link between psychological stress and cell aging," accessed April 10, 2015, http://www.ucsf.edu/news/2004/11/5230/ucsf-led-study-suggests-link-between-psychological-stress-and-cell-aging

"University of Maryland School of Medicine Study released on March 7, 2005 Shows Laughter Helps Blood Vessels Function Better," accessed March 10, 2015, http://umm.edu/news-and-events/news-releases/2005/school-of-medicine-study-shows-laughter-helps-blood-vessels-function-better

Ward, Elizabeth. "Health Concerns at Menopause: HRT Versus Natural Remedies for Relief," *Environmental Nutrition* (January 2002):4.

Wepfer, Scott T., R.Ph, FIACP. "The Science Behind Bioidentical Hormone Replacement Therapy," *International Journal of Pharmaceutical Compounding* (November/December 2001); 5(6): pages 10-11.

Wright, Jonathan V., M.D. and John Morgenthaler. *Natural Hormone Replacement for Women Over Age 45,* (1997):45-49, 67-69, 84-86. Smart Publications: Norman, Oklahoma.

CHAPTER 4

"Addyi, the New Pink Pill for Decreased Libido in Premenopausal Women," accessed October 18, 2015, https://www.nih.gov/health-information/menopausal-hormone-therapy-information and https://.drugs.com/addyi.html

Ahlgrimm, Marla, R.Ph., and John M. Kells. *The HRT Solution,* (2003):164-165. Avery Books: New York.

Barbach, L. *The Pause: Positive Approaches to Perimenopause and Menopause* (1993): Dutton: New York.

"Can You Improve Your Sex Life?" *WebMD, the Magazine* (March/April 2008):84.

Dodson, Betty, PhD. *Orgasms for Two: The Joy of Partnersex,* (2002): Harmony Books: New York.

"Dysfunction Junction. The American College of Obstetricians and Gynecologists Complete Guide to Midlife Health," *Pause* (Fall-Winter 2007):60-63.

"Is Your Sex Life Healthy?" *Web MD, the Magazine* (May/June 2008): 96.

Gotthardt, Melissa. "Leapin' Libido, Getting Your Motor Running the Natural Way. Navigator Health," *AARP Magazine* (July and August 2006): 20

Gultinan, Jane, N. D., Keesling, Barbara, Ph.D., and Northrup, Christiane, M.D. "How Can I rev up My Sex Drive," *Natural Health Magazine* (September 2006):26.

Jones, Marcia L., PhD and Theresa Eichenwald, MD. *Menopause for Dummies,* (2003): 104-105. Wiley Publishing: New York.

Kellogg-Spadt, Susan, PhD, CRNP. "Female Sexual Care Dysfunction: In Perspective, Part 1," *Monitor Magazine* (Summer 2009):9-11.

Northrup, Christiane, M.D. *The Wisdom of Menopause,* (2001): 267-277. Bantam Books: New York.

Oz, Mehmet, M.D. "Sex on the Brain," *AARP Magazine* (September/October 2011):26.

Redford, Gabrielle De Groot. "7 Reasons to Get Off the Couch Already! Increase Sexual Function," *Smart Fitness, AARP Magazine* (July and August 2006); (4):30.

Savage, Linda, PhD. *Reclaiming Goddess Sexuality,* (May, 1999):23. Hay House: Carlsbad, CA.

Slupik, Ramona, M.D., F.A.C.O.G., and Lorna Gentry. *The Everything Menopause Book,* (2003):131-141. Adams Media Corporation: Avon Massachusetts.

"Testosterone Improves Parameters of Sexual Function," *Clinical Reviews* (August 2015); 25 (8):49.

CHAPTER 5

"ACC/AHA Guideline on the Assessment of Cardiovascular Risk," accessed November 12, 2013, doi :01.1161.cir.0000437741.48606.98

"ACC/AHA Guideline on the Treatment of Blood Cholesterol to Reduce Atherosclerotic Cardiovascular Risk in Adults," accessed, November 12, 2013, doi: 1.01161/01. cir.0000437738.63853.7a

Albertazzi, P., et al., "The Effect of Dietary Soy Supplementation on Hot Flushes," *Obstetrics and Gynecology* (1998); 91(1):6-11.

"American Heart Association, 2016 Heart and Stroke Statistical Update, Dallas, Texas," American Heart Association, accessed February 15, 2016, https://www.heart.org/ HEARTORG/General/Heart-and-Stroke-Association-Statistics_UCM_319064_Sub HomePage.jsp

Aresnault, Benoit J., PhD, Rana, Jamal S., M.D., PhD., Stroes, Erik S. G., M.D., PhD., Despres, Jean-Pierre, PhD, Shah, Prediman K., M.D., Kastelein, John J. P., M.D. PhD, Wareham, Nicholas J.D., MBBS, PhD, Boekholdt, Matthijs, M.D. PhD, Khaw, Kay-Tee, MBBC. "Beyond Low-Density Lipoprotein Cholesterol," *Journal of the American College of Cardiology* (December 29, 2009-January 5, 2010); 55(1):35-41.

Basler, Barbara. "Taking it to Heart," *AARP Bulletin* (July-August 2007):12-14.

Ballantyne, CM, Hoogeveen RC, Bang H, Coresh J. Folsom AR, Heiss G, Sharrett AR. "Lipoprotein-Associated Phospholipase A2, High Sensitivity C-Reactive Protein and Risk for Incident Heart Disease in Middle-Aged Men and Women in the Atherosclerosis Risk in Communities (ARIC) study," *Circulation* (2004);109:837-842.

Beckman JA, Creager MA, Libby P. "Diabetes and Atherosclerosis," *JAMA* (2002); 287: 2570-2581.

Bradley, Jacqueline, M.D. and Bairey, C. Noel Merz. "Heart Disease in Women: What's New," *Consultant, Clinicians' Edition,* Vol. 51, No.5, (May 2011); 51(5):273-278.

"Consensus Panel Recommendation for Incorporating Lipoprotein-Associated Phospholipase A2 Testing into Cardiovascular Disease Risk Assessment Guidelines," *The American Journal of Cardiology, Supplement to the American Journal of Cardiology* (June 16, 2008); 101(12A)

"Controversy Surrounds New JNC 8 Guidelines," *The Clinical Advisor* (February 2014):71-73.

Committee on Cardiovascular and Metabolic Diseases, Considering... *Diet and Lifestyle, Seven Heart-Healthy Goals from the American Heart Association,* (Fall 2006).

Dayspring, Dr Thomas, Cardiologist in Poway, CA. Interview by author on October of 2012 discussing an overview of lipid disorders and how heart disease differs in menopausal women.

Ford ES, Giles WH, Dietz WH. "Prevalence of the Metabolic Syndrome Among US Adults," *JAMA* (2002);287:356-359.

Goldman, E. "Exercise Equals Estrogen for Lowering Heart Risk," *Internal News* (November 1, 1999):16.

Gondeck, Kari, DNP, APNP, FNP-BC. "LDL Particle Number and Size," *Advance Magazine for NPs and PAs* (January, 2012):26-28.

Herrington, DM, Reboussin, DM, Brosnihan, KB, et al., "Effects of Estrogen Replacement on the Progression of Coronary-Artery Atherosclerosis," *New England Journal of Medicine* (2000); 343: 522-529.

Hodis HN, Mack WJ, Azen SP, et al., "Hormone Therapy and the Progression of Coronary-Artery Atherosclerosis in Postmenopausal Women," *New England Journal of Medicine* (2003); 349: 535-545.

Hu FB, Bronner L, Willett WC, et al., "Fish and Omega-3 Fatty Acid Intake and Risk of Coronary Heart Disease in Women," *JAMA* (2002); 287:1815-1821.

Hu FB, Manson JE, Stampfer MJ., et al., "Dietary Fat Intake and the Risk of Coronary Heart Disease in Women," *New England Journal of Medicine* (1997);337:1491-1499.

"Intensive Blood Pressure Lowering May Provide Greater CVD Benefits," *The Clinical Advisor* (December 2015):18.

Kent, Ashley. "Innovations in the Treatment of Heart Disease," *PA Professional* (February 2011): 17-21.

Kirchheimer, Sid. "Ask the Experts," *AARP Bulletin,* (July/August 2012); 53(6):40.

Leaf, A., et al., "Cardiovascular Effect of n-3 Fatty Acids," *New England Journal of Medicine* (1998); 318(9):549-547.

Lloyd-Jones DM, Leip EP, Larson MG, et al., "Prediction of Lifetime Risk for Cardiovascular Disease by Risk Factor Burden at 50 Years of Age," *Circulation* (Feb 14, 2006);113(6):791-8. PMID 11368702.

"Migraines with Aura Associated With Increased Risk for Cardiovascular Disease," *Medscape Cardiology* (Sept 01, 2006); 10(2): c 2006 Medscape

Madsen T., Skou HA, Hansen VE, et al., "C-reactive Protein, Dietary n-3 Fatty Acids and the Extent of Coronary Artery Disease," *American Journal of Cardiology* (2001); 88: 1139-1142.

Manson, JE et al., "A Prospective Study of Walking as Compared With Vigorous Exercise in the Prevention of Coronary Heart Disease in Women," *New England Journal of Medicine* 341 (1999): 650-658.

Manson, JE et al., "A prospective Study of Obesity and Risk of Coronary Heart Disease in Women," *New England Journal of Medicine* (1990); 332(13): 882-889.

Manson, JE, et al., "Estrogen Plus Progestin and the Risk of Coronary Heart Disease," *New England Journal of Medicine* (2003); 349(6): 523-534.

"New Guidelines Change the BP Picture," *The Clinical Advisor* (May 2014):20.

Pearson, Tamera, Ph.D., F.N.P. and A.C.N.P. "Treating Hypertension-Losing Sight of the Forest for the Trees?" *The Clinical Advisor* (October 2013):55-60.

Taubes, Gary. *Why We Get Fat and What to do About It,* (2010):178-194. Anchor Books: New York.

Treister, Neil W., M.D, FACC. *Heartfulness, A Guide to Heart Health and Life Balance,* (February 2004): 31, 40-45, 96-98, 129, 180-181. Infinity Publishing: Haverford, PA.

"Numbers You Should Know by Heart," The American College of Obstetricians and Gynecologists Complete Guide to Midlife Health, *Pause* (Fall-Winter 2007):50-53.

Ozner, Michael, M.D., FACC, FAHA and Dale Kiefer. "The Clinically Proven Heart Healthy Diet," *Life Extension* (May 2008): 71-76.

Pradhan AD, Manson JE, Rossouw JE, et al., "Inflammatory Biomarkers, Hormone Replacement Therapy and Incidental Coronary Heart Disease," *JAMA* (2002); 288: 980-987.

Ridker, PM, et al., "C-Reactive Protein and Other Markers of Inflammation in the Prediction of Cardiovascular Disease in Women," *New England Journal of Medicine* (2000); 342(12): 836-843.

Ridker, PM, Rifai, N, Clearfield, M, et al., "Measurement of C-Reactive Protein for the Targeting of Statin Therapy in the Primary Prevention of Acute Coronary Events," *New England Journal of Medicine* (2001); 344:1959-1965.

Rimm, E B et al., "Folate and Vitamin B6 from Diet and Supplements in Relation to Risk of Coronary Heart Disease among Women, *JAMA* (1998);279(5): 359-364.

Sherman, Carl. "Reducing the Risk of Heart Disease in Women," *The Clinical Advisor* (January 2008): 49-53.

Stampfer, M., et al., "Primary Prevention of Coronary Heart Disease in Women Through Diet and Lifestyle," *New England Journal of Medicine* (2000); 343:16-22.

Von Schaky, C., et al., "The Effect of Dietary Omega-3 Fatty Acids in Coronary Atherosclerosis: A Randomized, Double-blind, Placebo Controlled Trial," *Annals of Internal Medicine* (1999); 130(7):554-562.

Ziajka, Paul M.D., Ph.D. "The VAP Cholesterol Test as a Replacement for the Traditional Lipid Profile, Clinical Summary (2007)," Atherotech Diagnostic Lab online, www.atherotech.com, August 18, 2012.

Zimmerman, Mike. "Heart Disease: Lifesaving News for Men and Women," *AARP, The Magazine* (April/May 2014):28-32.

CHAPTER 6

Ahlgrimm, Marla, R.Ph., and John M. Kells. *The HRT Solution,* (2003): 54-56. Avery Publishing: New York.

Arjamandi, B H. "The Role of Phytoestrogens in the Prevention and Treatment of Osteoporosis in Ovarian Hormone Deficiency," *Journal of American College of Nutrition* (2001); 20(5):398S-402S.

Einhorn, Dr Daniel. Interview by author in Poway, CA on July 11, 2011 discussing bone health and osteoporosis in menopausal women.

Goldstein, Steven R., M.D. and Laurie Ashner. *The Estrogen Alternative,* (1998):66-68. G.P. Putnam's Sons: New York.

Holick, M.F., Binkley, N.C., Bischkoff-Ferrari, H.A., et al., "Evaluation, Treatment and Prevention of Vitamin D Deficiency: An Endocrine Society Clinical Practice Guideline," *Journal of Clinical Endocrinology Metabolism* (2011);96(7):1911-1930.

Jones, Marcia L., PhD and Theresa Eichenwald, M.D. *Menopause for Dummies,* (2003):51-52, 63-66. Wiley Publishing: New York.

"Keeping Your Bones Strong After Menopause!" *Women's Health. Health Monitor* (December-January 2008); 5 (6):15-16.

Kessenich, Cathy R., DSN, ARNP. "Osteoporosis," *Healthy Body Magazine* (2004):80.

Nachtigall, Lila E., M.D. and Joan Rattner Helman. *Estrogen, The Facts Can Change Your Life!* (1991):112-132. Harper-Collins Publishers: New York.

"National Osteoporosis Foundation," accessed July 20, 2006 and August 15, 2015, https://www.niams.nih.gov/health_info/Bone/

"NIH Osteoporosis and Related Bone Diseases National Resource," accessed June 12, 2010, https://www.osteo.org

Northrup, Christiane, M.D. *The Wisdom of Menopause,* (2001):130-131, 376-384. Bantam Books: New York.

"Osteoporosis Fast Facts, Guide to Bone Health," *Health Monitor Magazine* (2013):4-5, 9, 12-15.

Podd, Daniel, MPAS, PA-C. *"*Hypovitaminosis D, a Common Deficiency with Pervasive Consequences," *Journal of the American Academy of Physician Assistants* (February, 2015); (28):20-26.

Singh, Shailendra, M. D. and Steven Gambert. "Health Practitioner Guide to Prescribing Vitamin D and Calcium," *Consultant Magazine* (March 2014) 54 (3):174-180.

Slupik, Ramona, M.D., F.A.C.O.G., and Lorna Gentry. *The Everything Menopause Book,* (2003):121-129. Adams Media Corporation: Avon, Massachusetts.

"Treating Osteoporosis," *Healthy Body, Every Woman Magazine* (Winter 2004):78-80.

"Unbreakable, Think That Calcium Supplements You're Taking Are Enough to Keep Your Bones From Breaking? Think Again," The American College of Obstetricians and Gynecologists Complete Guide to Midlife Health, *Pause* (Fall-Winter 2007): 54-58.

"Vitamin D for Fall Prevention," *The Clinical Advisor* Magazine (July 2012):21.

Wilczynski, Cory, M.D. "Secondary Osteoporosis: Are You at Risk?" *Empower Magazine* (2014)6(2):18-19.

CHAPTER 7

"American Cancer Society. Breast Cancer: Detailed Guide (2013)," accessed January 20, 2014, https://www.cancer.org/cancer/breast-cancer.html

"Breast Cancer Risk Reduction" (version 1.2013), accessed February 10, 2014, http://nationalcancernetwork.org/.

"Breast Cancer Information" accessed February 10, 2014, http://www.cancercenter.com/breast-cancer/learning

"Breast Health Information," accessed May 20, 2015, http://www.breasthealthcare.com

"Breast Cancer Screening and Diagnosis (version 2.2013)," accessed February 10, 2014, http://www.nationalcancernetwork.org

Chism, Lisa, DNP, APRN, BC, NCMP, FAANP. *"*Breast Cancer and Menopause," *Advance for NPs and PAs Magazine* (October, 2012); 3(10):21-24.

"Collaborative Group on Hormonal Factors in Breast Cancer. Breast Cancer and Hormone Replacement Therapy: Collaborative Reanalysis of Data from 51 Epidemiological Studies of Women With Breast Cancer and Women Without Breast Cancer," *Lancet* (1997):350(52)705:1047-1059.

Consultant Magazine, Clinician's Edition (April, 1, 2006); 46(4):407-414.

Goldstein, Steven R., M.D. and Laurie Ashner. *The Estrogen Alternative,* (1998):25-28. G.P. Putnam's Sons: New York.

Dalton, Katharina, M.D. *Once a Month,* (1999):79. Hunter House Publishers: Alameda, CA.

Greenwald, P. "Cancer Prevention Clinical Trials," *Journal of Clinical Oncology* (2002); 20: 14s-22s.

"Inflammatory Breast Cancer-Topic Overview-WebMD," accessed September 23, 2006, http://www.webmd.com/breast-cancer/tc/inflammatory-breast-cancer-topic-overview#1

"Inflammatory Breast Cancer (IBC)" accessed September 26, 2006 and September 30, 2006, https://www.cancer.org/cancer/breast-cancer/understanding-breast-cancer-diagnosis/types-of-breast-cancer/inflammatory-breast-cancer.html

"Introducing the Breast Cancer Risk Assessment Initiative," *Breast Cancer Risk Assessment.*

Jones, Marcia L., PhD and Theresa Eichenwald, M.D. *Menopause for Dummies,* (2003):162-167. Wiley Publishing: New York.

Kosmo, Dr Michael, Oncologist. Interview by author in Poway on May 24, 2011 discussing an overview of breast cancer diagnosis and treatment.

LaCross Salmans, Jessica, M.S., P.A.C., "Surgical Management of Breast Cancer," *Journal of the American Academy of Physician Assistants* (June 2015); 28(6):47-51.

"Mammograms-What's Best For You? Dixie Mills, M.D.," accessed September 23, 2006, https://www.womentowomen.com/breasthealth/mammograms.asp

"New Guidelines for Breast Cancer Screening in US Women," *JAMA* (2015); 314 (15):1569-1571.

Mctiernan, Anne., M.D., PhD. "Breast Cancer: Can Anything Help Prevent It," *Consultant Magazine* (April 1, 2006); 46(4):407-414.

"National Cancer Institute, Breast Cancer Patient Version," accessed September 23, 2006, https://www.cancer.gov/types/breast

"NCCN Clinical Practice Guidelines in Oncology," National Comprehensive Cancer Network (NCCN), accessed September 12, 2007, https://www.nccn.org/professionals/physician_gls/f_guidelines.asp

"NCCN Clinical Practice Guidelines in Oncology," National Comprehensive Cancer Network (NCCN), accessed April 10, 2014, https://www.nccn.org/professionals/physician/_gls/pdf/breast-blocks.pdf

"Newsletter, (Spring 2014)" accessed June 11, 2014, (Reach MD @info@email1), https://www.reachmd.com/

Northrup, Christiane, M.D. *The Wisdom of Menopause* (2001):423-427,437-439. Bantam Books: New York.

Slupik, Ramona, M.D., F.A.C.O.G., and Lorna Gentry. *The Everything Menopause Book,* (2003):83-84, 97. Adams Media Corporation: Avon, Massachusetts.

Smith, Marissa, MS, CGC, Jessica Mester, MS, CGC and Eng Charis, MD, PhD. "How to Spot Heritable Breast Cancer: A Primary Care Physician's Guide," *Cleveland Journal of Medicine* (January 2014); 81(1):31-38.

St. Lifer, Holly. "Fight Back Against Breast Cancer," *AARP, The Magazine* (October-November 2013):16-18.

"Updated Breast Cancer Information," accessed June 12, 2015, http://www.breastcancer.org/

US Preventive Services Task Force. "Screening for Breast Cancer: Recommendations and Rationale," *Annals of Internal Medicine* (2002):137:344-346.

US Preventative Services Task Force, "Screening for Breast Cancer: Recommendations and Rationale," *Annals of Internal Medicine* (2002); M137:344-346.

What Can You Expect During a Clinical Exam? Brochure from the Joan McLaughlin Women's Center in Poway, CA

Yamamoto S, et al., "Soy Isoflavones and Breast Cancer Risk in Japan." *Journal of National Cancer Institute* 2003; 95(12):906-913.

CHAPTER 8

"Thyroid Disease: Hypothyroidism Risk/Symptoms Checklist," accessed June 16, 2008, http://www.about.com

Adlersberg, M., & Burrow, G. 2002. "Focus on Primary Care. Thyroid Function and Dysfunction in Women," *Obstet Gynecol. Surv.* (2002); 57 (3):S1-S7, accessed May 13, 2012, https://www.ncbi.nlm.nih.gov/pubmed/12074547

Bailey Spitzer, T. 2010. "What the Obstetrician/Gynecologist Should Know About Thyroid Disorders," Obstet. Gynecol. *Surv.* (2010); 65(12); 779-785, https://www.ncbi.nlm.nih.gov/pubmed/21411022.

Campbell, Bryan. Have Faith: Actress Faith Ford's Struggle with Grave's Disease, *Empower Magazine* (2011); 3 (2): 6-7.

Chun, Hyun JI, P.A.C., BC-ADM. "Investigating Unstable Thyroid Function," *Clinical Reviews* (October 2015); 25(10):24-30.

Davies TF, Larsen PR., Kronenberg HM, Melmed S. Polonsky KS, Larsen PR, eds. *"Thyrotoxicosis," Williams of Endocrinology. 11th ed.* Philadelphia:PA: Saunders Elvsevier: 2008: chap 11.

Einhorn, Dr Daniel, Endocrinologist. Interview by author in Poway, CA on July 10, 2011, discussing thyroid disorders in menopausal women.

Goroll, Allan H. et al., *Screening for Thyroid Cancer in Primary Care Medicine. Office Evaluation and Management of the Adult Patient.* Philadelphia: Lippincott, Williams &Wilkins: 2000.

Leddy, Anne, M.D., FACE. "Is it My Thyroid?" *Empower Magazine* (2012); 4(4):14-15.

Marcelle Pick, OB/GYN NP. "Hypothyroidism in women," accessed September 23, 2006, https://www.womentowomen.com

Mason, G., et al., "Thyrotropin-Releasing Hormone. Focus on Basic Neurology," (2000), URL.

Nusynowitz, M.L. "Thyroid Imaging," *Lippincotts Primary Care Practice* 3 (November-December 1999): 546-55.

O'Connell, Claire Babcock and Zarbock, Sarah F. *A Comprehensive Review for the Certification and Recertification Examinations for Physician Assistants,* Lippincott Williams & Wilkins, (2010).

"Radioactive Iodine Uptake," *National Institutes of Health* (April 19, 2010), accessed September 28, 2013, https://www.nlm.nih.gov/medlineplus/ency/article/003689.htm

Rothfeld, Glenn S., M.D., M.A., & Deborah S. Romaine. *Thyroid Balance.* Adams Media, an F + W Publications Company (2003):4 and 76.

Sadler, Chris, MA, PA-C, CDE. "Thyroid Peroxidase Antibodies," *Clinical Reviews* (April 2012); 22(4):19.

Sandhu, A., et al., "Subclinical Thyroid Disease After Radiation Therapy Detected by Radionuclide Scanning," *International Journal of Radiation Oncology, Biology, Physics* (August, 2000); 48: 181-8.

Siberry, George K. et al., *The Harriet Lane Handbook: A Manual for Pediatric House Officers.* St. Louis: Mosby, 2000.

Thyroid and Menopause: Confusing the Symptoms, https://www.webmd.com/menopause/guide/symptoms-thyroid-vs-menopause

Hypothyroidism in Menopause-A Whole Body Perspective, accessed March 2, 2017, https://www.womenshealthnetwork.com/thyroid-health/hypothyroidism-in-menopause.aspx

"Thyroid Scan," (n.d.). *Harvard Health Publications*, accessed September 30, 2012, http://www.health.harvard.edu/diseases-and-conditions/thyroid-nuclear-medicine-tests-thyroid-scan-and-uptake

CHAPTER 9

Bakey, William M., DHSc, PA-C, MPH. "Predicting UTI in Symptomatic Postmenopausal Women. A Review of the Literature," *JAAPA* (August 2006); 19(8):48-54.

Bladder Leakage in Women, Healthy Advice. Pamphlet (2011).

Brown J, Vittinghoff E, Kanaya AM, et al., "Urinary Tract Infections in Postmenopausal Women: Effect of Hormone Therapy and Risk Factors," *Obstet. Gynecol.* (2001);98(6):1045-1052.

Chu FM, Dmochowski R. "Pathophysiology of Overactive Bladder," *American Journal of Medicine* (2006); 119:3s-8s.

"Could a Sweetener Be Causing My UTI's?" *First for Women Magazine* (September 14, 2009):102.

Crowe, Karen. *Bladder Matters, A Guide to Managing Overactive Bladder,* Astellas. US LLC (2008):30-36.

Frequent Bladder Urges and Leakage, Healthy Advice. Pamphlet (2011): Issue 12.

Lindahl, Sarah, PA-C. "How to Evaluate Urinary Incontinence? Just Ask!" *Monitor Magazine* (Summer 2009):7-10.

Hamlin, Amy S., MSN, FNP-BC, APRN and Robertson, Tamara M., DNP, FNP-BC, CUNP, APRN. "Incontinence in Women, Evaluation in the Primary Care Setting," *Advance for NPs and PAs Magazine* (October 2013); 4 (10):21-24.

Hu KK, Boyko EJ, Scholes D, et al., "Risk Factors for Urinary Tract Infections in Post-Menopausal Women," *Archives of Internal Medicine* (2004);164(9):989-993.

Jackson SL, Boyko, EJ, Sholes D., et al., "Predictors of Urinary Tract Infection After Menopause: A Prospective Study," *American Journal of Medicine* (2004); 117(12):903-911.

Martin, Dr. John, Urologist. Interview by author in Poway, CA on March 14, 2010 discussing urinary and kidney conditions commonly found in menopausal women.

Mishori, Ranit, M.D. "Oopsie Daisy, Many Women Live in Fear of Embarrassing Accidents. Here's How to Get Back in Control," *Health Report, AARP* (July-August 2006):34-38

Myrbetriq Prescribing Information. Northbrook, IL: Astellas Pharma US, Inc. (2012).

Najm, Wadie, M.D. "Cranberries Prevent UTI's, Data Show," *The Clinical Advisor* Magazine (December, 2005):16.

Nazareth I, King M. "Decision Making by General Practitioners in Diagnosis and Management of Lower Urinary Tract Symptoms in Women," *BMJ* (1993);306(6885):1103-1106.

Panzera, AK. "Interstitial Cystitis/Painful Bladder Syndrome," *Urology Nurses* (2007); 27(1):13-19.

Patrick, Frank, PA-C. "Keeping Women Dry, Uncovering and Treating Urinary Incontinence," *Advance Magazine for Physician Assistants* (October 2007); 15(10):32-36.

Pick, Marcelle, OB/GYN NP. "Urinary Incontinence-Help for Female Bladder Problems," accessed September 23, 2006, www.womentowomen.com/urinaryincontinence

Raz R, Gennesin Y, Wasser J, et al., "Recurrent Urinary Tract Infections in Postmenopausal Women," *Clinical Infectious Diseases* (2000); 30(1):152-156.

Stenson, Jacqueline. "5 Surprising Ways to Stay Dry," *Health Monitor* (June-July 2012); 10(3): 16.

Uribel (Methenamine, Sodium Phosphate Monobasic, Phenyl Salicylate, Methylene Blue, Hyoscyamine Sulfate), Mission Pharmacal Company 2012, prescribing information pamphlet.

"Urinary Tract Infections in Teens and Adults," accessed November 3, 2006, http://www.webmd.com

Watring, Nicole, M.D and Mason, Jon D., M.D. "Deciphering Dysuria, Diagnosing UTI's," *Emergency Medicine Update,* Clinical Reviews (December 2008); 18 (12):16-22.

CHAPTER 10

American Association of Clinical Endocrinologists. "The American Association of Clinical Endocrinologists Medical Guidelines for the Management of Diabetes Mellitus: The AACE System of Intensive Diabetes Self-Management," *Endocrine Practice* (2000); 6:43-84.

"American Diabetes Association Standards of Medical Care in Diabetes," *Diabetes Care* (2012); 35 (supplement 1):S11-S63.

Baggio LL, Drucker DJ. "Biology of Incretins: GLP-1 and GIP," *Gastroenterology* (2007); 132(6):2131-2157.

Centers for Disease Control and Prevention. National Diabetes Statistics Report: "Estimate of Diabetes and Its Burden in the United States, Atlanta, GA: U.S. Department of Health and Human Services (2014)," accessed July 7, 2015, https://www.cdc.gov/diabetes/data/statistics/2014/statisticsreport.html

Cholerton, B. Baker LD, Craft S. "Insulin Resistance and Pathological Brain Ageing," *Diabetic Med.* (2011); 28: 1463-1475.

"Clinical Diabetes and Primary Care Reports. Type 2 Diabetes, Insulin and You," *Health Monitor Magazine* (September-October 2006):25.

Einhorn, Dr. Daniel, Endocrinologist. Interview by author in Poway, CA on July 11, 2011, discussing diabetes in menopausal women.

Ettari, Mary, MPH, P.A. "Getting 'The Edge' in the Diabetes Epidemic," *The PA Professional Magazine* (November 2013):14-18.

Green, Mary. "A Tale for the Ages: How the Mystery of Diabetes Was Unraveled," *Empower Magazine* (2014)6(2):14-16.

Gerich, John E. M.D. "Contributions of Insulin-Resistance and Insulin-Secretory Defects to the Pathogenesis of type 2 Diabetes Mellitus," *Mayo Clinical Practice* (2003);78:447-456.

Griffith, Ceabert J., PA-C, ND. "An American Epidemic, Metabolic Syndrome," *Advanced Magazine* (November-December 2007); 15(11-12):28-32.

Moghissi, Etie, M.D., FACP, FACE. "Achieving A1c Goals: Back to the Basics," *Physician Weekly Updates* (December 2014):23.

Mueller, George, M.D., FACS, Medical Director of Bariatric Surgery at Sharp Memorial Hospital, Lecture, Sharp Annual Conference, Indian Wells, CA on Sunday, October 8, 2016 in.

Noorhasan, Marisela, M.D. "Managing Diabetes on A Budget," *Empower Magazine* (2014); 6 (2):4-6.

Ott A., Stolk R.P., van Harskamp F, et al., "Diabetes Mellitus and the Risk of Dementia. The Rotterdam Study," *Neurology* (1999); 53: 1937-1942.

Ronnemaa E., Zethelius B., Sundelof J., et al., "Glucose Metabolism and the Risk of Alzheimer's Disease and Dementia: A Population-Based 12 Year Follow-up Study in 71 Year Old Men," *Diabetologia* (2009);52: 1504-1510.

Ronnemaa E., Zethelius B., Sundelof J., et al., "Impaired Insulin Secretion Increases the Risk of Alzheimer's Disease," *Neurology* (2008); 71:1065-1071.

"This National Diabetes Month, Make a Change to Live Well: The NDEP Can Help You Take Small Steps for Better Health," *Empower Magazine* (2012); 4(4):10.

Trence, Dace, M.D., FACE. "Tools to Help You Manage Your Diabetes When Insulin Is Prescribed," *Empower Magazine* (2014); 6(2):7-9.

"Your Diabetes Information," accessed September 10, 2013, https://www.yourdiabetesinfo.org

CHAPTER 11

"Acid Reflux Disease, GERD," accessed September 2008, http://www.healthcentral.com/acid-reflux/

"Amitiza (Lubiprostone) Prescribing Information," Takeda Pharmaceuticals (2009), accessed May 2015, https://www.amitiza.com/

Carol Rees Parrish, R.D., M.S. *Diarrhea.* National Digestive Disease Information Clearinghouse (June, 2007).

Chey, W.D., Webster, L. Sostek, M., Lappalainen, J., Barker, P.N. and Tack, L. "Naloxegel for Opioid-Induced Constipation in Patients with Noncancer Pain," *New England Journal of Medicine* (2014); 370:2387-2396.

"Constipation: Diagnosis and Treatment," *The Clinical Advisor* (February 2016):16.

"Constipation: Exposing the Myths," The American Academy of Gastroenterology, *Health Monitor Magazine* (September-October 2006):32.

Constipation General Information patient handout, W.B. Saunders Company(1989).

"ConquerCandidaNaturally-NaturalNews.com,"accessedMay10,2011,http://www.natural news.com/032154_candida_solutions.html

Coping with Heartburn and Reflux, North County Internists. Patient handout, (2010).

Crook, William, M.D. *Eating When You Have Diarrhea. The Yeast Connection,* Professional Books (1983) online, www.yeastconnection.com, July 12, 2011.

"Digestive Diseases: Gastritis," accessed November, 2006, http://www.webmd.com/digestive-disorders/digestive-diseases-gastritis#1

Duggan C., Gannon J., Walker W.A. "Protective Nutrients and Functional Foods for the Gastrointestinal Tract," *American Journal of Clinical Nutrition* (May 2002); 75:789-808.

Heartburn & Acid Reflux Disease, TAP Pharmaceuticals. Healthy Advice Patient Pamphlet, Issue 12 (2006).

"Heartburn Cooldown," *AARP Magazine,* (July/August 2008):36-37.

Irritable Bowel Syndrome (IBS), A Patient's Guide. Glaxo Wellcome 2000. Pamphlet.

"Irritable Bowel Syndrome," National Digestive Diseases Information Clearinghouse (NDDIC), accessed July 2008, https://www.niddk.nih.gov/health-information/digestive-diseases/irritable-bowel-syndrome

"Irritable Bowel Syndrome Diet," Heather and Company, accessed November, 2006, http://www.helpforibs.com/

"Irritable Bowel Syndrome Overview," accessed November, 2006, http://health.usnews.com/health-conditions/digestive-disorders

"Irritable Bowel Syndrome, Rational Therapy," *Consultant Magazine,* (June 2011); 51(6):344-347.

Imperiale, Thomas F. M.D., David F. Ransohoff, M.D., Steven H. Itzkowitz, M.D., Theodore R. Levin, M.D., Philip Lavin, Ph. D., Graham P. Lidgard, Ph. D., David A. Ahlquist, M.D., and Barry M. Berger, M.D. "Multitarget Stool DNA Testing for Colorectal-Cancer Screening," *The New England Journal of Medicine* (April 2014); 370:1287-1297.

Johnson, David A. "A Promising New Treatment Option for IBS," accessed April 10, 2011, https://www.medscape.com/viewarticle/735490

Lembo, A and Camilleri M. "Chronic Constipation," *New England Journal of Medicine*, (2003); 349:1360-1368.

Movantik (naloxegol), AstraZeneca (2015), prescribing information pamphlet.

Pick, Marcelle, OB-GYN N.P. "Digestive Problems or Systemic Yeast," accessed September 2006, https://www.womentowomen.com/digestive-health/digestive-system-problems-causes-and-diagnostics/

"Probiotics Ease Antibiotic GI Side Effect, Diarrhea," *The Clinical Advisor* Magazine (July 2012):20.

Sharma, Arora A., M.P. "Use of Banana in Non-Ulcer Dyspepsia," *Lancet,* (1990); 335:612-613.

Snyder, Dr. Richard, Gastroenterologist. Interview by author in Poway, CA on September 11, 2010 discussing common gastrointestinal conditions and diseases that can occur in menopausal women.

Stomach Reflux (Heartburn) Parker Hill Associations, Inc. Patient Handout, 2006.

Trowbridge, John, M.D. and Morton Walker, DPM. "The Yeast Syndrome": 1986

Viberzi (eluxadoline), Actavis, Inc (2015), prescribing information pamphlet.

CHAPTER 12

"Anorexia Nervosa and Related Eating Disorders," accessed September 21, 2007 and November 12, 2008, https://www.anred.com/

"Anorexia: Overview and Statistics-National Eating Disorders," accessed March 5, 2017, https://www.nationaleatingdisorders.org/anorexia-nervosa

Anorexia nervosa-Part 1, Harvard Mental Health Letter (February 2008); 19 (8):1-4.

Berkseth, Kathryn, M.D. "Obesity, What Does the Brain Have to do with It?" *Empower Magazine* (2014)6(2):12-13.

"Bulimia nervosa: Overview and Statistics-National Eating Disorders," accessed March 5, 2017, https://www.nationaleatingdisorders.org/bulimia-nervosa

Fairburn, C.G. and Brownwell, K.D., *Eating Disorders and Obesity: A Comprehensive Handbook* (Second Edition). The Guilford Press: 2002.

Fleming, Shelley K., M.A. Edited by Matthew B.R. Nessetti, Ph. D., FPPR. "Prescribing Psychologists Register #18, PPR Home Course. Update on Eating Disorders: Diagnosis & Treatment of Bulimia and Anorexia."

Herrin M and Matsumoto N. *The Parent's Guide to Childhood Eating Disorders.* Owl Books: 2002.

National Eating Disorders Association, accessed June 14, 2007, https://www.nationaleatingdisorders.org/

National Association of Anorexia Nervosa and Associated Disorders, accessed July 12, 2008, http://www.anad.org/

National Eating Disorders Association (NEDA), accessed July 2008, http://www.wikepedia.org/wiki/National_Eating_Disorders

Polivy, J. and Herman, C.P. "Causes of Eating Disorders," *Annual Review of Psychology* (2002); 53: 187-213.

Practice Guideline for the Treatment of Patients with Eating Disorders, Second Edition. American Psychiatric Press (2000).

Sargent, J.T. *The Long Road Back: A Survivor's Guide to Anorexia.* North Star Publications: (1999).

Thorpe, Dr Shelby, Clinical Psychologist. Interview by author in Poway, CA on June 10, 2011 discussing diagnosis and treatment of Eating Disorders.

Vitiello, B. and Lederhendler, I. "Research on Eating Disorders: Current Status and Future Prospects," *Biological Psychiatry* (2000):47 (9):777-786.

"What Are Eating Disorders?," American Psychiatric Association, accessed March 5, 2017, https://psychiatry.org/patients-families/eating-disorders/what-are-eating-disorders

CHAPTER 13

"An Overview of Insomnia," WebMD, accessed November, 2006, http://www.webmd.com/sleep-disorders/guide/insomnia-symptoms-and-causes#1

"Are Women Sleeping Well?" *Health Monitor Magazine* (Spring 2007):24.

Abrams, Roberta B. "Finding Your Balance," *Every Women, the essential guide for healthy living, the nutritional issue* (2004): 93-96.

Blehar, Oren D.A., M.D. "Gender Differences in Depression," *Medscape Women's Health* (1997); 2:3.

Brem, Sabrina, D.N.P., F.N.P.-BC. "Insomnia: Using CBT in Primary Care," *The Clinical Advisor* (February 2015):42-45.

"Clinicians on the Front Line: Active Management of Depression and Anxiety in Primary Care," *JAPPA, A Supplement to the Journal of the American Academy of Physician Assistants* (July 2006):4-18.

Collazo, Susan, RN, MSN, APN-CNP. "Identifying Obstructive Sleep Apnea in Patients," *The Clinical Advisor* Magazine (September 2014):36-44.

Culpepper, Larry M.D., MPH, Catherine R. Judd, P,A-C, MPH, Mary D. Moller, DNP, ARNP, BC, CPRP, Charles B. Nemeroff, M.D., PhD., Mark H. Rapaport, M.D. "Depression and Anxiety in Primary Care," *A Supplement To The Journal of American Academy of Physician Assistants* (July 2006): 7-17.

Current Issues in Insomnia, Pri-Med Insomnia Pocket Guide. Pri-Med Institute. Spring 2006.

Depression. The National Institute of Mental Health. Patient Pamphlet. (2004).

Doghramji, Paul, M.D., FAAFP and Charles Moxin, MPAs, P.A.C. Treatment Options for Patients with Insomnia, *Advance Magazine for Physician Assistants* (May-June 2008):28-34.

"Do You Worry all the Time?" *Generalized Anxiety Disorder.* National Institute of Mental Health. Patient Pamphlet. (September 2002).

Farinde, Abimbola, Ph. D, Pharm D. Keep an Eye out for Depression, *The Clinical Advisor* Magazine (2014): 81.

Farinde Abimbola, Ph. D., Pharm D. Diagnosing Anxiety Disorders in Primary Care. *The Clinical Advisor* (October 2015):40-42.

"Generalized Anxiety Disorder (GAD)," accessed March 5, 2017, https:// www.adaa.org/understanding-anxiety/generalized-anxiety-disorder-gad

Healthy Advice Patient Handout. *Trouble Sleeping,* Issue 12 (2006). Sanofi-Synthelabo, Inc. New York.

Judd LL, et al., "Major Depressive Disorder. A Prospective Study of Residual Subthreshold Depressive Symptoms as Predictor of Rapid Relapse," *Affective Disorders* (1998):50(2-3):97-108.

Keeping a Lid on Stress. Dr. Andrew Weil's Guide to Living Longer and Better. Little Brown & Company (2013):78-81.

Marcia L. Jones, PhD., and Theresa Eichenwald, M.D. *Menopause for Dummies,* Wiley Publishing, New York, NY, (2003): 39.

Mackey, Ian, MS, PA-C. "Biological Markers and Depression," *Advance Magazine for NPs and PAs* (August 2013):29-30.

"Major Depression and Its Causes," accessed November 2006, http://www.webmd.com/depression/guide/major-depression#1

Quick, Ellen, PhD., *Anxiety Management ll: Behavioral Techniques.* Handout, 1994.

Ramona Slupik, M.D., F.A.C.O.G., with Lorna Gentry. *The Everything Menopause Book,* F&W Publications. Inc., Avon, Massachusetts:(2003): 276-277.

"Restless Leg Syndrome," WebMD, accessed November 2006, http://www.webmd.com/brain/restless-legs-syndrome/restless-legs-syndrome-rls#1

Sklar, Debbie, L. "Alternatives to Living with Stress," *Image Magazine* (2006); 2:14-16.

"Sleep Disorders," accessed May 15, 2007, https://sleepfoundation.org/

Teodorescu, Mihai, M.D. "Sleep Disruptions and Insomnia in Older Adults," *Consultant Magazine* (March 2014) 54(3):166-172.

Thorpe, Dr Shelby, Clinical Psychologist. Interview by author in Poway, CA on June 10, 2011 discussing Anxiety Disorders, Depression and Sleep Disorders that can commonly occur in menopausal women.

"Updates on Antidepressant Use," *Clinical Reviews* (October 2015); 25(10):22-23.

What You Should Know About Anxiety, An Informational Guide. Forest Pharmaceuticals, Inc., Pamphlet (2004).

"Women's International Pharmacy, Good Night, Sleep Tight," *Connections.* (April 2007); 14(1):1-5.

CHAPTER 14

Amen, Daniel, G. M.D. and William Rodman Shankle, M.S., M.D. *Preventing Alzheimer's: Ways to Help Prevent, Delay, Detect, and Even Halt Alzheimer's Disease and Other Forms of Memory Loss* (Kindle Edition). The Berkeley Publishing Group, New York, (2004).

Blumenfeld, Dr Andrew, Neurologist. Interview by author in Poway, CA on June 15, 2012 discussing different types of common headaches that occur in menopausal women.

Blumenfeld, Dr Andrew, Neurologist. Interview by author in Poway, CA on June 15, 2012 discussing disorders of the brain and cognition.

"Depression—An Early Sign of Dementia?" *The Clinical Advisor* (February 2015):32.

"Eating to prevent Alzheimer's disease," *Annals of Neurology and Health Monitor Magazine* (December 2007-January 2008); 5(6):7.

Ferber, Dan, PhD. "Brain Powered: A Wave of New Advances Shows How the Mind Affects Health in Ways We Never Imagined," *Registered Dietician* (March 2007):116-121.

Hertoghe, Thierry M.D. *The Hormone Solution,* Harmony Books, New York (2002): 87-89.

Howard, Beth Age-Proof Your Brain, AARP Magazine (February/March 2012): 43-46.

Laux's, Dr. Marcus. "Diabetes of the Brain," *Naturally Well Today, Healing with Nature's Medicine* (May 2006); 3 (11): 1-3.

Laux's, Dr. Marcus. "Brain Eating Proteins Are Back," *Naturally Well Today, Healing with Nature's Medicine* (May 2006); 3(11): 3-5.

"Modifiable Risk Factors for Alzheimer's Disease," *Clinical Advisor* (October 2015):22.

Penne-Myers, Cherri, PA-C, MSCS. "Seven Stress Relievers for Your Brain Which Will Help Improve Your Brain, Health and Life," *CAPA News* (January-February 2006):14.

Weil, Andrew, Dr. *Brain Boosters that Really Work.* Guide to living longer & better. Little Brown and Company (2013):114-121.

"Your Brain at 50 plus," *AARP, The Magazine* (March-April 2010):48-49.

"Your Brain Craves Challenges," *AARP, The Magazine,* (June-July 2012):53.

Zazula, Pauline A. "Am I Losing My Mind?" *Every Woman, the essential guide for healthy living, the nutritional issue* (2004): 101-102.

CHAPTER 15

Bousser MG, Welch KM. "Relationship Between Migraine and Stroke," *Lancet Neurology Journal* (2005); 4: 533-542.

"Butterbur Overview Information," WebMD, accessed March 5, 2017, https://www.webmd.com/vitamins-supplements/ingredient-649-butterbur.aspx?activeingredient id=649&activeingredientname=butterbur

"Diet for the Migraine Patient," *Modern Medicine.* Palomar Pomerado Health Centers, Pamphlet. (July, 1986):82.

Drugs for migraine. *Treatment Guidelines from the Medical Letter* (2011); 9 (102): 7-12.

Eross, E. M.D. Gliacin for the Prophylactic Treatment of Migraine: Review of an Initial Case Series. *Headache* (2014); 54 (8): 1418-1434.

Eross, E. M.D. The Efficacy of Gliacin, a Derivative of Boswellia Serrata Extract, on Indomethacin Responsive Headache Syndromes, *Cephalgia* (2011); 31 (Sup):47.

Hammond, Allexa, MS3 and Maura Holcomb, M.D. Exploring Treatment Options for Migraine Headache, *The Clinical Advisor* (August 2015):35-42.

"Healthy Advice Patient Pamphlet," Ortho-McNeil Neurologics, Inc. *Migraines,* Issue 12 (2006).

Imaging Studies Overused for Headaches. *The Clinical Advisor* (2014):30.

Kurth T., Gaziano, J.M., Cook N.R., Logroscino G., Diener, H.C, Buring, J.E. Migraine and Risk of Cardiovascular Disease in women, *JAMA* (2006); 296:283-291.

Menstrual Migraines, *Monitor Magazine* (Summer 2009):6-8.

"Nerve Blocks For Headaches," American Migraine Foundation, accessed March 5, 2017, https://americanmigrainefoundation.org/nerve-blocks-for-headaches/

Scher A.I., Gudmundsson L.S., Sigurdsson S., Ghambaryan, A., Aspelund, T., Ericiksdottir, G., et al., "Migraine Headache in Middle Age and Late-Life Brain Infarcts," *JAMA* (2009); 301:2563-2570.

Scher, A.I., Terwindt, G.M., Picavet, H.S., Verschuren, W.M., Ferrari M.D., Launer LJ. "Cardiovascular Risk Factors and Migraine: The GEM population-based study," *Neurology* (2004); 64:614-620.

Shurks, M., Rist, P.M., Bigal, M.E., Buring, J.E., Lipton RB, Kurth, T. "Migraine and Cardiovascular Disease: Systemic Review and Meta-Analysis," *BMJ* (2009); 339:3914.

CHAPTER 16

"ABCDEs of Melanoma," American Academy of Dermatology, accessed May 21, 2015, https://www.aad.org/public/spot-skin-cancer/learn-about-skin-cancer/detect-what-to-look-for

"Cancer Basics," American Cancer Society, accessed March 5, 2017. https://www.cancer.org/cancer/cancer-basics.html

"Cancer Facts and Figures 2010," American Cancer Society, accessed May 29, 2010, https://www.cancer.org/research/cancer-facts-statistics/all-cancer-facts-figures/cancer-facts-figures-2010.html

"Cancer Facts and Figures 2015," American Cancer Society, accessed April 12, 2016, https://www.cancer.org/research/cancer-facts-statistics/all-cancer-facts-figures/cancer-facts-figures-2015.html

"Cancer of the Skin," Harrisons online, 18th Edition, 2012. McGraw-Hill Medical, accessed May 30, 2013, http://accessmedicine.mhmedical.com/

Carlson, Karen J., M.D. and Co-editors-in-Chief Aronson, Mark D., M.D., Fletcher, Robert H. and Suzanne W., M.D. *"Up To Date in Adult Primary Care and Internal Medicine," Screening for Ovarian Cancer.* Pamphlet. (June 2006):1-16.

Felker, Lori, MPAS, PA-C, Eric Felker, PA-C and Donnita Scott, M.D., FACEP. "Long-Standing Invasive Squamous Cell Carcinoma in a 55 Year Old Man," *Journal of the American Academy of Physician Assistants* (December 2103); 26 (12):31-34.

Fife, Annie, WHNP-C, MSN. "Ovarian Cancer, This 'Silent Killer' Does Make Noise," *Clinical Reviews* (September 2007)17(9):11-12 and 16.

Foundation for Women's Cancer, accessed May 27, 2014, http://www.wcn.org/

Foundation for Women's Cancer-Types of Gynecological Cancers, https://www.foundationforwomenscancer.org/types-of-gynecologic-cancers/

Jacobson, Abby A., M.S., P.A.C. *"Save a Life with Early Detection of Melanoma," The Clinical Advisor* (2014):32, 41-48.

Kosmo, Dr Michael, Oncologist/Hematologist. Interview by author in Poway, CA on May 24, 2011 discussing an overview of the diagnosis and treatment of different cancers.

Najjir, Talib, DMD,MDS, PhD. "Cutaneous Squamous Cell Carcinoma," Medscape, accessed June 15, 2016, https://www.emedicine.medscape.com/article/1965430-overview

National Cancer Institute: Cancer Statistics, accessed May 29, 2014, https://seer.cancer.gov/statistics/summaries.html

National Cancer Institute: Cancer Types, accessed May 29, 2014, https://www.cancer.gov/types/uterine

National Cancer Institute: Menopause Hormone Therapy and Cancer, accessed June 10, 2014, https://www.cancer.gov/about-cancer/causes-prevention/risk/hormones/mht-fact-sheet

Skin Cancer Facts. Sun Protection Zone. Pamphlet (2014).

Trouskova, Olga, BS, PA-S and Alexander, Beth, Pharm D, BCPS, CGP, R.Ph. "Early Detection of Ovarian Cancer," *Advance for NPs and PAs.* (January 2012); 3(1):21-25.

"Screening Colonoscopy Linked to 50% Lower Colorectal Cancer Rate," *The Clinical Advisor* (August 2015):16.

Routt, Meghan, GNP, ANP, ACCNP. "Improving Geriatric Cancer Survivorship," *The Clinical Advisor* (August 2013):48-64.

"United States Cancer Statistics," Centers for Disease Control and Prevention, accessed May 22, 2013, https://nccd.cdc.gov/uscs/

U.S. Cancer Statistics Working Group. *United States Cancer Statistics: 1999-2012 Incidence and Mortality Web-based Report.* Atlanta (GA): Department of Health and Human Services, Centers for Disease Control and Prevention and National Cancer Institute; 2015.

Vierra, Dr Elizabeth. Interview by author in Poway, CA on May 12, 2012 discussing an overview of skin conditions and cancer.

CHAPTER 17

"Antidepressants Ease Fibromyalgia Complaints," *Clinical Advisor Magazine* (March 2009):12.

"Arthritis: Ask the Experts," *Health Monitor Magazine* (Spring 2007):23.

"Arthritis Plus Aging Equals Disability?" *Health Monitor Magazine* (Spring 2007):19-20.

Aumiller, Wade, D., Ph.D and Harry Anderson Dollahite, M.D. "Advances in Total Knee Arthroplasty," *Journal of the American Academy of Physician Assistants* (March 20160; 29(3):27-28.

Becker, Aaron, Associate Director. "Study Assesses Behavioral Therapy for Fibromyalgia," *Arthritis Practitioner* (September-October 2007):11.

Cianflocco, A.J., MD, FAAFP. "Advances in Chronic OA Management, Using Treatment Guidelines," *Primary Care Practice Magazine* (December 2013); 2(4):3-8.

Cook, C., Pietrobon R. and Hegedus E. "Osteoarthritis and the Impact on Quality of Life Health Indicators," *Rheumatol. Int.* (2007); 27: 315-321.

"Dermatologic Look-Alikes: Discoid Lupus Erythematosus," *The Clinical Advisor* Magazine (July 2012):55-56.

"Exercise Will Not Cause Knee Arthritis," *The Clinical Advisor* (2013):24.

Fibromyalgia. Arthritis Foundation. Pamphlet, (2004):2-6.

Fibromyalgia Syndrome (FMS): A Patient's Guide. American College of Rheumatology. Brochure.

Gout. Arthritis Foundation. Pamphlet (2004):2-9.

Lupus. Arthritis Foundation. Pamphlet (2004):2-6.

Osteoarthritis. Arthritis Foundation. Pamphlet (2004):2-14.

Rakesh, Jain, M.D., MPH, and Shailesh Jain, M.D., MPH. "Fibromyalgia: Management Strategies for the Primary Care Practitioner," *Advances in Primary Care Medicine, Clinical Update.* (December 2008):15-18.

Reddy, Dr Smitha, Rheumatologist. Interview by author in Poway, CA on April 10, 2011 discussing an overview of connective tissue disorders and conditions that can occur in menopausal women.

Rheumatoid Arthritis. Arthritis Foundation. Pamphlet (2004):209.

Sherman, Alexa Joy. "Strong in the Knees," *Natural Health Magazine* (September 2006):45-48.

Sego, Sherril, FNP-C, DNP. "Alternative Meds Update," *The Clinical Advisor* (July 2012):51-52.

Wei, Nathan, M.D., Clinical Director. "Key Strategies for Addressing Treatment with RA," *Arthritis Practitioner* (September-October2007):12-13.

"Say Ahh… The Tongue Has Many Stories to Tell," *Clinical Reviews* (January 2016):19.

CHAPTER 18

Anderson, William D. III, M.D., DABFM, FAAFP, Treister, Nathaniel S., DMD, DMSc, Mayeaux Jr., E.J., M.D., DABFM, FAAFP and Nalliah, Romesh P., DMD. "Oral Lesions You Can't Afford to Miss," *Clinical Reviews* (September 2015):44-53.

Astroth, Jeffrey, DDS, MSPH. "The Link Between Oral and Systemic Health," *The Clinical Advisor* (March 2009):19-23.

"Burning Mouth Syndrome," *JADA* (August 2005); 136:1191, accessed March 1, 2016, http://www.ada.org/en/publications/jada?source=VanityURL

"Diabetes, Exploring a Periodontal Connection," *Journal of the American Academy of Physician Assistants,* (July 2012); 5(7):18.

Genco, R., Chadda, S. and Grossi, S. "Periodontal Disease is a Predictor of Cardiovascular Disease in a Native American Population," *J Dent Res.* (1997);76:408.

Herman, Christopher, DDS. Interview by author in Vista, CA on August 27, 2013 discussing an overview of oral health and diseases of the mouth.

Lysander, Tracey, DDS. Interview by author in Rancho Bernardo, CA on September 14, 2010 discussing an overview of oral health and diseases that can occur in menopausal women.

Nagel, Maria A., M.D., "Burning Mouth Syndrome Due to Herpes Simplex Virus Type 1," *BMJ Case Reports* (April 1, 2015); doi10.1136/bcr-2015-209488.

Oral Care, Gum Disease. Colgate-Palmolive Company. Pamphlet (March 2009).

"Periodontal Disease and Cardiovascular Disease," *Journal of Periodontology* (October 1996); 67(10):1123-1137, accessed March 1, 2016, http://www.joponline.org/doi/abs/10.1902/jop.1996.67.10s.1123

Periodontal Diseases: Preventing Tooth Loss. American Dental Association, Pamphlet, (2003).

"Preventing and Treating Periodontitis," *The Clinical Advisor* (March 2015):35-40.

Rodrigues, Janette. "Good Oral Health, A Key to Good Overall Health," *PA Professional Magazine* (February 2011):28.

Understanding Dry Mouth. GlaxoSmithKline. Pamphlet (2006).

CHAPTER 19

American Cancer Society, accessed March 12, 2016, https://www.cancer.org/

"New Screening Guidelines for Cervical Cancer," American Cancer Society, accessed April 5, 2016, https://www.cancer.org/latest-news/new-screening-guidelines-for-cervical-cancer.html

"American Cancer Society Recommendations for Colorectal Cancer Early Detection," accessed April 5, 2016, https://www.cancer.org/cancer/colon-rectal-cancer/early-detection/acs-recommendations.html

American Heart Association, accessed March 28, 2016, http://www.heart.org/HEARTORG/

"At-Home Stool Test Can Help Halt Colon Cancer," February 15, 2010, accessed March 29, 2016, http://www.nbcnews.com/id/35407223/ns/health-cancer#.WJjVphDprO0

Centers for Disease Control and Prevention, accessed March 29, 2016, https://www.cdc.gov/ www.coloncancerscreeningguidelines.org , September 2005.

Cancer Facts and Figures 2006, accessed October, 2007, http://cancerfactsandfigures.org/

Colorectal Cancer Screening-Colon Cancer Facts, accessed March 14, 2107, https://www.cdc.gov/cancer/colorectal/basic_info/screening/index.htm?_cid+sfl_sem_010&g-clid+CNPFoqi-1tICFRB2fgodBaQBhA

Polymedco Cancer Diagnostics Products, LLC, accessed March 28, 2016, http://www.polymedco.com/

National Institutes of Health of Health, accessed March 29, 2016, https://www.nih.gov/

National Women's Health Information Center, accessed March 29, 2016, https://www.womenshealth.gov/

"Updated Screening Guidelines for Mammogram Screening," *The Clinical Advisor* (November 2015):24.

U.S. Department of Health and Human Services, accessed March 28, 2016, https://www.hhs.gov/

U.S. Preventive Services Task Force (USPSTF), accessed March 29, 2016, https://www.uspreventiveservicetaskforce.org/Page/Name/tools-and-resources-for-better-preventive-care

U.S. Preventive Services Task Force (USPSTF), accessed April 5, 2016, https://www.uspreventiveservicetaskforce.org/Page/Name/recommendations

INDEX